The Genetics of Alcoholism

Alcohol and Alcoholism

Edited by Henri Begleiter and Benjamin Kissin

1. *The Genetics of Alcoholism,* 1995

The Genetics of Alcoholism

Edited by

Henri Begleiter

and

Benjamin Kissin

New York   Oxford

OXFORD UNIVERSITY PRESS

1995

Oxford University Press

Oxford   New York
Athens   Auckland   Bangkok   Bombay
Calcutta   Cape Town   Dar es Salaam   Delhi
Florence   Hong Kong   Istanbul   Karachi
Kuala Lumpur   Madras   Madrid   Melbourne
Mexico City   Nairobi   Paris   Singapore
Taipei   Tokyo   Toronto

and associated companies in
Berlin   Ibadan

Copyright © 1995 by Oxford University Press, Inc.

Published by Oxford University Press, Inc.,
200 Madison Avenue, New York, New York 10016

Oxford is a registered trademark of Oxford University Press

Library of Congress Cataloging-in-Publication Data
The genetics of alcoholism / edited by Henri Begleiter and Benjamin Kissin.
p. cm. — (Alcohol and alcoholism ; 1)
Includes bibliographical references and index.
ISBN 0-19-508877-8
1. Alcoholism—Genetic aspects.   I. Begleiter, Henri.
II. Kissin, Benjamin, 1917–   .   III. Series: Alcohol and alcoholism
(New York : N.Y.) ; 1.
[DNLM: 1. Alcoholism—genetics.   WM 274 G32857 1994]
RC565.G38   1995
616.86′ 1042—dc20   DNLM/DLC
for Library of Congress   93-35497

9 8 7 6 5 4 3 2 1

Printed in the United States of America
on acid-free paper

PREFACE

This volume introduces a new series, Alcohol and Alcoholism, to be published over the next several years. These volumes are intended to offer a comprehensive and systematic review of recent research on the nature of alcoholism, and of advances in diagnosis and treatment. Like our previous series, The Biology of Alcoholism, this series is broadly conceptualized, so that the two may appear superficially similar; because of the tremendous advances in the field, however, the differences are much greater than the similarities. The first volume in our previous series was published in 1971, the last in 1983. Since that time, there have been sufficient new developments in most fields of alcohol research and in the nature of the illness to make many of the old findings and conclusions obsolete. This inaugural volume in the new series is a case in point; its main subject was barely touched upon in all seven volumes of the previous series. Similar, though somewhat less dramatic advances have been made in the neuropharmacology of alcoholism, in the toxic effects of alcohol on metabolism and organ system functions, and in our understanding of the underlying dynamics of alcoholism. As a result, there is a vast new body of knowledge to be presented.

Equally significant is our editorial decision to change the organization of the volumes within the series. Each volume will address a specific topic, such as the genetics of alcoholism, rather than a diffuse discipline (e.g., *Biochemistry,* the first volume of the previous set). In addition, the chapters in each volume will be grouped into parts to indicate how they relate to each other. To give each volume further coherence, an introductory chapter will present an overview of the material in the various sections.

We have adopted a theoretical model that will provide the frame of reference for all of the volumes in the series. This model is the disease concept of alcoholism, in which we assume that etiological factors may be biological, psychological, or social, but that there is almost always some combination of the three. Some types of alcoholism may be more biological in origin, some more psychological, and some more social, but in every instance the other influences also are present. Biological influences may be endogenous (genetic) or exogenous (the effects of heavy alcohol ingestion); psychological effects may be endogenous (genetic) or exogenous (largely parental); and social or cultural effects, although generally considered exogenous, when sufficiently internalized may also become endogenous. Thus, to adopt a strictly genetic or environmental explanation for any human characteristic is misleading, except perhaps in a rare case like Huntington disease, which is essentially biological in origin, or the ability to speak French (as opposed to English), which is entirely the result of environmental influences.

Jellinek first seriously introduced the disease concept of alcoholism in 1960[1]; in one form or another, it has dominated thinking in the field ever since. Seevers (1968)[2] extended the theory to other drug addictions as well. The basic mechanisms underlying each of the clinical syndromes, whether resulting from the abuse of CNS depressants, stimulants, or hallucinogens are essentially similar.

Our view, based on Jellinek's and Seevers' work, is that with alcohol, as with other depressants, the individual's experience may be determined by multiple factors involving various effects, e.g., anxiolytic (the anxiety-reducing effect in anxious individuals); energizing (the paradoxical "stimulatory" effect of alcohol in some low-functioning individuals); anesthetic (the numbing effect of alcohol on agitated individuals); escapist (the liberating effect on depressed patients); or disinhibitory (the extraverting effects on introverts). Each of these responses involves the interaction of a particular pharmacologic effect of alcohol, in a given situation, with an individual's particular psychological and physical makeup. From this interaction comes the concepts of predisposing factors and of a greater or lesser vulnerability to alcohol abuse.

If one or another of these tendencies exists in a given individual, each positive experience with alcohol is reinforcing, and the individual may develop what Seevers labeled "primary psychological dependence." This is the essential element in all addictions and applies even to use of some stimulant and hallucinogenic drugs in which physical dependence does not develop. (The phenomenology of psychological dependence will be described in Volume 3 of this series.) After psychological dependence develops, acquired tolerance may rapidly occur, in which increasingly larger amounts of alcohol are necessary to produce a given effect. Over time, physical dependence develops, which entails an additional need for alcohol to suppress the occurrence of withdrawal symptomatology. Subsequently, according to Seevers, secondary psychological dependence ensues, characterized by an almost continuous drinking pattern to avoid the terrifying experience of withdrawal. Brain pathology and other organic disease ultimately exacerbate the downward spiral.

---

[1]Jellinek, E. M. (1960). *The Disease Concept of Alcoholism.* New Haven: Hillhouse Press.

[2]Seevers, M. H. (1968). Psychopharmacological elements of drug dependence. *J. Amer. Med. Assoc.* **206**:1263–1266.

None of these concepts are new, yet they form the basis of much of this volume on recent genetic research. For example, Part II on laboratory studies involves experimental considerations including sensitivity to alcohol, alcohol metabolism, alcohol preference, physical dependence, and brain function. All of these processes are elements of the alcohol-addictive cycle just described. The topic of genetics as a whole fits directly into the disease model, in terms of the endogenous biological factors that predispose a given individual to alcohol addiction. The connections of ensuing volumes in the series to this underlying disease model will be equally clear.

There are, of course, alternatives to the disease concept. These include biological, social, anxiety reduction, and other models that will be fully described in later volumes. However, it is our conviction that the disease concept of alcoholism encompasses these other models that consider only one aspect or another of the total syndrome. In this series, we provide a comprehensive review of the biological, psychological, and social evidence on which the various models are based. By this strategy we hope to give readers state-of-the-art information about alcoholism that will advance scientific or clinical work and sharpen thinking about theoretical questions concerning the nature of alcoholism.

Organization of the Series

The series will consist of nine volumes: the first four will deal with basic theoretical and experimental issues, and the last five will be more clinical in orientation. "More clinical" need not mean less scientific, however; these later volumes will continue to maintain critical standards of scholarship and experimental reliability, even as the emphasis shifts from laboratory studies of underlying mechanisms in animals to clinical studies of humans suffering from alcoholism.

The next three volumes on fundamental mechanisms will deal with neuropharmacology and physical dependence, psychological dependence, and neurotoxicity. The fifth volume of the series will review the clinical aspects of alcoholism. The following two volumes will deal with medical complications and treatment, including psychotherapy as well as medical therapy. The eighth volume on social issues will provide a useful backdrop to the final volume on the disease concept of alcoholism and its medical and social implications.

CONTENTS

The Genetics of Alcoholism

Introduction

It has long been observed that alcoholism runs in families, but whether for genetic or environmental reasons has depended more on current ideology than on any firm evidence in one direction or the other. Although there was much speculation about hereditary influences in the transmission of alcoholism, the first solid evidence came from Kaij's twin study in 1960 and later from the 1973 Danish Adoption Study by Goodwin et al. The Goodwin study suggested that although genetic factors might be very important in the pathogenesis of both alcoholism and problem drinking, environmental factors appear to have greater influence on problem drinking. The Swedish Adoption Study (Cloninger et al., 1981) provided support for the strong clinical impression that there are several different types of alcoholism and offered the additional insight that genetic factors might exert a greater influence in some types than in others. Thus epidemiologic studies not only provided substantial evidence for the role of heredity in the transmission of alcoholism but shed light on some of the problems to be expected in attempting to assess the interaction of genetic and environmental effects.

Research on the genetics of alcoholism is still in the formative stages; nevertheless, a tremendous amount of work has been accomplished, and many tentative conclusions appear not only possible but reasonable. The authors in this volume have reviewed their evidence in depth, presenting data to support their conclusions and opposing findings as well. Given these caveats, a discernible image of hereditary influences in alcoholism is beginning to emerge.

Part I: Epidemiologic Studies

In Chapter 1, "The Genetic Epidemiology of Alcoholism," Victor Hesselbrock reviews the data from the dominant approaches in this field, twin studies and adoption studies.

3

He concludes that "taken collectively . . . the body of evidence provides a powerful demonstration of the influence of genetic factors on the risk for alcoholism." Regarding the genetic effects on drinking patterns, his conclusions are less definite. On one hand, he writes of the Goodwin et al. (1973) Danish Adoption Study that "these data are consistent with several twin studies (cf. Kaij 1960; Pickens et al., 1991) and suggest that genetic factors are important for the transmission of alcoholism, but not for problem drinking." On the other hand, in his section on "Twin Studies in Normal Drinking," his review of the literature supports the view that there are also significant hereditary influences on drinking patterns, although probably not of the same magnitude as those involved in the development of alcoholism. This interpretation is supported by the findings of Heath in Chapter 4.

Hesselbrock raises the issue of the heterogeneity of alcoholic populations as it complicates the effort to obtain reliable statistical results in epidemiological studies. This question is addressed in detail by Michie Hesselbrock in Chapter 2, "Genetic Determinants of Alcoholic Subtypes." The well-established existence of different types of alcoholism creates problems in considering whether these apparently different syndromes represent different underlying mechanisms or, as in tuberculosis and syphilis, a condition caused by a single etiologic agent that manifests itself in multiple forms. Current evidence appears to support the hypothesis that many different influences operate in the various subtypes of alcoholism.

Michie Hesselbrock's comprehensive review of alcoholic typologies begins with the psychoanalytically oriented studies of Knight (1938) and Fleeson and Gildea (1942). Knight distinguished among three groups of alcoholics: essential (psychopathic), reactive (neurotic), and symptomatic. Fleeson and Gildea also identified three groups that matched fairly closely with those of Knight: endogenous primary addicts, endogenous symptomatic drinkers, and exogenous drinkers.

Hesselbrock also reviews the typologies of Bowman and Jellinek (1941) and Jellinek (1960). In general, these typologies appear more to classify drinking patterns than to distinguish among basically different types of alcoholics. Jellinek's description of alpha, beta, gamma, and delta patterns of drinking is still generally used today.

The last sections of Hesselbrock's chapter address two central questions: Are there significantly different types of alcoholism that can be reliably identified as such? Do genetic factors play a significant role in that differentiation? Hesselbrock describes Cloninger's classification of Type 1 and Type 2 alcoholics, in which Type 2 resembles Knight's essential alcoholic, showing early onset and a strong family history of alcoholism. Type 1 resembles Knight's so-called neurotic alcoholic, with late onset and a weak family history for alcoholism. Hesselbrock reviews the predisposing conditions to Type 2 alcoholism, which are hyperactivity and conduct disorder, antisocial personality, and Cloninger's personality traits. Although the evidence is not yet complete, it appears that all three elements contribute to what constitutes a fairly homogeneous group. Particularly interesting is the fact that Cloninger's personality factors for Type 2 or essential alcoholics are basically the same as his personality profiles for the antisocial personality (ASP). The role of childhood hyperactivity and conduct disorder in these associations, which remains unclear, is reviewed from a neurophysiologic perspective by Begleiter and Porjesz in Chapter 11.

The role of genetics in differentiating between Type 1 (neurotic) and Type 2 (essential) alcoholics is at issue. Cloninger postulated a strong family history of male alcoholism as a correlate of the personality traits of Type 2 alcoholics. Some of the early negative reports on his work may have resulted from the inability of others to find such a relationship. When Cloninger's personality traits were related to clinical alcoholic patterns (early onset, acting out, etc.) rather than to heredity, however, more positive confirmation was reported. Thus, the origins of Type 2 alcoholism and antisocial personality appear to be related but not identical.

In Chapter 3, "Familial Transmission of Psychiatric Disorders Associated With Alcoholism," Cadoret explores the association of genetic factors in the transmission of alcoholism with those of the several psychiatric conditions in which alcoholism is a common complication. He reports on the coincidence of alcoholism with other psychiatric disorders and not unexpectedly finds it very high for the antisocial personality (ASP). Incidence is also significantly high in schizophrenia, panic disorder, phobia, bipolar disorder, and major unipolar depression. Cadoret systematically reviews the evidence for genetic concordance between each of these syndromes and alcohol abuse or dependence. He concludes that in general, genetic transmission of psychiatric disorders is separate and distinct from that of alcoholism.

Cadoret examines the typologies of alcoholic ASPs, alcoholic depressives, and alcoholic ASP/depressives. He agrees with Hesselbrock that the genetics of ASP and alcoholism are quite different. However, he raises the possibility that alcoholic ASPs may be of two types, analogous to primary and secondary sociopaths, and that genetic influences may be greater in one than in the other. He also reviews the literature on depression and alcoholism, e.g., the linkage studies of A. F. Wilson (described in more detail by Wilson and Elston in Chapter 14), which supports his conclusion that the genetic origins are different. Finally, he suggests that the interaction of various psychiatric disorders (e.g., depressive ASPs) may result in a more serious form of alcohol abuse or dependence.

Cadoret explores the relationship between genetically and environmentally determined personality traits and the development of alcohol abuse. He concludes that genetic factors show a stronger influence. He mentions the effects of temperament, maturation, and environment on personality development and on their relation to alcohol abuse. In this connection he stresses the work of Tarter and his associates (see Chapter 12).

Chapter 4, "Genetic Influences on Drinking Behavior in Humans," deals with normal drinking patterns rather than alcohol abuse and dependence. Heath stresses epidemiologic methods in his chapter; most of the studies he reviews were based on data derived from questionnaires. One exception is Martin et al.'s study (1985), which involved the administration of alcohol and the subsequent determination of "sensitivity" with psychomotor tests. Heath finds that normal drinking patterns show both significant genetic and environmental influences, but whether the genetic influences are the same as those that predispose to alcoholism is not clear. Heath doubts that the genetic influences that favor abstinence, mild to moderate drinking, or heavy drinking are the same and suggests that they probably involve different mechanisms. He concludes on the basis of the Martin et al. study that decreased sensitivity to the effects of alcohol in humans is more a function of prior drinking level than of any discernible genetic influence.

Wilson and Laffan describe their Colorado Alcohol Research on Twins and Adoptees (CARTA) study in Chapter 5, "Alcohol Metabolism, Sensitivity and Tolerance: Testing for Genetic Influences in Humans." In addition to their epidemiologic data, Wilson and Laffan measure the gradual development of behavioral tolerance to alcohol over a 3-hour period and provide a detailed analysis of alcohol metabolism. Many group differences were demonstrated in these studies, mainly in sensitivity levels, alcohol metabolism, and drinking patterns. Women showed no greater sensitivity than men but did have faster alcohol clearance rates and lower drinking patterns, and developed less tolerance over the period of the experiment. Older individuals showed somewhat different patterns of responsiveness when compared to younger subjects, as did Orientals when compared with Europeans. (The origins of the differences in Orientals are explored in depth by Crabb and his colleagues in Chapter 8.)

Less clear in CARTA was the evidence, in terms of both Mz/Dz comparisons and familial patterns, for significant genetic influences. In most of these analyses, the findings in alcohol metabolism sensitivity and tolerance showed no significant differences among the groups tested. The authors suggest that this inconclusiveness might be due to the instability of these processes as indicated by their low test-retest reliability. Thus, even positive findings might be obscured by instability of testing procedures.

Chapters 4 and 5 are a bridge between Parts I and II. For example, how do normal drinking patterns in humans relate to alcohol preference in rodents, and how do both relate to sensitivity to alcohol? The complexity and variability of human responses makes it very difficult to explore these questions directly. Yet some such genetic influences almost certainly do exist, or it would not have been possible to develop through selective breeding rodent strains with high and low alcohol preference and high and low sensitivity. Thus, the laboratory studies discussed in Part II offer approaches to the questions raised in the chapters on genetic epidemiology in humans.

Part II: Selective Breeding Studies

Part II focuses on research that involves the selective breeding of rodents. This method has produced homogeneous strains exhibiting specific behavioral response patterns that are considered significant in the development and maintenance of alcohol dependence. The four major aspects of human responses to alcohol measured in the CARTA studies were alcohol preference (normal alcohol intake), sensitivity to the soporific effect of alcohol, acquired tolerance to alcohol, and the rate of alcohol metabolism. All these reactivities have similar analogues in animal models: high and low alcohol preference (P and NP); high and low sensitivity, i.e, long-sleep (LS) and short-sleep (SS); high and low acquired tolerance; and high and low adaptive increases in alcohol metabolism. In addition, strains with characteristics not readily addressed in humans, e.g., the tendency to develop convulsions or physical dependence and withdrawal (severe and mild ethanol withdrawal, SEW and MEW), have also been bred, thus expanding the research possibilities.

In Chapter 6, "Genetic Influences on Alcohol Metabolism and Sensitivity to Alcohol in Animals," Deitrich and Baker show that responses to alcohol can be studied in much greater depth in animal models than in humans. Phenomena such as sensitivity and acute tolerance can be separated more easily, and the genetic homogeneity of a large group of subjects rather than pairs of twins permits valid statistical analyses. Alcohol preference in rodents is almost certainly biologically determined, whereas regular drinking patterns in humans (the accuracy of which is itself open to question) are subject to social influences. Test-retest reliability for these parameters is far greater in animals than in humans, eliminating what Wilson and Laffan found to be the greatest problem in their studies. Finally, the biological correlates of a particular behavior, the major goal of all this research, can be studied in both the intact and the sacrificed animal, providing a much broader range for research.

Deitrich and Baker have used the LS–SS dichotomy as their major index of sensitivity to alcohol. They found that LS and SS strains of rodents differed in the activity of brain GABA and that these differences were probably genetically determined. There was also a strong correlation between alcohol preference and acute tolerance, a finding resembling Heath's in humans. However, Heath's correlation was between chronic tolerance and drinking patterns, and he concluded that high alcohol intake in humans causes chronic tolerance. Wilson and Laffan, on the other hand, could find no significant correlation between acute tolerance (for which they tested specifically) and drinking pattern, but their work was contaminated by poor test-retest reliability and by the unreliability of the drinking pattern data. Neither of these objections applies to the animal data, nor was there any question of chronic tolerance since the animals were alcohol-naive. Since both acute tolerance and alcohol preference show strong genetic influences, as Chapter 7 makes clear, the correlation may prove to be highly significant.

In Chapter 7, "Genetic Influences on Alcohol Preference in Animals," Lumeng, Li, and McBride attempt to synthesize the various etiologic strands into a comprehensive view of the pathogenesis of alcoholism. They review Cicero's six criteria for the use of selectively bred alcohol-preferring lines of rats as valid animal analogues to human alcoholism:

1. Alcohol drinking exceeds 5 g/kg/day.
2. BACs reach >100 mg% during free-choice alcohol drinking.
3. Ethanol is reinforcing as shown by operant responding or other measures.
4. Metabolic tolerance develops with chronic free-choice drinking.
5. Behavioral or neuronal tolerance develops with chronic free-choice drinking.
6. Physical dependence (withdrawal) develops with chronic free-choice drinking.

The authors' alcohol-preferring (P) rats but not their nonpreferring (NP) rats exhibit all six of these responses and thus constitute a valid animal analogue to the biological, if not the psychosocial, model of human alcoholism. The final level of alcohol preference in these animals is determined by the interaction of two conflicting influences. The hedonic, positively reinforcing effects of ethanol are usually associated with low dosage, and the aversive effects are associated with high dose alcohol administration. The significant factors contributing to the disparate influences for alcohol intake in P and NP rats are as follows.

1. Ethanol is more positively reinforcing to P than to NP rats, i.e., they are more willing to perform tasks to obtain it.
2. In alcohol-naive animals, aversive affects of ethanol appear at BACs that are significantly lower in NP than P rats.
3. Acute tolerance development to a single high (aversive) dose of ethanol is more robust and more persistent in P than NP rats.
4. Chronic tolerance to the higher dose and the aversive effects of ethanol develop in P rats (but not NPs) during chronic free-choice alcohol drinking. This effect can lead to a progressive increase in alcohol intake with time in the P rats.

Items 2, 3, and 4 confirm the conclusion in Chapter 6 that the development of acute tolerance is an important element in alcohol preference. In addition, Lumeng et al. identify alcohol-naive, alcohol-preferring animals as naturally more resistant to the aversive effects of alcohol; delineate the development of acute tolerance in alleviating the aversive effects of high doses of alcohol; and demonstrate that this effect carries over even more strongly into chronic tolerance. Finally, the strong, positively reinforcing hedonic effect of ethanol in alcohol-preferring animals (item 1, above) is manifested by increased motor activation with low doses, by increased lever pressing in a positively reinforcing operant-conditioning situation, and by increased cortical arousal.

Lumeng et al. review neurotransmitter differences in P and NP rats. Reduced levels of both serotonin and dopamine metabolism were consistently found in P rats, serotonin more or less throughout the brain and dopamine mainly in the nucleus accumbens. Antagonists that inhibit the activities of either of these neurotransmitters increase alcohol preference further, and agonists conversely decrease alcohol ingestion.

Chapter 8, "Genetic Factors That Reduce Risk for Developing Alcoholism" by Crabb et al., continues the analysis begun in Chapter 7 of reactions to the aversive effects of alcohol. In an interesting reversal, the findings in humans have been more detailed and revealing than those in animals because the major natural aversive reaction to alcohol in humans, the Oriental flush, has been the object of study for many years. The original report of von Wartburg et al. (1964) identified an atypical alcohol dehydrogenase isoenzyme in Orientals that metabolizes alcohol more rapidly, resulting in higher levels of circulating acetaldehyde; these levels in turn were presumed to produce the flush. More recent work has pinpointed a deficiency in the aldehyde dehydrogenase isoenzyme (ALDH2), the dominant catalyst for the breakdown of acetaldehyde, as the major mechanism in the Oriental flush. Nevertheless, the atypical alcohol dehydrogenase isoenzyme also plays an important if lesser role.

Crabb et al. discuss in detail the various alcohol and aldehyde dehydrogenase enzymes, their incidence in a variety of populations (mostly Asian), and the correlation between the presence of atypical isoenzymes and the incidence of alcoholism. They describe the molecular structure of the specific RNA and proteins involved in the production of the enzymes and identify the amino acid mutations that differentiate between alleles for the typical *(ALDH2*1)* and atypical *(ALDH2*2)* enzymes. Finally, they report that individuals who are heterozygous for *ALDH2*2* show mild to moderate flush reactions to alcohol, while those who are homozygous show such severe reactions that they seldom drink.

The authors found a similar difference in *ALDH2* isoenzymes in P and NP rats, including a change in the amino acid structure of the antecedent alleles. However, preliminary investigation did not show these isoenzymes to differ in their catalytic properties; certainly it is too early to predict how large a role, if any, these variants play in the aversive effects of ethanol in NP rats. On the other hand, if the aversive effects of alcohol in NP rats can be shown to result from mechanisms other than differences in *ALDH2* isoenzymes, it would be helpful in understanding aversive reactions in Caucasians, among whom isoenzymes for either alcohol dehydrogenase or aldehyde dehydrogenase are atypical.

Chapter 9, "Genetic Influences on the Development of Alcohol Physical Dependence and Withdrawal" by Kosobud and Crabbe, introduces a clinical parameter that is central to the disease concept of alcoholism and to an understanding of the dynamics of the illness. As mentioned in the preface to this book, the original addictive mechanism in the disease model is "primary psychological dependence," a somewhat misleading term since the mechanisms underlying that dependence are presumably physical as well. Whatever the nature of the dependence, it leads to increased alcohol intake that in turn leads to increased tolerance and still greater intake, and then finally to physical dependence. New mechanisms are superimposed with the advent of physical dependence; the nature of the syndrome changes from alcohol abuse to "alcohol dependence," drinking to *suppress* withdrawal symptomatology, and to "secondary psychological dependence," drinking to *prevent* withdrawal symptomatology. With these new developments, the full-blown picture of alcoholism appears.

Given this background, it is easy to see the utility of an animal model that would permit further exploration of the genetic and neurobiological mechanisms underlying the development of physical dependence. Kosobud and Crabbe describe the major methods for developing such a model: selective breeding for alcohol withdrawal severity, and the use of recombinant inbred mouse strains. Selective breeding for specific responses to alcohol was the method used to develop the LS/SS and P/NP strains and has the advantage of producing the greatest behavioral extremes for the particular variables to be tested. The use of recombinant inbred (RI) strains has other advantages that are alluded to in Chapter 9 and discussed in depth by McClearn and Plomin in Chapter 13.

Kosobud and Crabbe describe three strains selectively bred for severity of alcohol withdrawal: the severe (SEW) and mild (MEW) ethanol withdrawal mouse lines, the high (HA) and low (LA) addictability mouse lines, and the withdrawal seizure-prone (WSP) and seizure-resistant (WSR) mouse lines. The three lines differ in mode of induction and in the scope of their responses to alcohol, but in general are more similar than different. The WSP and WSR strains have been studied most comprehensively. Alcohol metabolism measured in terms of both blood ethanol levels and elimination rates were comparable in early generations of WSP and WSR mice even though there were already significant differences in withdrawal severity. In later generations, WSP mice did achieve higher blood concentrations but this was assumed to have been the effect of increased drinking rather than the cause of increased severity of withdrawal.

More significant was the finding that WSP mice differed from WSR mice in a variety of brain GABA receptors. These differences were evidenced mainly in expression of whole-brain levels of RNA specific for GABA-receptor subunits, both in naive animals and after prolonged administration of ethanol. In each case there was a significant decrease in GABA activity levels in the brain concomitant with withdrawal. This finding parallels the differentiation between LS and SS mice, where the SS strain also shows significantly lower GABA levels. When LS and SS strains were tested for withdrawal symptomatology, SS mice also showed more severe reactions, further evidence for the role of GABA deficiency in withdrawal convulsions. On the other hand, as Kosobud and Crabbe observe, WSP and WSR strains do not differ in ethanol-induced sleep time, a GABA effect. This discrepancy suggests that some mechanism other than GABA deficiency may be involved in the greater sensitivity to convulsions in WSP mice.

Part III: Phenotypic Studies

The investigation and analysis of phenotypic markers that serve as correlates to the genotypic determinants of alcoholism characterize many of the studies in Part III. Phenotypic markers can be defined as molecular, biochemical, physiological, or behavioral patterns of response to alcohol that are not necessarily directly related to alcoholism but that can be shown to be genetically *associated* or *linked* with the types of alcoholism mechanisms described in the studies of Part II.

The advantages of using phenotypic markers are several. As in the electrophysiological studies of humans described in Chapter 11 by Begleiter and Porjesz, they sometimes suggest underlying genetic mechanisms in the pathogenesis of alcoholism that might otherwise not have been suspected. In addition, they provide a broader context for the interpretation of similar studies in animals, such as the investigations of electrophysiological responses in P and NP rats by Morzorati et al. (1988) and Ehlers et al. (1991). The suggestion by Tarter et al. (Chapter 12) that disturbances in cortical arousal in alcoholics may be of a temperamental nature (i.e., genetic) fits into this same paradigm.

Even more significant is the fact that genetic loci, specific locations on specific genes in specific chromosomes, have been identified for many biochemical, physiological, and behavioral traits. As Wilson and Elston state in Chapter 14,

> The normal variation, or polymorphism, that is found in the phenotypes of well-characterized marker loci is used in linkage analysis to map other traits to the human genome. The cosegregation of a trait and a marker locus suggests that there is a genetic locus physically near the location of the marker locus that is responsible, at least in part, for the expression of the trait.
>
> There are currently thousands of genetic polymorphisms distributed throughout the human genome that can be used as markers. . . .

The first three chapters of Part III respectively identify biochemical, neurophysio-logic, and behavioral phenotypic markers; the last two chapters attempt to locate such markers on specific chromosomes. Chapter 13 uses various behavioral markers to iden-tify specific genetic loci for alcohol-related behavior in rodents. In Chapter 14, Wilson and Elston use biochemical markers to identify the genetic loci of other biochemical responses presumably related to the pathogenesis of alcoholism in humans.

In Chapter 10, "Biochemical Phenotypic Markers for Genetic Alcoholism," Dia-mond and Gordon review biochemical and molecular effects at the intracellular level that are thought to be involved in the pathogenesis of alcoholism. Some of these effects predate exposure to ethanol; others appear to be the direct outcome of such exposure. Increased vulnerability to the effects of alcohol is presumably related to some geneti-cally influenced preexposure condition, which makes the identification of such factors in active alcoholics difficult. For this reason, such conditions are sought in the alcohol-naive relatives of alcoholics, the so-called high risk (HR) probands. Although this approach is the best available for the study of physiological and behavioral factors, it is less satisfactory for biochemical studies where so many other externally produced effects are involved.

Diamond and Gordon have devised a technique in which the lymphocytes of alco-holics and nonalcoholics are cultured in the laboratory over several generations, during which time environmental influences are gradually eliminated and only genetic mecha-nisms remain. Using that method, the authors have found significant differences in cyclic AMP signal transduction and adenosine transport between alcoholics and nonal-coholics, both before and after exposure of the cultured lymphocytes to alcohol. This methodology is fairly new, but the early findings are extremely interesting. The lym-phocytes of high risk and low risk (LR) alcohol-naive offspring are now being tested in attempt to corroborate the genetic origin of these effects. In addition, this technique represents an important advance toward direct genetic analysis. As the authors state, "Cultured lymphocytes will prove useful in cloning the gene(s) responsible for the cel-lular phenotype. Once the genes for the specific candidate proteins responsible for the phenotype are cloned, e.g., adenylyl cyclase, $G\alpha_s$, and the nucleoside transporter, they can be used for RFLP analyses in families with alcoholism."

Chapter 11, "Phenotypic Markers for the Development of Alcoholism," by Begleiter and Porjesz, describes electrophysiological phenotypic markers that differentiate alco-holics and their naive offspring from nonalcoholic adults and their offspring. The most consistent of the findings is decreased height of the P3 wave of the event-related poten-tials (ERP) on discriminatory tasks. This response is also characteristic of hyperactive attention-deficit children.

Begleiter and Porjesz also describe psychophysiological and neuropsychological differences in the HR and LR offspring of alcoholic and nonalcoholic parents in regard to the effects of alcohol. In particular, HR subjects characteristically show greater psy-chophysiological reactions to stress than do LR subjects, suggesting that they have higher levels of cortical arousal. Consistent with this interpretation is the fact that HR subjects tend to be more hyperactive than LR subjects. Paradoxically, HR subjects return to normal levels of physiological responsivity with smaller doses of alcohol than do healthy LR subjects.

This apparent discrepancy may be explained by the studies of Cohen et al. (1993), in which an increase in slow alpha activity on the rising arm of the alcohol metabolic curve was significantly greater in HR than in LR subjects, indicating a stronger arousal-reducing effect. If these interpretations are valid, then they suggest that HR subjects do have increased levels of cortical arousal and that lower doses of alcohol decrease them.

In Chapter 12, "Genetic Behavior and the Etiology of Alcoholism," Tarter et al. describe the behavioral differences between HR and LR children. They address the temperamental (personality) characteristics antedating the development of Cloninger's Type 2 alcoholism, as well as the interaction of such characteristics with environmental influences that may either foster or suppress the development of alcoholism. They use the six dimensions of temperament extracted by Rowe and Plomin (1977) from other studies:

1. Behavior activity level
2. Attention span-persistence
3. Emotionality
4. Reaction to food
5. Sociability
6. Soothability

Tarter systematically describes these parameters in HR subjects before the onset of drinking by reviewing both the data on HR children of alcoholics and self-reports of drinking history from alcoholics.

Of these six dimensions of temperament, all except "reaction to food" (on which there were no significant findings) were fairly consistent with regard to the characteristics that differentiate HR from LR subjects. HR subjects are more hyperactive than LR subjects; have shorter attention spans; and are more emotional and sociable, and less soothable. Soothability is measured as the rate of return to a normal psychophysiologic state after exposure to stress. Each of these response patterns fits the general picture of the temperament of the essential alcoholic outlined in other studies. The relationship of essential alcoholism in adulthood to hyperactivity in childhood was discussed by Hesselbrock in Chapter 2. Short attention span is characteristic of both conditions. One interpretation has been that in alcoholics, short attention span may be due to the toxic effects of alcohol on hippocampal and frontal lobe function. However, the fact that this response has also been demonstrated in the HR children of alcoholics before exposure to alcohol makes this interpretation less likely. Furthermore, the diminished P3 in both alcoholics and their HR children points to attention deficits in these individuals before such exposure (Chapter 11).

Chapter 13, "Strategies for the Search for Genetic Influences in Alcohol-related Phenotypes" by McClearn and Plomin, addresses the optimal method for identifying the genetic loci of certain alcohol-related characteristics in animals. McClearn and Plomin describe the technique of recombinant inbreeding (RI) that results in the highest level of separateness for such characteristics as ethanol acceptance (EA) or preference; low dose activation (LDA), a measure of positive reinforcement; and withdrawal severity (WS). They then describe the quantitative trait loci (QTL) method of analysis that permits localization of traits at specific loci on specific chromosomes.

McClearn and Plomin found in the recombinant-inbred rat strain a cosegregation of EA and LDA on two separate loci on chromosome 4, of LDA and WS on chromosome 13, and of EA and WS on chromosome 1. Each of these traits had independent loci on other chromosomes where they did not cosegregate at all. If valid, these findings indicate that at least in rats, each trait related to alcoholism has a different genetic pattern than the others. Thus, not only is the genome of alcoholism in rats polygenic, but indeed so are the genomes for the various traits that may contribute to the development of alcoholism. The cosegregation of traits on a single genetic locus, as described above, may or may not be a necessary event for alcoholism to develop.

In contrast to the behavioral traits discussed by McClearn and Plomin, in Chapter 14, "Linkage Analysis in the Study of the Genetics of Alcoholism," Wilson and Elston address chemical phenotypes. In large studies of families with and without alcoholism they have found linkages between alcoholism and the genetic sites of various alcohol-related enzymes and neurotransmitters that may be masked in alcoholism. The loci for alcohol dehydrogenase Class I are on the long arm of chromosome 13, tryptophan oxygenase on chromosome 4, dopamine-B-hydroxylase (DBH) on chromosome 9, aldehyde dehydrogenase on the long arm of chromosome 9, and the serotonin 5 HT 2 receptor site on chromosome 13. The evidence that clinical alcoholism appears to be associated genetically with enzymes and neurotransmitters that may be involved in the pathogenesis of alcoholism, i.e., alcohol dehydrogenase and aldehyde dehydrogenase, and in the neurotransmitters serotonin and dopamine, suggests a rewarding area for investigation.

In summary, the chapters of this volume review much of the major work that has been done on the genetics of alcoholism. They muster evidence, delineate methodologies, and present a comprehensive overview of the research in each particular area. We as editors have found it gratifying that despite the great variability in approach, there is a general internal consistency among the findings and interpretations that enhances one's sense of the validity of the entire body of work.

Epidemiologic Studies

The Genetic Epidemiology of Alcoholism

VICTOR M. HESSELBROCK

Genetic epidemiology is a relatively new discipline that seeks to unravel the sources of family resemblance. It focuses on the etiology, distribution, and control of diseases in biologically related individuals and on the inherited causes of diseases in populations. Both biological and cultural inheritance are subsumed under the rubric of "inherited." Cultural inheritance is defined to include any social, behavioral, nutritional, or other factor that is nonrandomly distributed among families. Further, the set of relatives investigated may be as closely related as twins or as extended in relationship as a particular ethnic group (Morton, 1982). As such, genetic epidemiology provides a strong theoretical and methodological background for the study of the genetic basis of alcoholism, including the transmission of alcohol-related problems from affected parents to their offspring.

Although the debate over genetic versus environmental transmission of alcoholism has raged for many years, this chapter concentrates on the evidence for a genetic basis of the transmission of the disorder. Evidence that genetic factors contribute to a disease of unknown etiology usually comes from four different types of studies: studies that show a familial aggregation of the disorder (i.e., family studies of biologically related individuals); studies showing a higher concordance of the disorder among monozygotic twins compared to dizygotic twins (i.e., twin studies); studies showing a higher prevalence of the disorder (regardless of rearing environment) among biologically related offspring of a parent affected with alcoholism (i.e., adoption studies, half-sibling studies); and genetic linkage of the disorder with an identifiable allele at a marker locus (Merikangas, 1987). The genetic linkage studies are reviewed elsewhere in this volume (Chapter 14). Family studies can demonstrate the "familial" nature of a disorder by determining whether the prevalence of that disorder is higher among the biological relatives of an affected individual than would be expected from known rates within the general population. Higher than expected lifetime prevalence rates demonstrate that the disorder is "familial" in nature, but cannot separate the genetic and environmental sources of variation responsible for this difference. Monozygotic twins have identical genotypes, while dizygotic twins share, on average, half of their genes in common. Higher concordance rates of the disorder found among monozygotic twins compared to dizygotic twins would be suggestive of genetic factors for the disorder. Studies of adoptees separated from their biological parents at birth and reared in a foster home provide a natural experiment to examine both genetic and environmental factors. The degree of resemblance in affectional status of the child with both the biologic and adoptee parents can be compared to determine the relative contribution of genetic and of environmental factors. Finally, family pedigrees can be examined with a variety of statistical methods, such as segregation and linkage analysis. Segregation analysis is used to determine the mode of transmission of the disorder, while linkage analysis is used to assign a putative disease locus to a region of a chromosome.

Familial/Genetic Studies

The familial nature of alcoholism has been repeatedly observed since the time of the ancient Greeks. Systematic investigation of biologically related individuals has consistently documented the higher prevalence of alcoholism among the family members of alcoholic patients compared to the general population (cf. Amark, 1951; Goodwin, 1976; Cotton, 1979). A review of several studies by Goodwin (1976) indicates that about 25% of fathers and brothers of an alcoholic are also affected with alcoholism, while one study has reported that 80% of a sample of treated alcoholics had at least one biological first- or second-degree relative also affected with alcoholism (Hesselbrock et al., 1992). The familial nature of the disorder seems to hold regardless of the nationality of the samples (Cotton, 1979) or whether the proband has an additional comorbid psychiatric disorder such as depression (Merikangas et al., 1985), heroin addiction (Kosten et al., 1991), or antisocial personality disorder (Reich et al., 1981). The familial nature of alcoholism has also been reported for nonclinical samples of persons with alcoholism drawn from the community (Webster et al, 1989). However, traits or disorders that are familial in nature are not necessarily influenced or transmitted by genetic factors alone. Evidence for the importance of genetic factors in the transmission of any psychiatric disorder, including alcoholism, is usually derived from a variety of sources such as twin and adoption studies.

Twin Studies

Twin Studies in Alcoholism

Several investigators have used the strategy of comparing the concordance rates for alcoholism in monozygotic (MZ) and dizygotic (DZ) twins. The first reported study of alcoholism in twins was that of Kaij (1960).

Based on data derived from interviews of the twins and from the Swedish Temperance Board, Kaij examined the concordance of drinking styles, including alcoholism, in male twin pairs ($n = 174$). Even though this study was conducted over 30 years ago, Kaij's definition of alcoholism is consistent with current conceptualizations of alcohol dependence. His definition included (1) a pathological desire for alcohol; (2) regular blackouts, and (3) evidence of physiological dependence. Persons who admitted two of these symptoms, persons who were continually intoxicated, and those persons with cirrhosis or alcohol psychosis were classified as chronic alcoholics. Kaij found that the concordance rate among MZ twins increased with increasing levels of alcohol abuse. For chronic alcoholism, a concordance rate of 71.4% of MZ twins was found compared to 32.3% of DZ twins. However, this concordance rate was based on a relatively small number of alcoholic MZ twins (10/14).

Hrubec and Omenn (1981) examined the concordance of male twin veterans in the National Academy of Science–National Research Council (NAS–NRC) Twin Registry for both alcoholism and its biological end points. Among the 15,924 white male pairs in the study, the overall prevalence rate for alcoholism was 29.6% for alcoholism, 4.1% for liver cirrhosis, and 2.1% for pancreatitis; these rates did not vary for MZ or DZ twins. Within the cases, twin concordance for alcoholism was 26.3% for MZ twins ($n = 41$ pairs) versus 11.9% for DZ twins ($n = 28$ pairs). The concordance rate for alcoholic psychosis among MZ twins was 21.1% compared to 6.0% for the DZ twin pairs, while the rate for liver cirrhosis was 14.6% in MZ pairs and 5.4% in DZ pairs. No twin pairs were concordant for pancreatitis. Upon further examination of the data, the higher MZ twin concordance rates for psychosis and cirrhosis could not be explained by the difference in alcoholism rates between the MZ and DZ twin pairs. Hrubec and Omenn concluded that the data provide evidence supporting a genetic predisposition to organ-specific complications of alcoholism.

This study has been faulted for using records (military medical records, Veterans Administration computerized records) to determine alcoholism and its biological sequelae. Both the medical and psychiatric diagnoses used in the analyses were based on information abstracted from these records. While it is likely that milder forms of alcohol abuse were not documented, as suggested by Hrubec and Omenn, twins with alcoholism were identified through hospital admission records and many also had medical complications attributable to chronic alcohol use. It is also important to note that the medical and psychiatric diagnoses made from the records were based on standardized criteria (ICD-8) and not on clinical judgment. The zygosity of the twin pairs has been questioned, since blood grouping methods were used in only about 5% of the twin pairs. Responses to questionnaire items indicating similarity in childhood or physical similarity of fingerprints were used for zygosity determination of the remaining 95% of the twin pairs. Although not perfect, these methods have an accuracy rate of 85%+ compared to laboratory methods.

Another twin study of alcoholism was conducted by Gurling and Murray (1981, 1987). Their sample, derived from a register based at the Maudsley psychiatric hospital in London, contained 20 male and 15 female MZ twins, and 33 male and 11 female same-sexed DZ twins. Reliable data have been reported on 56 twin pairs. Twins who met ICD-8 criteria for either alcoholism or habitual excessive alcohol use were traced by using national health records. Information on alcohol use and abuse was based on searches of the health and hospital records, a standardized psychiatric interview, and a standardized alcohol interview schedule. Zygosity was determined using blood group methods in 54% of the sample, by resemblance questionnaire in 27% of the sample, by fingerprints in 4%, and by case notes/reports in 12% of the cases. Gurling and Murray's data do not support a genetic predisposition hypothesis for alcoholism. Pairwise concordance rates for alcoholism, based on Research Diagnostic Criteria (Spitzer et al., 1978) were 29% for MZ twin pairs compared to 33% for DZ twin pairs. When the criteria for the alcohol dependence syndrome (Edwards and Gross, 1976) were used, similar rates were found: 21% MZ (33% males; 8% females) compared to 25% DZ (30% males; 13% females) twin pairs.

Several questions are raised by this study, however. First, the sample was ascertained through a psychiatric hospital register. It is possible that the alcoholism present in the identified twins is a complication of another psychiatric disorder and not a heritable form. Second, the sample was relatively young; about 38% were below 40 years of age. Since the age of risk for developing alcoholism extends into middle age, additional subjects are likely to have become affected over time. The concordance rate may rise as the number of affected individuals in the sample increases. Finally, approximately one-third of the total sample was female. Previous studies were based on samples of males only. Gender-specific factors not considered in their analyses may differentially influence the concordance rate for alcoholism in females compared to males.

A study of the heritability of substance abuse (including alcohol-related problems) among monozygotic twins reared apart has been reported by Grove et al. (1990). The MZ twin reared apart method avoids several of the problems regarding the potential sources of twin similarity due to environmental factors. This method, then, has an advantage over studies that examine twins reared together. However, the frequency of such identifiable twin pairs in the population is relatively low, limiting the utility of this approach. Grove et al. (1990) studied 31 pairs of MZ twins and one set of triplets; 68.7% of the sample were female with a median age of 43 years. Mean age at separation was .6 years and mean age when reunited was 34.0 years. Subjects were interviewed using a standardized psychiatric diagnostic interview schedule, the NIMH-DIS. Due to the low number of subjects meeting DSM-III criteria (American Psychiatric Association, 1980) for alcohol abuse/dependence, signs and symptoms from the NIMH-DIS (Robins et al, 1981) counting toward DSM-III, RDC, and Feighner (Feighner et al, 1972) criteria sets were summed into a quasi-continuous variable. The probandwise concordance rate for alcohol disorders (abuse and/or dependence) was 33%, for drug abuse/dependence 36%, and for antisocial personality disorder 29%. Grove et al. found a modest heritability for alcoholism (.13) and a modest phenotypic correlation of alcoholism with drug abuse (.25), childhood conduct problems (.27), and adult antisocial behavior (.28). Yet, a high genetic correlation was found for the combination of alcohol and drug problems (.78). They interpret their data as indicating a strong overlap between the genes that contribute to both drinking behavior and to drug use.

As with the Gurling and Murray twin study, Grove et al. found a relatively modest concordance rate for alcoholism in their MZ twin pairs. It should also be noted, however, that the samples of the two studies were small and were similar with respect to having both a significant proportion of female subjects and subjects still young enough to be in the period of risk for developing alcoholism.

Pickens et al. (1991) examined a sample of males and females from the United States for the genetic risk of alcoholism. The sample included $n = 50$ MZ and $n = 64$ DZ male (same-sexed) pairs and $n = 31$ MZ and $n = 24$ DZ (same-sexed) female pairs. The probands were identified via a retrospective examination of treatment records. After being recruited, probands and their cotwins completed a series of questionnaires and were directly interviewed using the NIMH-DIS. Lifetime DSM-III diagnoses for Alcohol Abuse and for Alcohol Dependence were made from the NIMH-DIS responses. Zygosity was determined using blood markers for 159 pairs; questionnaires were used for the remaining 10 pairs. For the male sample, significant differences in concordance rates were found between the MZ and DZ twins for Alcohol Abuse (74% vs. 58%), for Alcohol Dependence (59% vs. 36%) and for the combined category of Alcohol Abuse and/or Dependence (76% vs. 61%). For the female twin pairs, however, differences in concordance rates were found only for Alcohol Dependence (25% vs. 5%). The concordance rates observed for Alcohol Abuse (26.7% vs. 27.3%) and Alcohol Abuse and/or Dependence (35.5% vs. 25%) were not statistically different. Heritability estimates of .35 for male subjects and .24 for female subjects were rather modest when examined without regard to the severity of the alcohol problems present. For Alcohol Abuse, familial risk was largely due to environmental factors (i.e., approximately 50% of the liability variance) for both male and female subjects. Risk for Alcohol Dependence, however, appeared to be more largely due to genetic factors, with heritability estimates of .596 for male subjects and .420 for female subjects.

Using a larger sample that partially overlaps the Pickens et al. study, McGue et al. (1992) examined both same-sexed and opposite-sexed twin pairs with respect to their concordance for DSM-III-defined Alcohol Abuse and/or Alcohol Dependence. The proband twin was ascertained from an alcohol treatment center. Twin pairs included 268 same-sex (85 MZ males, 44 MZ females; 96 DZ males, 43 DZ females) and 88 opposite-sex pairs (65 with male probands, 23 with female probands). Data on the subjects' alcohol/drug use history, reported conduct problems, and psychiatric treatment history were obtained via a mailed survey. Zygosity was determined using responses to a physical resemblance questionnaire and by serological methods. Consistent with the Pickens et al. study, significant concordance was found for the male twins (MZ males, 77% DZ males, 54%), but not for the female twin pairs (MZ females, 39%; DZ females, 42%). The heritability of liability for alcoholism was significantly higher for males ($h^2 = .54$) compared to females ($h^2 = .00$). Further, the heritability of early onset ($h^2 = .73$), compared to late onset ($h^2 = .30$), alcoholism was significantly greater among males, while no differences were found for the female sample. It should also be noted that for the male DZ cotwins, the rate of alcoholism was higher when the proband was female rather than male. A similar, but nonsignificant, trend in the same direction was noted among female DZ cotwins. These data are consistent with those reported in several of the preceding studies, i.e., greater heritabilities are often found for males with more severe alcoholism (including alcohol dependence) compared to more milder forms of alcohol abuse.

For the female twins, heritability estimates did not vary in relation to the age of onset of alcohol problems in the proband. Genetic influences were minimal in the pooled heritability estimates, while shared environmental factors were substantial for both early ($h^2 = .732$) and late ($h^2 = .525$) onset alcohol problems in the female twins. The reasons for the failure to find genetic effects in the heritability of alcohol problems among the female twins are not obvious. The sample of female twin pairs was small ($n = 44$ MZ; $n = 43$ DZ; $n = 23$ OS) and a large percentage of the probands (65.5%) had also been treated for depression (compared to 27.4% of the male probands). Further, more female probands reported drug use than male probands (60.9% vs. 46.3%). Yet, male and female probands did not differ with respect to the number and type of alcohol-related symptoms (including dependence) reported, the age of onset of first intoxication or first symptom, the length of their illness, or in the number of reported conduct problems.

Kendler et al. (1992), using a population-based sample of female twins (Virginia Twin Registry) examined the heritability of alcoholism according to three different definitions of alcoholism. These definitions were conceptualized as representing different levels of severity on a dimension of liability for alcoholism. The dimensions were defined in terms of *DSM-III-R* (American Psychiatric Association, 1987) criteria as alcoholism with or without tolerance-dependence or problem drinking (broad definition); alcoholism with or without dependence-tolerance (*DSM-III-R* definition of dependence) (intermediate definition); and alcoholism with dependence-tolerance (narrow definition). The average age of the sample was about 30 years, with a range from 17 to 55 years. From a sample of $n = 2060$ directly interviewed subjects, $n = 128$ met criteria for the narrow definition of alcoholism, $n = 57$ fit the intermediate definition, and $n = 172$ met criteria for the broad definition. Probandwise concordance for alcoholism was consistently higher in MZ than in DZ twin pairs and increased in relation to the broadening of the definition of alcoholism. The heritability of alcoholism also varied according to the narrow definition of alcoholism used: narrow $h^2 = .50$, intermediate $h^2 = .56$, broad $h^2 = .61$. The heritability estimates decreased only slightly when frequency of contact with cotwin (a social environment factor) was considered. Given that the onset of alcoholism is somewhat later for women than for men, it is likely that these heritability estimates may increase as more of the subjects enter and pass through the age of risk for alcoholism. However, this study, using a population-based sample, provides evidence of the importance of genetic factors in the liability for developing alcoholism among women.

Few data on ethnic minority twin pairs are available. A twin study reported by Caldwell and Gottesman (1991) is notable in that approximately 30% of the sample is black. The probands were ascertained from inpatient and outpatient psychiatric facilities and were, on average, approximately 35 years of age. The sample included $n = 95$ same-sex twin pairs (28 MZ males, 17 MZ females, 26 DZ males, and 24 DZ females) and $n = 59$ opposite-sex pairs of twins (40 male probands; 19 female probands). Zygosity was determined using physical similarity methods; if inconclusive, serological methods were employed. Alcohol abuse/dependence was assessed using the

NIMH-DIS, and diagnoses were made according to DSM-III criteria. Concordance for alcoholism (abuse and/or dependence) differed by zygosity for males (MZ = 68% vs. DZ = 46%), but not for females (MZ = 46% vs. DZ = 42%). A MZ/DZ ratio of concordances for alcohol abuse and/or dependence was 1.5 for males, but this increased to 3.1 when only alcohol dependence was considered. Again, genetic factors seem to be greatest for the more severe form of the disorder. Male heritability of liability was estimated to be .70 compared to only .08 for females. Neither age of onset of the disorder nor race appeared to moderate the reported effects.

The heritability of alcoholism and other types of psychopathology were examined in $n = 12,884$ twin pairs in Sweden by Allgulander et al. (1991). Physical similarity was used to determine zygosity; information with respect to the presence of alcoholism was obtained via hospital registrations. The prevalence of alcoholism, based on ICD-8 criteria hospital discharge diagnoses, was found to be less than 2% among the males and less than .5% among the females. Tetrachoric correlations (rather than concordance rates) were reported as .40 and .36 for MZ and DZ male twins, respectively, compared to .62 and .51 for MZ and DZ twin females. A heritability estimate of only .16 was reported for alcoholism. This finding is not too surprising, however given the rather low prevalence rates for alcoholism in this sample and the use of a broad definition of alcoholism that also included both alcohol dependence and alcohol abuse.

A number of studies comparing the drinking styles, rather than drinking-related problems, of MZ and DZ twins have also been conducted. Such studies, particularly when based on large-population-based samples, are useful for estimating the variance in aspects of drinking behavior (but not necessarily alcohol-related problems or alcoholism) that is due to additive genetic effects, shared family environment affecting both members of the twin pair, and specific environmental factors that are unique to one of the twins.

Twin Studies of Normal Drinking

In a study drawn from the Finnish Twin Registry based on the general population, Partanen et al. (1966) reported on 902 (MZ $n = 172$; DZ $n = 577$) pairs of male twins. Three aspects of drinking behavior were examined: density—the frequency and regularity of drinking; amount—the volume of ethanol consumed per occasion; and loss of control—an inability to control alcohol intake and to stop drinking. Concordances for abstinence and for heavy drinking were higher among MZ compared to DZ twin pairs. Heritabilities of .39 for density and .36 for amount were found, suggesting the influence of heredity on normal drinking habits, but only .14 for loss of control. However, the heritabilities of the consequences of heavy drinking (addictive symptoms, arrests for intoxication, and social complications) were low. It should be noted, however, that when loss of control and heavy consumption were considered together (i.e., approximating alcoholism), the heritability was 66%. This figure is similar to the heritability estimates reported for the male twin samples of Kaij (1960), Hrubec and Omenn (1981), and more recently, by Pickens et al. (1991).

Carmelli et al. (1990) examined the heritability of substance use in adult male twins from the NAS–NRC Twin Registry. Cigarette smoking, and alcohol and caffeine consumption were studied in $n = 2390$ MZ and $n = 2570$ DZ twin pairs. Before adjusting for sociodemographic factors (e.g., socioeconomic status, age, etc.), genetic effects accounted for 36% of the variance in the total number of drinks consumed weekly. After adjustment for these factors, the heritability estimate was reduced to 29%. These figures approximate those for "density" (regularity of drinking) and for amount of drinking reported by Partanen et al. (1966).

Various aspects of alcohol-use behavior (rather than alcoholism per se) have also been examined using subjects from the Australian Twin Register. The sample contains complete data on the responses of $n = 3810$ twin pairs to a mailed questionnaire that assessed alcohol consumption and other health-related habits. The resulting sample represented approximately a 64% pairwise response rate and contained $n = 1233$ MZ female, $n = 567$ MZ male, $n = 751$ DZ female, $n = 352$ DZ male, and $n = 907$ opposite-sex DZ pairs. At the time of this assessment, the average age of the sample was approximately 35–36 years of age. A genetic analysis by Jardine and Martin (1984) of the amount of alcohol consumed weekly and the amount consumed in the past week revealed that individual environmental factors accounted for 44% of the variance for both sexes. No evidence for shared environmental effects were found for females, however, with 56% of the variance due to genetic factors. Among the male twins, 20% of the variance in drinking behavior was accounted for by common environmental effects, while 36% of the variance could be attributed to genetic factors. The age of the proband for females did not affect these analyses. For male twins under 30 years of age, however, more than 60% of the variance in drinking behavior was attributable to genetic factors. In male twins over 30 years old, the variation in drinking behavior was due to either individual or shared environmental differences.

In a subset of these twins, genetic and social factors associated with abstinence and with onset of alcohol use among those who drank were examined (Heath and Martin, 1988). Variability in the concordance for teenage abstinence was explained by additive genetic effects (35%) and by shared environmental effects (32%) among females compared to 47% and 48% of the variance in the male twins liability. Their analysis, which tested several different models of transmission, suggests that the age of onset of drinking of male twins was strongly influenced by the social environment, while genetic effects appeared to play an important role in determining the age of onset of drinking among the female twins.

A more recent analysis of the Australian twin data focused on the contribution of genetic factors to the risk for developing problem drinking in both males and females and an examination of the correlation between genetic effects and alcohol consumption (Heath and Martin, 1994). Both average weekly consumption of alcohol and problem drinking history were found to be associated with genetic factors. Approximately 58% of the variation in females' average weekly consumption of alcohol was accounted for by genetic factors, compared to 45% of the variance in the male twins. However, heritability estimates of problem drinking were quite model-dependent. For females, estimates of the genetic correlation for problem drinking ranged from 8 to 44%, versus 10 to 50% in males.

Other twin studies have also examined the transmission of drinking behavior rather than alcoholism. Cederlof et al.'s (1977) study of $n = 13,000$ Swedish twin pairs concluded that normal drinking was not greatly influenced by heritable factors. This conclusion is supported by a small study ($n = 34$ MZ, $n = 43$ DZ) of Italian twin pairs (Conterio and Chiarelli, 1962). Pederson's 1981 study of 137 Swedish twin pairs reported a heritability of .71 for heavy drinking, but did not distinguish genetic and environmental influences. The genetic influence on the heritability of alcohol consumption may decrease with age. Kapprio et al.'s (1981) study of Finnish twins found an overall heritability of alcohol consumption for males of .37, but this value ranged from .53 for 20--24-year-olds to $-.04$ for 70--74-year-old males. The overall heritability of female alcohol consumption was .25.

Further, sibling similarity in alcohol consumption patterns does appear to be associated with their level of social contact over time. In a reanalysis of alcohol consumption data derived from twins in the United Kingdom (Clifford et al., 1984), Australia (Heath et al., 1989), and Finland (Kaprio et al., 1987), Rose et al. (1990) found that twins (both MZ and DZ) who cohabit longer into adult life and who maintain closer social contact after leaving the home of rearing are more alike in their alcohol consumption than those twins who do not. However, the estimates of heritable genetic effects were unchanged, and only the proportion of variance attributable to shared and unshared environmental factors varied according to amount of social contact.

Adoption Studies

Although the separation of genetic and environmental/familial influences on the transmission of alcoholism from an affected parent to biological offspring can be disentangled to some extent by using mathematical models, the distinction often relies heavily on imprecise measures of these two constructs. A more elegant method of study has been developed based on a naturally occurring experiment: the adopted child separated at (or near) birth from the affected parent. A basic assumption of this method is that the genetic trait present in the affected biological parent will still be expressed in adoptees, regardless of the genotypic status and environmental/familial circumstances of the adoptive parents. There are four basic separation study methods: (1) adoptive family method—alcoholic proband adoptees compared to control adoptees with respect to the prevalence of alcoholism in both the biological and adoptive relatives; (2) adoptee study method—compares the prevalence of alcoholism among the adopted-away children of an alcoholic parent to either adoptees of controls or to the general population; (3) adoptive parents' method—begins with alcoholic probands and compares the prevalence of alcoholism in their biological and adoptive parents; and 4) the cross-fostering method—identifies two groups of adoptees (e.g., children of an alcoholic parent raised by a nonalcoholic adoptive parent and children of a nonalcoholic biological parent raised by an alcoholic parent) and then compares them with respect to the preva-

lence of alcoholism in each group. The adoptee study method can provide direct estimates, then, of both genetic effects and of environmental/familial effects with respect
to the transmission of alcoholism.

An Early Report

The first known published followup study of adopted-away children of an alcoholic
parent was by Roe in 1944. This study, which used the adoptee study method, compared $n = 36$ adoptees (21 males, 15 females) of fathers said to be "heavy drinkers
with syndrome" to $n = 25$ adoptees (11 males, 14 females) whose parents had no
known psychiatric or criminal record. When followed into young adulthood neither
group was found to be heavy drinkers nor to have alcohol problems. It should be noted
that both the proband and control adoptees were adopted away in early childhood (at
5.6 vs. 2.6 years of age) rather than immediately after birth. This study's failure to find
differences due to parental alcohol problems has been attributed to its low statistical
power due to a small sample size and to the relatively few males included in the sample. Further, a higher portion of the "high-risk" sample (67%) were also placed in rural
areas or small towns compared to the control group (28%). These types of environments typically are considered to attenuate the risk (familial or otherwise) for the
development of alcoholism. It should also be noted that a large percentage (25%) of
the putative fathers had a criminal arrest record and that 81% had been charged with
child abuse/neglect. These data suggest that a substantial number of the heavy drinking
fathers may have had a primary diagnosis of antisocial personality disorder rather than
alcoholism. If so, the offspring of these fathers, then, would be more likely to develop
conduct or antisocial problems other than alcoholism (Reich et al., 1981; Cloninger
and Reich, 1983; Cadoret et al., 1985).

The Danish Adoption Study

The most widely cited series of studies of adopted-away children of a biologic parent
were based on samples derived from the Copenhagen, Denmark, Adoption Registry.
This study also used the adoptee study method. Goodwin et al. (1973) reported on
three groups of sons: $n = 55$ adoptees with an alcoholic biologic parent (85% of whom
were fathers); $n = 50$ control adoptees with no known psychiatric problems (registrations) among either biologic parent; $n = 28$ control adoptees with one biologic parent
hospitalized for psychiatric problems other than alcoholism. The adoptee probands
were placed with nonbiological relatives before six weeks of birth and were between
22 and 45 years of age at followup. Alcoholism in the biologic parent was based on a
hospital chart diagnosis of alcoholism or alcohol abuse. Interestingly, 13% of the
probands' adoptive fathers met criteria for possible or definite alcoholism, compared to
22% of the adoptive fathers of the controls, but being reared by an alcoholic father was
not associated with the offspring's risk for developing alcoholism. When the lifetime
drinking patterns of the adoptees were examined, 18% of the proband group versus

only 5% of the combined control group met criteria for a lifetime diagnosis of alco-holism. For the problem drinker and heavy drinker classifications, however, the preva-lence rates tended to be higher for the controls (36%; 14%) compared to the probands (22%; 9%). When the adopted-away sons of an alcoholic parent were compared to their brothers who had been raised by the alcoholic biologic parent, the rate of alco-holism was similar in the two groups (Goodwin et al., 1974). Taken together, these data are consistent with several twin studies (cf. Kaij, 1960; Pickens et al., 1991) and suggest that the genetic factors are important for the transmission of alcoholism, but not for problem drinking.

Data from the Danish adoptee female sample were reported in a second publication (Goodwin et al., 1977). Using a methodology similar to that used to study the adoptee sons, $n = 49$ adopted-away daughters of a biologic alcoholic parent were compared to $n = 47$ control adoptees. The lifetime prevalence of alcoholism for the proband daugh-ters was 2% compared to 4% in the controls. This difference in the direction contrary to expectation was not significant. Although the reported rates of alcoholism in both groups were higher than the population prevalence rate (.1%–1.0%) for women in Denmark at the time, over 90% of the remaining samples reported themselves to be either abstainers or very light drinkers. Thus, inadequate exposure to heavy drinking may help account for the lack of expression of alcoholism in the biologic daughters of the alcoholic parent.

The Swedish Adoption Study

More recently, a cross-fostering study of Swedish adoptees of a biologic alcoholic par-ent was reported by Cloninger and colleagues (1981). The first report examines the inheritance of alcohol abuse in $n = 862$ Swedish men adopted before three years of age by nonrelatives. At the time the last information was available, subjects ranged in age from 23 to 43 years of age. Archival information was obtained from several national registries, including the Temperance Board, the National Health Insurance, and the criminal register. Mild alcohol abuse in the adoptee and the biologic parent was defined as having one temperance board registration and no history of alcohol abuse treatment; moderate abusers had 2–3 registrations and no treatment of alco-holism. Severe abusers had four or more registrations and a history of compulsory treatment for alcohol problems or a psychiatric hospitalization with a diagnosis of alcoholism. Higher lifetime rates of alcohol abuse (i.e., at least one registration) were found among the reared-away sons of alcoholic (22.4%) versus nonalcoholic (14.7%) fathers and among alcoholic (28.1%) versus nonalcoholic (14.7%) mothers. The great-est heritability was found among the moderate abusing sons ($h^2 = .90$) compared to adoptee sons with either mild ($h^2 = .38$) or severe ($h^2 = .25$) alcohol abuse. These data led Cloninger et al. to posit two separate types of alcoholism: Type I is only moder-ately heritable and characterized by a late age of onset (after age 25), loss of control when drinking, and guilt about drinking; Type II is viewed as the highly heritable form of alcoholism and is characterized by an early onset of problems (before age 25), an inability to abstain, and fighting and arrests when drinking. Similar to Goodwin et al. (1973), Cloninger et al. found that being reared in an alcoholic family was not related to the risk for the more severe type of alcoholism.

Data from the $n = 913$ females in the sample were reported by Bohman et al. (1981). In general, adopted-away daughters of a biologic alcoholic parent demonstrated an increased risk for alcoholism compared to the adopted away daughters of nonalcoholic parents. A fourfold increase in risk was found if the biologic mother (but not the father) was alcoholic compared to women whose biologic parents were not alcoholic (10.3% vs. 2.8%). Similarly, a fourfold increase in risk was noted when both biologic parents of the female adoptee were alcoholic compared to women whose biologic parents had no history of alcoholism (9.8% vs. 2.8%). If only the biologic father abused alcohol, however, no excess of alcoholism was found among the female adoptees compared to women with no family history of alcoholism (3.5% vs. 2.8%). Thus, an excess of alcoholism was found among the daughters of alcoholic mothers (9.8%), but not among the daughters of alcoholic fathers (3.9% vs. 2.8%). Being reared by an alcoholic adoptive father did not modify the daughter's risk for developing alcohol abuse.

In a further analysis of this data set, Bohman et al. (1987) identified three types of families with alcoholism. These types differed with respect to the frequency of alcohol abuse in the family, to the presence of somatoform disorders in the female family members, and in relation to the frequency of antisocial behaviors in the male adoptees. The development of the most frequent type of alcoholism by both the male and female adoptees, milieu-limited alcoholism, was characterized by both genetic and environmental factors. A less common type of male-limited family vulnerability was characterized by a highly heritable form of alcoholism among the male adoptees, while the female relatives typically had multiple somatic complaints (but seldom had alcohol abuse). The third type of vulnerability was associated with violent criminality and recurrent alcohol abuse in the male family members and a high frequency of somatic complaints and disability among the female relatives. They conclude that these three types of alcoholism are relatively discrete. Thus, the likelihood of developing a disorder and its type seems to depend on social/environmental factors.

The Iowa Adoption Studies

The use of the adoption paradigm to study the genetic basis of alcoholism in the United States has been limited. Unlike Scandinavia or Japan, no national registries exist and available records (particularly on the biologic parents) are often scant. The single exception is a series of published adoption studies from Iowa based on samples derived from two children's social service agencies in Des Moine. The initial study of adoptees from the Children's and Family Services reported by Cadoret and Gath (1978) was of $n = 84$ adoptees over the age of 18 who had been separated at birth from their biologic parents. Diagnoses of the adoptees were made following a direct interview of the adoptee and the adoptive parent using Feighner criteria (1972) for alcoholism. Diagnoses of the biologic parents was made following a record review; a diagnosis of alcoholism was made if two or more social or medical complications associated with alco-holism or hospitalization for detoxification were reported. Heavy drinking was defined if one social or medical complication of alcohol was reported or if the individual was described as a heavy drinker or "drinks too much for own good." Primary alcoholism occurred more frequently among the adoptees of alcoholic or heavy drinking biologic parents (3/6) than among the control group (1/78). Of the seven adoptees with a diag-nosis of secondary alcoholism, none had a biologic parent affected with alcoholism. Adoptee alcoholism was not associated with any other psychiatric diagnosis in the bio-logic parent nor with any environmental variable (e.g., socioeconomic status of adop-tive parents, adoptive parents psychiatric status, time in foster care, adoptee's age). Due to the small sample size, no gender comparisons could be made.

A later report, using a similar methodology and based on an expanded sample, examined $n = 92$ male adoptees over the age of 18 years old (Cadoret et al., 1980). Using logistic regression methods, a significant association was found between adoptee alcoholism and an alcoholic background (i.e., the presence of alcoholism among first- and/or second-degree biological relatives). However, the relative contri-bution of affected first-degree and second-degree biologic relatives in the predictive model could not be distinguished. Further, the addition of environmental variables to the equation did not improve the prediction of adoptee alcoholism.

Reporting on the Lutheran Social Services adoptee sample ($n = 127$ males; $n = 87$ females), Cadoret et al. (1985) examined the interrelationship of alcoholism and anti-social personality disorder. The adoptees were in their midtwenties at the time of the assessment. Adoptee diagnoses of alcohol abuse or dependence were assigned blindly based on DSM-III criteria (1980) using composite information gathered from adoptee and adoptee parent interviews (using either the SADS-L or NIMH-DIS) and from school and psychiatric records. Definite alcoholism in the biologic family member was defined as having one or more social, legal, work, or medical consequences in addition to heavy drinking or a hospitalization for detoxification. Possible alcoholism was defined based on a report of heavy drinking or drinking too much for their own good. For both male and female adoptees, the rates of adoptee alcohol abuse were signifi-cantly higher when a biologic first-degree relative had alcohol problems (males = 61.6%, females = 33%) than when no family background of alcoholism was present (males = 23.9%; females = 5.3%). Drinking problems in the adoptive home con-tributed to the prediction of adult alcohol abuse problems among the male, but not the female, adoptees. A biologic background of antisocial personality disorder did not con-tribute to the risk for alcohol abuse for either the male or female adoptees, suggesting that antisocial personality disorder and alcoholism are separately transmitted disorders. This finding is consistent with several other previous studies (cf. Cloninger et al., 1978; Reich et al., 1981; Cloninger and Reich 1983)

Half-sibling Studies

Although not formally an adoption study, half-sibling studies provide another method of examining the prevalence of alcoholism in a sibship in which only one biologic parent is shared. These types of studies can contribute additional evidence for the separate roles of genetic and environmental factors in the transmission of alcoholism, particularly when the child was reared apart from the alcoholic parent. Schuckit et al. (1972) examined $n = 69$ probands, aged 22–54 years old, admitted to an alcoholism treatment unit. Patients with a history of serious antisocial or drug-related behavior were excluded. Data were obtained via a structured interview regarding the psychiatric status of the biologic parents, stepparents, and full and half-siblings. Collateral information from relatives was obtained for confirmatory purposes when possible; information was available on $n = 164$ subjects (including the probands). Living with an alcoholic parent was defined as living with that parent for six or more years prior to the age of 17. The rate of alcoholism among half-siblings with a biologic parent was similar whether raised with an alcoholic parent (46%) or not (50%); similarly, the rate of alcoholism among half-siblings with no biologic parent affected with alcoholism was similar whether raised with an alcoholic parent (14%) or not (8%). Further, living with an alcoholic parent or parent surrogate for six or more years or having lived in a broken home did not distinguish the half-siblings who developed alcoholism from those who did not, suggesting that alcoholic rearing was unrelated to the rate of alcoholism among the half-siblings.

The Gene Versus Environment Controversy

There have been a number of challenges to the role of genetic factors in the transmission of alcoholism (cf. Murray et al., 1983; Peele, 1986; Searles, 1988). A principal issue behind the controversy is the inconsistency across studies with respect to the amount of variation in the heritability of alcoholism explained by genetic factors. One reason for the lack of convergence in the extant literature may have to do with the heterogeneous nature of the disorder under investigation. Indeed, the search to identify subtypes has spanned several decades of alcoholism research. The majority of these efforts have been based on clinical observation [cf. Knight's (1937) "Essential—Reactive" types; Jellinek's (1960) "Alpha, Delta, Epsilon; Gamma" subtypes], while the empirically derived subtypes of alcoholism [cf. Morey and Blashfield (1981); Babor et al. (1992)] have also included a variety of other psychosocial factors. However, none of these proposed subtypes include heredity or genetic factors in their conceptualization, instead focusing primarily on the drinking history, drinking-related behaviors, and/or associated personality traits of the proband. The single exception is Cloninger et al. (1981) who discussed the importance of genetic factors for both the development and transmission of Type I/Type II alcoholism.

This lack of agreement in describing the clinical phenomenon of "alcoholism" is also manifest in terms of existing formal diagnostic criteria. While most criteria sets [e.g., Feighner et al (1972); National Council on Alcohol (1972); ICD-9 (1980); DSM-III-R (1987)] share common features (e.g., incapacitation in several aspects of life due to alcohol consumption), the criteria sets vary with respect to the duration of problem drinking necessary to become a case, the types of symptoms (including the importance of biological sequelae) required, and the clustering of symptoms. Consequently, different diagnostic systems may identify different groups of patients as alcoholic. Since different individuals will be identified as being affected using different diagnostic systems, variations in their genotype and, therefore, in the explanatory power of genetic factors in the transmission of alcoholism should be expected. A major step forward in resolving the gene versus environment issue is likely to result when the phenotype of alcoholism to be studied is more precisely defined. In addition to presenting symptomatology, the definition of the phenotype could be improved by including gender of the proband, age of onset of alcoholism, and possibly, response to biological and psychotherapeutic treatments as part of the definition.

A second, related point that may cloud the gene–environment issue is the presence of an additional comorbid psychiatric disorder in the proband, in addition to alcohol abuse/dependence. Other psychiatric disorders such as major depressive disorder and antisocial personality disorder are also strongly familial in nature and may have genetic factors contributing to their heritability. Studies of samples of alcoholic probands drawn from both clinical settings (cf. Hesselbrock et al., 1985) and from the community (cf. Helzer and Pryzbeck, 1988; Regier et al., 1990) have found a variety of other psychiatric disorders coexisting with the alcoholism. As many as 80% of persons with alcoholism may have at least one other coexisting psychiatric condition (Hesselbrock et al., 1985) that is relatively stable over time (Penick et al., 1988). Major depressive disorder is the most common additional problem among females with alcoholism, while depression and antisocial personality disorder are frequently found among alcoholic males. The presence of an additional psychiatric disorder may complicate the specification of the alcoholic phenotype since symptoms of these disorders often mimic those associated with alcoholism. For example, persons with alcoholism often feel dysphoric and display antisocial behavior. Conversely, persons with either depression or antisocial personality disorder frequently drink heavily. Failure to distinguish symptoms arising from alcohol use from those due to a separate psychiatric disorder could lead to diagnostic confusion (Schuckit, 1973), particularly for those less severely affected cases. In this situation, such cases could be misidentified as affected when in fact they are not (i.e., false positive). The inclusion of false positives in genetical analyses can falsely attenuate the size of any genetic effects found.

Major depressive disorder and antisocial personality are frequently found in families with alcoholism, yet both appear to have different etiologies and to be genetically distinct (cf. Cadoret et al., 1985; Merikangas et al., 1985). While certain comorbid conditions, such as depression or antisocial personality disorder, are neither necessary nor sufficient causes of alcoholism, their presence may increase a person's vulnerability for developing alcohol problems. Unless clear diagnostic distinctions are made with respect to both the proband and their biological relatives, misattributions regarding the presence and the magnitude of genetic effects for the heritability of either disorder may be made.

The age of the proband and the proband's biological family members at the time of ascertainment may also influence estimates of genetic heritability. The age at which a person is likely to become affected (i.e., the age of risk) varies across psychiatric disorders. Therefore, the proportion of family members who are either not yet at risk, who are currently in the period of risk, or who have passed through the period of risk varies according to the psychiatric disorder of interest and the age of the individual family members at the time of assessment. Failure to find genetic effects may arise, for example, when the sample contains a number of youthful probands. Thus, families showing little or no familial alcoholism at the initial assessment may show substantial familial aggregation when followed years later after the majority of the biologically related individuals have passed through the period of risk. A further related complication is the possibility that some psychiatric disorders may show secular trends in their age of onset and the lifetime prevalence rates. Reich et al. (1988) found that more recently born cohorts, compared to older cohorts, had higher than expected lifetime prevalence rates of alcoholism and decreased ages of onset. Age corrections can be applied to the rates of the disorder (e.g., alcoholism) found among biological relatives—for example, using the Stromgren method (Slater and Cowie, 1971), which involves weighing the number of persons at risk by the proportion of the risk period through which they have passed. Such a correction is often necessary in order to make accurate comparisons of samples spanning several generations or from different populations.

The method used to establish the presence of alcoholism in the proband and the biological family members may also influence estimates of genetic effects. Data collected via direct interview methods, family history methods, and from records often lead to different conclusions regarding the presence and severity of alcohol problems present in any given individual. Undoubtedly, the most accurate method of obtaining information regarding psychiatric diagnoses (including alcoholism) is through the use of a direct interview of the subject. When direct interviews are conducted, the reliability and validity of the resulting diagnoses are often enhanced when the information is obtained using a structured interview schedule, e.g., SCID, CIDI, SSAGA, NIMH-DIS, DIGS.

In large-scale family studies, however, all relatives may not be available for a direct interview, or conducting direct interviews may be too time-consuming or too costly. One solution is to use the family history or family story method. With the family history method, one (or preferably more) family member provides as much information as possible about the psychiatric status of the unavailable relative. Systematic interviewing methods and specific criteria (cf. Andreasen et al., 1977) have been developed to enhance the reliability of this method. The economy of the family history method is often obtained at the expense of the reliability of the diagnoses made. Studies comparing the diagnoses obtained via direct interview methods to diagnoses made using family history methods report only a modest level of agreement for most psychiatric conditions. Informants generally tend to underestimate the level of psychiatric illness in relatives, but this varies in relation to the disorder under consideration and the relationship of the informant to the relative. The reliability of the more prevalent psychiatric disorders is usually higher than for those that occur less frequently. The concordance of the diagnosis of alcoholism made using direct interview methods with those made using family history methods, however, is quite good, with kappas as high as .70 reported (Andreasen et al., 1977; Hesselbrock et al., 1985). Reliability also improves when collateral information is collected from more than one informant (Hesselbrock, 1986).

Many published studies of the heritability of alcoholism have used hospital, health service, or registry records to obtain information on the psychiatric status of the proband and/or the family members. Records seldom contain the information necessary to meet formalized diagnostic criteria (e.g., DSM-III-R; ICD-9), requiring a compromise in the criteria used for the identification of a case. The use of a reduced diagnostic criteria set often results in reduced sensitivity (i.e., the number of true positives) and specificity (i.e., the number of true negatives). The inability to accurately identify a true case can dramatically reduce the ability of many statistical analytic methods.

Conclusions

To date, no single study has convincingly established the role of genetic factors in the transmission of alcoholism. This is not surprising given the number of methodological issues discussed earlier that may attenuate the finding of possible genetic effects on the risk for alcoholism. Taken collectively, however, the body of evidence provides a powerful demonstration of the influence of genetic factors on the risk for alcoholism. This relationship is not unconditional, and some caveats need to be offered. First, the contribution of genetic factors to the risk for alcoholism seemingly varies according to gender. The data from the male twin studies reviewed previously found higher concordance of alcoholism rates for MZ compared to DZ twin pairs. The two apparent exceptions are the studies by Gurling et al. (1984) and Allgulander et al. (1991). Gurling et al.'s sample of twin pairs was somewhat small, and comorbid psychiatric conditions were not considered, while Allgulander et al.'s reliance on records for identifying affectional status may have led to a significant under ascertainment of the number of affected cases. The twin studies provide estimates indicating that genetic effects may account for 40–60% of the variance in liability for the development of alcoholism. Similarly, the studies of male adoptees reviewed earlier [excepting Roe (1944)] found that a biological background of alcoholism (usually the biological father) was an important predictor of the adoptee son's risk for developing alcoholism.

Second, the evidence supporting the influence of genetic factors on the risk for females developing alcoholism is rather modest. There are however, few published studies of the heritability of alcoholism for females, and even fewer studies have employed sufficiently large samples of well-characterized female probands. At this time, data supporting the importance of genetic factors for the liability of alcoholism for females come from two pedigree, one twin, and two adoption studies. Data from the two family pedigree studies (Cloninger et al., 1978; Hall et al., 1983) reported similar prevalence rates of alcoholism among the biological relatives of male and female alcoholic probands, supporting the possibility of genetic influences for women's vulnerability to alcoholism. Only the twin study of Pickens et al. (1991) and two studies of female adoptees (Bohman et al., 1981 and Cadoret et al., 1985) were able to find significant genetic effects in the liability for alcoholism of females. It should also be noted that in one twin study, cross-sex transmission of the risk for alcoholism was found. McGue et al. (1992) found a rate of alcohol abuse/dependence of 30.7% among the female cotwins of DZ male probands compared to an age-corrected ECA population prevalence estimate of 6.3%. The male cotwins of DZ female probands had a rate of alcohol abuse/dependence of 78.3% (compared to an age-corrected population estimate of 26.3%). While the dearth of evidence at this time does not conclusively prove the absence of genetic effects for the liability for alcoholism among women, it is possible that only the liability for the most severe form of alcoholism among females is influenced by genetic factors. The samples of females studied by Hall et al. and Pickens et al. met criteria for DSM-III alcohol dependence rather than for alcohol abuse or other less stringent criteria for alcoholism. Further, there are few data to suggest that either the etiology of alcoholism (cf. Hesselbrock et al., 1984; Hesselbrock et al., 1986) or the response to treatment (cf. Rounsaville et al., 1988) substantially varies according to gender. If genetic factors in the liability for alcoholism are absent for females, greater differences in the course and outcome of the disorder would be expected.

The studies reviewed also suggest that environmental factors provide a significant influence on both the male and female risk for alcoholism. Of the twin studies of alcohol abuse/dependence reviewed, the proportion of alcoholism liability attributable to shared (e.g., socioeconomic status of the family of rearing) and nonshared (e.g., friends) environmental factors is often quite large. For males, the amount of variance attributable to shared and nonshared environmental factors in the liability for the severe forms of alcoholism including alcohol dependence tended to be small relative to the amount of variance attributable to genetic factors. When less severe forms of alcoholism were examined, however, the amount of variance attributable to environmental (shared + nonshared) factors approached or exceeded that explained by genetic factors. For females, regardless of the severity of the disorder, environmental (shared + nonshared) factors accounted for more of the variance in the liability for alcoholism than genetic factors. Further, aspects of alcohol use behavior such as age of onset of drinking, abstinence, and similarity of sibling's drinking styles appear to be strongly influenced by environmental factors, although this may vary by gender. According to the findings of the adoption studies, however, being reared by an alcoholic parent does not by itself appear to be critical to the development of alcoholism. Only Cadoret et al. (1987) and Cadoret and Wesner (1990) reported a similarity in alcoholism between adoptees and adoptive parents. No adoptive parent–adoptee resemblance in terms of alcoholism was found in the studies reported by Goodwin et al. (1973), Cloninger et al. (1981), Bohman et al. (1981), or the half-sibling study of Schuckit et al. (1973).

Summary

The familial nature of alcoholism is well documented, and a variety of studies have described the influence of genetic and environmental factors on the transmission of drinking behavior and the pathological use of alcohol. Collectively, family pedigree studies, studies of MZ and DZ twins, and studies of adoptees (and half-siblings) of alcoholic parentage attest to the influence of genes in the liability for the development of alcoholism. However, no single study has clearly demonstrated the importance of genetic factors for either males or females. While this is somewhat discouraging, a variety of methodological issues related to identifying a clear phenotype and problems related to the sampling of the proband cloud many of the studies failing to demonstrate genetic effects. While the evidence grows that the liability for developing severe forms of alcoholism (such as DSM-III-R-defined alcohol dependence) has a strong genetic component, it is also clear that environmental factors play an important role in the development of different aspects of drinking behavior, including heavy drinking. Further, environmental factors including comorbid psychopathology and the level of exposure to alcohol may be responsible for the gender differences in the population prevalence rates of alcoholism. Thus, the interaction of genetic and environmental factors plays an important role in both the etiology and transmission of alcohol-related problems, including the more severe forms of alcohol dependence.

Acknowledgments: This work was supported by National Institute of Alcohol Abuse and Alcoholism Grants P50 AAA3510 and U10-AA08403/06.

References

Allgulander, C., Nowak, J., and Rice, J. P. (1991). Psychopathology and treatment of 30,344 twins in Sweden. II. Heritability of estimates of psychiatric diagnosis and treatment in 12,884 twin pairs. *Acta Psychiatr. Scand.* **83**:12–15.

Amark, C. (1951). A study in alcoholism: Clinical, social-psychiatric and genetic investigations. *Acta Psychiatr. Neurol. Scand.* **70**(suppl.):1–283.

American Psychiatric Association (1980). *Diagnostic and Statistical Manual of Mental Disorders,* 3d ed. Washington, DC.

American Psychiatric Association (1987). *Diagnostic and Statistical Manual of Mental Disorders,* 3d ed., rev. Washington, DC.

Andreasen, N. C., Endicott, J., Spitzer, R. C., and Winokur, G. (1977). The family history method using diagnostic criteria. *Arch. Gen. Psychiatr.* **34**:1229–1235.

Babor, T., Hofmann, M., Del Boca, F., Hesselbrock, V., Meyer, R., Dolinsky, Z., and Rounsaville, B. (1992). Types of alcoholics. I: Evidence for an empirically-derived typology based on indications of vulnerability and severity. *Arch. Gen. Psychiatr.*

Bohman, M., Sigvardsson, S., and Cloninger, C. R. (1981). Maternal inheritance of alcohol abuse: Cross-fostering analysis of adopted women. *Arch. Gen. Psychiatr.* **38**:965–969.

Bohman, M., Cloninger, C. R., Sigvardsson, S., and von Knorring, A. L. (1987). The genetics of alcoholisms and related disorders. *J. Psychiatr. Res.* **21**:447–452.

Cadoret, R. J., and Gath, A. (1978). Inheritance of alcoholism in adoptees. *Br. J. Psychiatr.* **132**:252–258.

Cadoret, R. J., Cain, C. A., and Grove, W. M. (1980). Development of alcoholism in adoptees raised apart from alcoholic biologic relatives. *Arch. Gen. Psychiatr.* **37**:561–563.

Cadoret, R. J., O'Gorman, T., Troughton, E., and Heywood, E. (1985). Alcoholism and antisocial personality: Interrelationships, genetic and environmental factors. *Arch. Gen. Psychiatr.* **42**:161–167.

Cadoret, R. J. and Wesner, R. B. (1990). Use of the adoption paradigm to elucidate the role of genes and environment and their interaction in the genesis of alcoholism. In *Genetics and Biology of Alcoholism,* C. R. Cloninger and H. Begleiter, eds. Cold Spring Harbor, NY: Cold Spring Harbor Laboratory Press, pp. 31–42.

Caldwell, C. B., and Gottesman, I. I. (1991). Sex Differences in the Risk for Alcoholism: A Twin Study. Paper presented at the 21st annual meeting of the Behavior Genetics Association, St. Louis, MO, June.

Carmelli, D., Swan, G. E., Robinette, D., and Fabsitz, R. R. (1990). Heritability of substance use in the NAS-NRC twin registry. *Acta Genet. Med. Gemellol.* **39**:63–71.

Cederlof, R., Friberg, L., and Lundman, T. (1977). The interactions of smoking, environment, and heredity. *Acta Med. Scand.* **202**(suppl):1–128.

Clifford, C. A., Hopper, J. L., Fulker, D. W., and Murray, R. M. (1984). A genetic and environmental analysis of a twin family study of alcohol use, anxiety, and depression. *Genet. Epidemiol.* **1**:63–79.

Cloninger, C. R., and Reich, T. (1983). Genetic heterogeneity in alcoholism and sociopathy. In *Genetics of Neurological and Psychiatric Disorders,* S. Kety, L. P. Rowland, R. L. Sidman, and Matthysse, S. W. eds. Raven Press, New York, pp. 145–163.

Cloninger, C. R., Christinsen, K. O., Reich, T., and Gottesman, II. (1978). Implications of sex differences in the prevalence of antisocial personality, alcoholism, and criminality for models of familial transmission. *Arch. Gen. Psychiatr.* **35**:841–851.

Cloninger, C. R., Bohman, M., and Sigvardsson, S. (1981). Inheritance of alcohol abuse: Cross-fostering analysis of adopted men. *Arch. Gen. Psychiatr.* **38**:861–868.

Conterio, F., and Chiarelli, B. (1962). Study of the inheritance of some daily life habits. *Heredity* **17**:347–359.

Cotton, N. (1979). The familial incidence of alcoholism. *J. Stud. Alcohol* **40**:89–116.

Edwards, G., and Gross, M. (1976). Alcohol dependence: Provisional description of a clinical syndrome. Br. Med. J. **1**:1058–1061.

Feighner, J. P., Robins E., Guze, S. B., Woodruff, R. A., Winokur, G., and Munoz, R. (1972). Diagnostic criteria for use in psychiatric research. *Arch. Gen. Psychiatr.* **26**:57–63.

Goodwin, D. W. (1976). *Is Alcoholism Hereditary?* New York: Oxford University Press.

Goodwin, D. W., Schulsinger, F., Hermansen, L., Guze, S., and Winokur, G. (1973). Alcohol problems in adoptees raised apart from alcoholic biologic parents. *Arch. Gen. Psychiatr.* **28**:238–243.

Goodwin, D. W., Schulsinger, F., Moller, N., Hermansen, L., Winokur, G., and Guze, S. (1974). Drinking problems in adopted and nonadopted sons of alcoholics. *Arch. Gen. Psychiatr.* **31**:164–169.

Goodwin, D. W., Schulsinger, F., Knop, J., Mednick, S., and Guze, S. (1977). Alcoholism and depression in adopted-out daughters of alcoholics. *Arch. Gen. Psychiatr.* **34**:751–755.

Grove, W. M., Eckert, E. D., Heston, L., Bouchard, T. J., Segal, N., and Lykken, D. T. (1990). Heritability of substance abuse and antisocial behavior: A study of monozygotic twins reared apart. *Biol. Psychiatr.* **27**:1293–1304.

Gurling, H. M. D., Clifford, C. A., and Murray, R. M. Genetic contributions to alcohol dependence and its effect on brain function. In *Twin Research,* vol. 3, L. Gedda, P. Parisi, and W. A. Nance, eds. New York: A. R. Liss, pp. 77–88.

Gurling, H. M. D., and Murray, R. M. (1987). Genetic influence, brain morphology and cognitive deficits in alcoholic twins. In *Genetics and Alcoholism,* H. W. Goedde, and D. P. Agarwal, eds. New York: Allan R. Liss, pp. 71–82.

Gurling, H. M. D., Oppenheim, B. E., and Murray, R. M. (1984). Depression, criminality and psychopathology associated with alcoholism: Evidence from a twin study. *Acta Genet. Med. Gemellol.* **33**:333–339.

Hall, R. L., Hesselbrock, V. M., and Stabenau, J. R. (1983). Familial distribution of alcohol use: I. Assortative mating in the parents of alcoholics. *Behav. Gen.* **13**:361–372.

Hrubec, Z., and Omenn, G. S. (1981). Evidence of genetic predisposition to alcoholic cirrhosis and psychosis. Twin concordances for alcoholism and its biological endpoints by zygosity among male veterans. *Alcohol.: Clin. Exp. Res.* **5**:207–212.

Heath, A. C., Jardine, R., and Martin, N. G. (1989). Interactive effects of genotype and social environment on alcohol consumption in female twins. *J. Stud. Alc.* **50:**38–48.

Heath, A. C., and Martin, N. G. (1988). Teenage alcohol use in the Australian twin register: Genetic and social determinants of starting to drink. *Alcohol.: Clin. Exp. Res.* **12:**735–741.

Heath, A. C. and Martin, N. G. (1994). Genetic influences on alcohol consumption patterns and problem drinking: Results from the Australian NH and MRC Twin panel follow-up survey. In: T. Babor, V. Hesselbrock, and R. Meyer (eds). *Genetic Susceptability, Biological Markers.* of Vulnerability and alcoholic subtypes. Annals New York Academy of Sciences, pp. 72–85.

Helzer, J., and Pryzbeck, T. (1988). The co-occurrence of alcoholism with other psychiatric disorders in the general population and its impact on treatment. *J. Stud. Alcohol* **49:**219–224.

Hesselbrock, V. M. (1986). Family history of psychopathology in alcoholics: A review and issues. In *Psychopathology and Addictive Disorders,* Meyer, R. E. ed, New York: The Guilford Press, pp. 41–56.

Hesselbrock, M., Meyer, R., and Keener, J. (1985a). Psychopathology in hospitalized alcoholics. *Arch. Gen. Psychiatr.* **42:**1050–1055.

Hesselbrock, V., Stabaneu, J. R., and Hesselbrock, M. N. (1985b). Subtyping of alcoholism in male patients by family history and antisocial personality. *J. Stud. Alcohol* **49:**89–98.

Hesselbrock, M., Hesselbrock, V., Babor, T., Stabenau, J., Meyer, R., and Weidenman, M. (1984). Antisocial behavior, psychopathology and problem drinking in the natural history of alcoholism. In *Longitudinal Search in Alcoholism,* D., Goodwin, K. Van Dusen, and Mednick, S. eds. Boston: Kluwer-Nijhoff, pp. 197–214.

Hesselbrock, V., Meyer, R., and Hesselbrock, M. (1992). Psychopathology and addictive disorders: A specific case of antisocial personality disorder. In *Addictive States,* C. P. O'Brien, and J. H. Jaffe, eds. New York: Raven Press, pp. 179–191.

Jardine, R., and Martin, N. G. (1984). Causes of variation and drinking habits in a large twin sample. *Acta Genet. Med. Gemellol. (Roma)* **33:**435–450.

Jellinek, E. M. (1960). *The Disease Concept of Alcoholism.* New Haven: Hillhouse Press.

Kaij, L. (1960). *Alcoholism in Twins.* Stockholm: Almquist and Wiksell.

Kaprio, J., Koskenvuo, M., and Sarna, S. (1981). Cigarettes, smoking, use of alcohol and leisure-time, physical activity among like-sexed adult male twins. *Prog. Clin. Biol. Res.* **69C:**37–46.

Kaprio, J., Koskenvuo, M., Langinvainio, H., Romanov, K., Sarna, A. S., and Rose, R. J. (1987). Social and genetic influences in drinking patterns of adult men. A Study of 5,638 adult Finnish twin brothers. *Alcohol.* **1**(suppl.):373–377.

Kendler, K. S., Heath, A. C., Neale, M. C., Kessler, K. C., and (1992). A population-based twin study of Alcoholism in women. *JAMA* 268:1877–1882.

Knight, R. P. (1937). The dynamics and treatment of chronic alcohol addiction. *Bull. Menninger Clin.* **1:**233–250.

Kosten, T. R., Rounsaville, B. J., Kosten, T. A., and Merikangas, K. R. (1991). Gender differences in the specificity of alcoholism transmission among the relatives of opioid addicts. *J. Nerv. Ment. Dis.* **179:**392–400.

McGue, M., Pickens, R. W., and Svikis, D. S. (1992). Sex and age effects on the inheritance of alcohol problems: A twin study. *J. Abnorm. Psychol.* **101:**3–17.

Merikangas, K. R., (1987). Genetic epidemiology of psychiatric disorders. In *American Psychiatric Association Annual Review,* Vol. 6, Psychiatry Update. A. J. Francis and Hales, R. E. eds. Washington, DC: American Psychiatric Association Press, pp. 625–646.

Merikangas, K. R., Leckman, J. F., Prusoff, B. A., Pauls, D. L., and Weissman, M. M. (1985). Familial transmission of depression and alcoholism. *Arch. Gen. Psychiatr.* **42**:367–372.

Morey, L. C., and Blashfield, R. C. (1981). Empirical classification of alcoholism: A review. *J. Stud. Alcohol* **42**:925–937.

Morton, N. E. (1982). *Outline of Genetic Epidemiology.* New York: Karger.

Murray, R. M., Clifford, C. A., and Gurling, H. M. D. (1983). Twin and adoption studies: How good is the evidence for a genetic role? In *Recent Developments in Alcoholism,* M. Galanter, ed. New York: Plenum Press, pp. 25–48.

National Council on Alcoholism Criteria Committee (1972). Criteria for the diagnosis of alcoholism. *Am. J. Psychiatr.* **129**:127–135.

Partanen, J., Bruun, K., and Markkanen, T. (1966). *Inheritance of Drinking Behavior.* Helsinki: The Finnish Foundation for Alcohol Studies.

Pederson, N. (1981). Twin similarity for usage of common drug. In *Twin Research 3 Part C Epidemiological and Clinical Studies,* L. Gedda, P. Parisi, and Mance, W. E. eds. New York: Allan R. Liss, pp. 53–59.

Peele, S. (1986). The implications and limitations of genetic models of alcoholism and other addictions. *J. Stud. Alcohol* **47**:63–73.

Penick, E., Powell, B., and Liskow, B. (1988). The stability of coexisting psychiatric syndromes in alcoholic men after one year. *J. Stud. Alcohol* **49**:395–405.

Pickens, R. W., Svikis, D. S., McGue, M., Lykken, D. T., Heston, L. L., and Clayton, P. J. (1991). Heterogeneity in the inheritance of alcoholism: A study of male and female twins. *Arch. Gen. Psychiatr.* **48**:19–28.

Regier, D., Farmer, M. E., Rae, D. S., Locke, B. Z., Keith, S. J., Judd, L. L., and Goodwin, F. K. (1990). Comorbidity of mental disease with alcohol and other drug abuse. *JAMA* **264**:2511–2518.

Reich, T., Winokur, G., and Mullaney, J. (1975). The transmission of alcoholism. In *Genetic Research in Psychiatry,* R. R., Fieve, D. Rosenthal, and H. Brill, eds. Baltimore: Johns Hopkins University Press, pp. 259–272.

Reich, T., Cloninger, C. R., Lewis, C., and Rice, J. (1981). Some recent findings in the study of genotype-environment interaction in alcoholism. In *Evaluation of the Alcoholic: Implications for Research, Theory and Treatment,* R. E. Meyer ed. NIAAA Research Monograph 5. Washington, DC: GPO, pp. 145–166.

Reich, T., Cloninger, C. R., Van Eerdewegh, P., Rice, J. P., and Mullaney, J. (1988). Secular trends in the familial transmission of alcoholism. *Alcohol.: Clin. Exp. Res.* **12**:458–464.

Robins, L. N., Helzer, J., Croughan, J., and Ratclif, K. (1981). National Institute of Mental Health Diagnostic Interview Schedule. *Arch. Gen. Psychiat.* **38**:381–389.

Roe, A. (1944). The adult adjustment of children of alcoholic parents raised in foster homes. *Q. J. Stud. Alcohol* **5**:378–393.

Rose, R. J., Kaprio, J., Williams, C. J., Viken, R., and Obremski, K. (1990). Social contact in sibling similarity: Facts, issues and red herrings. *Behavr. Genet.* **20**:736–778.

Rounsaville, B. J., Dolinsky, Z. S., Babor, T. F. and Meyer, R. E. (1988). Psychopathology as a predictor of treatment outcome in alcoholics. *Arch. Gen. Psychiatr.* **44**:505–513.

Schuckit, M. A. (1973). Alcoholism and sociopathy—diagnostic confusion. *Q. J. Stud. Alcohol* **34**:157–164.

Schuckit, M. A., Goodwin, D., and Winokur, G. (1972). A study of alcoholism in half siblings. *Am. J. Psychiatr.* **128**:1132–1136.

Searles, J. S. (1988). The role of genetics in the pathogenesis of alcoholism. *J. Abnorm. Psychol.* **97**:153–167.

Slater, E., and Cowie, V. (1971). *The Genetics of Mental Disorders.* London: Oxford University Press.

Spitzer, R. L., Endicott, J., and Robins, E. (1978). Research Diagnostic Criteria (RDC) for a selected group of functional disorders. *Arch. Gen. Psychiatr.* **35:**713–718.

Webster, D. W., Harburg, E., Gleiberman, L., Schork, A., and Di Franceisco, W. (1989). Familial transmission of alcohol use: I. Parent and adult offspring alcohol use over 17 years in Tecumseh, Michigan. *J. Stud. Alcohol* **50:**557–565.

World Health Organization (1980). *International Classification of Diseases,* ninth rev. Geneva.

2

Genetic Determinants of Alcoholic Subtypes

MICHIE N. HESSELBROCK

It is generally accepted that not all alcoholics are alike. Alcoholics are heterogeneous in terms of the etiology of their disorder, their demographic characteristics, alcohol use patterns and history, presence of comorbid psychiatric disorders, and patterns of other substance use. Different family backgrounds, different rearing environments, and a variety of biological, social, and psychiatric problems are also associated with chronic alcohol use. These factors may influence treatment-seeking behavior, treatment outcomes, and the life course of alcoholism. Over the years researchers and clinicians have sought ways to describe and synthesize the wide range of behavior patterns and the variety of problems resulting from alcohol abuse in a systematic and structured manner.

Many attempts have been made to describe alcoholism by classifying affected individuals into discrete categories or typologies. By systematically categorizing alcoholics according to certain common characteristics, clinicians have sought to identify and provide appropriate and effective treatments for alcoholics, while researchers have attempted to predict treatment outcomes for groups of alcoholics classified according to common characteristics. The term "typology," as used in this chapter, is defined as "systematically classifying alcohol dependent individuals according to the methods which are derived from logical rules and conceptual clusters based on one or more combinations of biological, psychological, social and cultural characteristics" (Babor and Dolinsky, 1988).

Traditionally, efforts to classify alcoholics into distinct typological classifications were limited to descriptions of the phenomenology of alcoholism. Little consideration was given to the association between etiology, alcohol-related variables, and the prediction of treatment outcomes. Recent developments in research on the genetics of alcoholism strongly indicate that typological classifications of alcoholism should consider potential genetic contributions to both the etiology and the natural history of alcoholism. This chapter examines various typological classifications identified in the literature and their relationship to genetic factors.

Early Typologies

Current typological classification systems have their roots in the late nineteenth century. Babor and Lauerman (1986) reviewed 39 scientific articles describing typological classifications of alcoholics that were published between 1850 and 1941 in France, Germany, England, and in the United States. They included 24 typologies summarized by Bowman and Jellinek (1941) and 15 additional typologies found in the *International Bibliography of Studies on Alcohol* (Jordy, 1966). According to their paper, the published French typologies were concentrated in the late nineteenth century; the German and British typologies in the 1920s and 1930s; while the American typologies were concentrated in two stages, the era of the American Association for the Study and Cure of Inebriety (1870–1916) and from post-Prohibition to the beginning of World War II (1933–1941).

These typological classifications were based mainly on drinking patterns, chronicity, and severity of dependence and/or addiction (Babor and Lauerman, 1986). The classifications based on etiology included hereditary, psychological, and social/environmental causes. While all typological classifications dealt with drinking patterns, variations in the criteria of classification were observed across the four countries in terms of etiology. The French and German classification schemes considered heredity an important etiological factor, while the German classifications also attached importance to psychological factors. British typological theory focused on psychological factors, with little attention to heredity. Early American typologists also considered heredity, but psychological theories of etiology dominated after Prohibition (Babor and Lauerman, 1986).

The description of alcoholism in early American typology was influenced by the organizations that brought together scientists and other medical practitioners interested in the scientific study of alcoholism (Babor and Dolinsky, 1988). Alcoholics were subclassified into several groups according to their drinking patterns: chronic heavy drinkers (termed chronic inebriates and dipsomania), periodic drinkers, and binge drinkers. In terms of etiology, the type of alcoholism associated with heredity tended to be more chronic, out of control, and had a more severe course than those types not associated with heredity. The hereditary type was thought to be less curable; thus these individuals were regarded as the best candidates for asylums. Some recommended that they be segregated from society to keep them from reproducing, and thus to eliminate this type of inebriate from society (Babor and Lauerman, 1986).

Early American typologies published before Prohibition, like the European typologies, seemed to consider genetic factors important in the etiology of alcoholism, but provided little empirical support. These typologies also lacked a clear description of how genetic factors were linked to their specific classifications. Rather, heredity was viewed as an etiologic subtype of alcoholism in and of itself. Perhaps this was because the concept of a "typology" developed from loosely organized observation of patients who sought treatment for alcoholism (Babor and Dolinsky, 1988).

Another problem with the early typologies was that the concept of heredity was not well defined. Genetically transmissible factors and social and environmental factors were included in these early discussions of hereditary factors, but biological factors were not distinguished from environmental factors. Consequently, the separate and independent contributions of genetic and environmental factors were not discussed. With the dominance of psychoanalytic theories after Prohibition, the hereditary aspects of alcoholism became less important in the explanation of typologies and the etiology of alcoholism.

Interest in alcoholism declined during the Prohibition years between 1919 and 1933, but the concept of addiction did not disappear from American society (Levine, 1978). Typologies of alcoholism proposed after Prohibition reflected psychoanalytic theory, explaining the etiology of alcoholism in terms of stages of psychosexual development. While Knight (1937) acknowledged that few psychoanalysts had written about alcoholism due to the small number of alcoholics seeking psychoanalysis, he proposed that "alcohol addiction is a symptom, rather than a disease . . ." He added that "There is always an underlying personality disorder evidenced by obvious maladjustment, neurotic character traits, emotional immaturity or infantilism . . ." in alcoholics. He did find a "certain parental constellation" in the etiology of alcoholism. However, these parental characteristics were not genetic factors, but rather were related to the way the parents (especially the mother) raised their children, i.e., overindulgence, overprotectiveness. Knight (1938) proposed three types of alcoholism based on the observation of 30 alcoholics who sought treatment at the Menninger Clinic. He subclassified alcoholics according to how far they had progressed in their psychosexual development. *Essential* or *true* alcoholics were labeled as fixation addicted, or alcoholic personality, and were considered to have a poor prognosis without complete abstinence. Knight thought they should be institutionalized since they missed appointments because of drinking, came to the therapeutic hour intoxicated, and did not remember the session as outpatients. Their excessive use of alcohol was thought to begin in adolescence. In terms of psychoanalytic etiology, essential alcoholics were also characterized as not having progressed beyond the oral stage so that they had an oral dependence, a craving for drink and food.

Reactive or *regressive* alcoholism were characterized as being similar to secondary alcoholism, in which heavy drinking developed after precipitating events. Reactive alcoholics were thought to have a later onset of alcoholism, to be better adjusted socially than essential alcoholics, and likely to have better treatment outcomes. Reactive alcoholics seemed to have character traits indicative of progression beyond the oral stage, e.g., perseverance, retention and mastery of the object. The third type, the *symptomatic* alcoholic, was considered to have prominent neurotic or psychotic symptoms, and drinking was considered an extension of these problems.

Fleeson and Gildea (1942) studied the records of 280 abnormal drinkers (220 men and 60 women) who were admitted to the New Haven Psychiatric Clinic. They classified three groups of abnormal drinkers: 28% of the men and 20% of the women as endogenous, primary addicts; 18% of the men and 23% of the women as endogenous, symptomatic drinkers; and 44% of the men and 55% of the women as exogenous drinkers. The *primary addicts* or *true addicts* were characterized as suffering from addiction at the start of their use of alcohol, due to factors within their personality structures. Thus, the development of alcoholism in primary addicts was thought to be influenced very little by external factors (endogenously determined). The primary addicts were also found to have a high rate of psychopathic personalities. *Symptomatic drinkers* were also determined endogenously, but unlike primary addicts, drinking was only one of many clinical symptoms, principally depression. *Exogenous drinkers* were considered to constitute the majority of abnormal drinkers, and were thought to be influenced mainly by environmental factors.

Knight's (1937, 1938) essential alcoholism and Fleeson and Gildea's endogenous, primary addict resembled an earlier subtype that was often considered to have a genetic etiology, but neither Knight's nor Fleeson and Gildea's studies implied heredity as a factor in the etiology of essential or primary alcoholism. Instead, several other psychoanalytically based typologies were proposed though most were similar to the essential and reactive types in terms of drinking styles and underlying psychopathology (Babor and Dolinsky, 1988).

The psychoanalytic view of an alcoholic typology had limited utility because the conceptualizations were based on a limited number of observations stemming from the few middle-class alcoholics who sought psychoanalysis. The etiology of alcoholism was narrowly defined, only in terms of psychosexual developmental stage. No consideration was given to biological or environmental factors that might have contributed to the etiology of alcoholism, which meant that the psychoanalytic perspective in general represented the dominant approach to the conceptualization of psychiatric disorders during that era. The psychoanalytic descriptions of alcoholism also marked the beginning of a loss of interest among alcohol theorists in the possible genetic contributions to etiology.

Bowman and Jellinek's Typology

The post-Prohibition era also saw a change in the concept of addiction. Alcohol was socially acceptable again, and the "rediscovery" in the 1930s and 1940s by A. A. and the Yale Center of Alcohol Studies of alcoholism as an addiction and as a disease began to shift views toward a medical model of alcoholism, the "disease concept of alcoholism" (Levine, 1978). A comprehensive theory on the typology of alcoholism was published by Bowman and Jellinek in 1941. Their classification scheme was hierarchical, branching out from a general classification based on drinking patterns to etiology and personality factors. They divided alcoholics into two broad groups, steady and intermittent drinkers, according to their alcohol use pattern. These classifications were further subdivided several times, branching to seventeen different subtypes. Four subtypes labeled as "decadent, discordant, compensating, and poverty" were considered to be "primary" addicts. The remaining subtypes were thought to represent "potential secondary addicts and chronic addicts."

Although Bowman and Jellinek's notion of primary addicts or true addicts implicated a biological mechanism in the development of alcoholism, they defined true addicts as

> actually not a type but a group of types with the common characteristic that alcohol is a definite need for them, that it has a definite function in their scheme of things and that their dependence on the intoxicant and their inability to give it up are not determined by habit and physiologically processed. . . . True addicts all come to their addiction on an endogenous basis and they are steady drinkers. (Bowman and Jellinek, 1941, p. 132)

Thus, the process of addiction was not explicitly connected to hereditary factors in their scheme.

However, Bowman and Jellinek (1941) did not overlook heredity as a contributory factor in the development of alcoholism, but they discussed it in terms of personality factors and constitutional disposition, although these factors might only be implicitly expressed. In their review of typological classifications based on personality types in the early literature, Bowman and Jellinek found that certain psychopathies were often based on the hereditary aspects of constitution. Their review included subtypes in which the inherited disposition to alcoholism was a very important factor, and others in which it was not.

Bowman and Jellinek (1941) also reviewed other work in which a hereditary influence was associated with "only a small part of the alcoholic population." For most forms of alcoholism, Bowman and Jellinek state that "heredity plays no part," and hereditary factors were important in only one small group, a certain type of "dipsomania." Jellinek and Jolliffe (1940) reviewed and postulated alcoholic subtypes based on constitutional forms, drinking patterns, reasons for drinking, and personality types. They included two basic constitutional forms among drinkers. The "instincto-motrice sphere" type was characterized by continuous drinking without physical harm. This type mainly displayed neurotic personality traits, i.e., impulsiveness or apathy, hypochondria, paranoia, and recurring but curable subacute episodes of confusion and hallucination. The other type, "emotivo-motrice sphere," was characterized by a poor prognosis, psychomotor instability, obsession, and schizoid states. These subtypes, however, were not mutually exclusive and often clinically difficult to separate.

Generally, the literature Bowman and Jellinek (1941) reviewed dealt with two hereditary factors, a psychopathic disposition and hereditary liability. Two major conceptualizations were proposed in terms of a psychopathic constitution. First, they suggested that "addiction grows on the ground of a weak personality organization which may be purely congenital or may be the expression of nonspecific heredity." Secondly, they considered that "tolerance is widely regarded as being an element of constitutional disposition." In terms of tolerance, they described the importance of heredity in determining how much drinking is sufficient. While a psychopathic disposition and hereditary liability were emphasized in alcohol addiction, they also considered social and environmental factors to be important. These factors included "traumatic disorders, other uninheritable mental disorders, migraine and petty deviations occurring in the families of alcoholic patients" (Bowman and Jellinek, 1941).

In the investigation of different cross sections of alcoholic patients admitted to general hospitals, Bowman and Jellinek (1941) found "35 to 40 percent hereditary liability and an incidence of psychopathic dispositions in these patients." Their critique stated that "some investigations have been based entirely on heredity or on the prepsychotic psychopathies of patients with alcoholic psychoses inclusive of those not of alcoholic origin."

Bowman and Jellinek thus considered heredity a contributory, or indirect, factor in the development of alcoholism, i.e., constitutional disposition. While they acknowledged the heritability of certain biological factors, such as psychopathic personality or tolerance, they considered only a small group of alcoholics to have been affected by a genetic predisposition to alcoholism. "Psychopathic disposition, and perhaps hereditary liability, may be expected in the symptomatic drinkers, who are probably the farthest removed from the problem of addiction and in the group which constitutes a relatively small part of the alcoholic population." They further stated "that the large group which furnishes the secondary addict is generally free from hereditary liability, as well as from psychopathic disposition, according to the evidence available." While "symptomatic drinkers" were thought to be at risk, in part, due to heritable factors, their description of this type of alcoholism lacks clarity and detail. Further, none of the work they reviewed describes in detail possible patterns of transmission of alcoholism across generations.

Jellinek (1945) later placed more emphasis for the development of alcoholism on environmental than on genetic factors within alcoholic families. In a study of 4372 alcoholics, he found 2799 (52%) who had either an inebriate father or mother. However, he considered his findings as "evidence of the great risks to which the offspring of alcoholics are exposed through example and neglect."

One limitation of Bowman and Jellinek's formulation is the vagueness of the presentation of "evidence." They did not provide a methodological description of their data source in terms of sample size, sample description, or research design. Further, while they considered hereditary factors to be associated with certain types of symptomatic drinkers, the types were not specified in their grand scheme of typologies. It is often assumed, however, that "dipsomania" was the one classification related to hereditary factors. Another limitation of their study is that their classifications were not mutually exclusive categories. It is thus difficult to separate each typology, since several characteristics are common across types.

Jellinek's Typology

Jellinek (1960) later proposed several types of alcoholism based on the progression of the disease process. Using the Greek alphabet, his classifications included four types (Alpha, Beta, Gamma, and Delta), each determined by the variety and the severity of the consequences experienced and the alcoholic's drinking patterns. He also proposed a separate category of drinker, Epsilon, to denote a certain type of dypsomania, binge drinking. In terms of applying the disease concept, only Gamma and Delta types were considered to be appropriate. Jellinek's typological classification was an important step beyond his earlier classification system because it considered several important conceptual factors in the description of alcoholism: dependence, withdrawal, drinking patterns, loss of control, physical as well as psychological and social consequences, and the application of the disease concept. Consideration of genetic contributions to the etiology of alcoholism is, however, even further removed than in his earlier typologies.

Jellinek (1960) considered that Alpha and Beta drinkers were not severely affected by the disease of alcoholism. He judged the "Alpha" type to have a purely psychological dependence on alcohol, i.e., they drank to relieve bodily pain or emotional disturbance. Consequently, the damage caused by drinking was limited to interpersonal relations, problems with family budgets, or occasional absences from work.

Beta alcoholism is similar to Alpha alcoholism except in terms of the experienced consequences. A possible consequence for the Beta type is physical damage, i.e., polyneuropathy, gastritis, or cirrhosis. However, the physical symptoms may not be due to the direct effects of prolonged heavy drinking, but might result from poor nutrition or poor health in the prealcoholic state. Neither the Alpha nor the Beta type was characterized by symptoms considered to be associated with severe forms of addiction, i.e., loss of control, inability to abstain, or withdrawal symptoms.

The most serious type of alcoholism according to Jellinek's conceptualization was the Gamma type. The Gamma type was considered to be the most predominant type of alcoholism in the United States and Canada at that time. Gamma alcoholics were thought to develop physical dependence to alcohol in which physiological adaptations are indicated by acquired tissue tolerance and adaptive cell metabolism. They also experience withdrawal symptoms and develop craving. In terms of consequences, the Gamma alcoholic experiences all of the physical, psychological, and social problems that are experienced by both Alpha and Beta alcoholics, but to a greater degree. The hallmark of Gamma alcoholism is "loss of control"; persons with Delta alcoholism may not experience loss of control, but an inability to abstain is a characteristic symptom. Delta alcoholics were also considered to be dependent on alcohol and to experience craving. For Delta alcoholics the damage caused by alcoholism was similar to, but not as severe as that experienced by Gamma alcoholics.

Jellinek applied the disease concept to both Gamma and Delta alcoholism, but not to Alpha and Beta alcoholism. He described persons in these latter categories as problem drinkers, even though he preferred not to use this term. Jellinek did not believe Epsilon alcoholism fit the disease concept of alcoholism either. "Pseudoperiodic alcoholism or pseudoepsilon alcoholism is a relapse into a disease, but I must add that the occasion for the relapse is a voluntary one and does not form a part of the disease process, except perhaps in a psychopathological sense" (Jellinek, 1960, p. 41).

Jellinek's typology was based on drinking patterns and the consequences of drinking, not on etiology. He considered the etiology of alcohol addiction applicable only to Gamma and Delta alcoholism. While Jellinek acknowledged the physiological aspects of alcohol addiction, he placed greater importance on the social and psychological factors in the development of alcoholism. The addiction process was pharmacological and part of the disease process, but possible genetic contributions were not mentioned. "When the addictive process is on its way, the role of the person diminishes and alcohol takes the upper hand as the nervous tissue becomes gradually conditioned by that substance." Jellinek admits, however, that psychological and psychiatric etiologies of alcoholism as explanations of heavy drinking might not be sufficient to explain the progression of disease or loss of control in Gamma alcoholism. Enzymes, vitamin anomalies, liver injuries, and other biochemical factors could affect the resistance to adaptation to alcohol. He was not sure whether these anomalies were due to heredity or to the stresses caused by prolonged heavy drinking. He was also unable to explain individual variability in the length of the addictive process: "some 3 years or less while in others only after 7, or as long as 18 years." He suspected that "heredity may play a role in the time necessary for alcohol to exert serious stresses on the system to which anomaly attaches" (p. 155).

Jellinek only recognized the role of genetics when he was unable to explain the process of addiction in terms of psychological and sociological etiology. He did consider prealcoholic psychological vulnerability, but the specific roles of this vulnerability were not discussed. He was unable to establish a causal relationship between hereditary and Gamma alcoholism. Instead, he mentions heredity only in the form of a hypothesis, which he never tested in relation to the available evidence.

Jellinek's formulation of a typology was well accepted by both clinicians and alcohol researchers because "the work of this extraordinary individual has framed most aspects of the current debate on the nature of alcoholism and its treatment" (Lender, 1979). While his conceptualization represents a significant attempt to classify alcoholism, it was too general to be adapted for empirical testing. Consequently, it was not widely utilized by modern researchers. Further, Jellinek considered Gamma-type alcoholics to be a relatively homogeneous group and did not adequately address the heterogeneity and multidimensional nature of alcoholism within this type. (Hesselbrock, 1986a).

Statistical Applications to Typology

An increase in the development of empirical classification systems of alcoholism was associated with the development and application of computer-based statistical packages in the late 1960s and early 1970s. Such studies make use of a variety of parametric statistical techniques, such as cluster analysis, factor analysis, and discriminant function analysis. Because of the underlying assumptions required for these statistical methods, these empirical studies have included a large number of subjects, and the data examined were measured on an interval level scale. Consequently, the variables included in the analyses were limited to those with known psychometric properties such as those derived from the Minnesota Multiphasic Personality Inventory (MMPI).

With statistically derived typologies, alcoholic subjects are often classified along several dimensions or categories with varying degrees of correlation or geometric distance among the variables examined. Unlike dichotomous classifications (e.g., the DSM III-R), which classify subjects into one or two categories, the empirical approach attempts to classify subjects with respect to several dimensions or categories. Each dimension or factor is often described in terms of the degree or severity of involvement with alcohol. Meyer and Babor (1986) suggest standards and criteria for typological classifications based on an empirical model. These criteria include "homogeneity within categories, heterogeneity between categories, and stability of the groupings." Most studies reviewed in this section appear to follow these standards.

Depending on the type of statistical methods utilized, alcoholic subjects can be classified into either categorical classifications (e.g., based on cluster analysis) or dimensional classifications (e.g., dervived by factor analysis) (Morey and Skinner, 1986). The most often cited empirically derived typological classifications are based on descriptions of personality types derived from the MMPI. Goldstein and Linden (1969) applied a cluster analysis of the MMPIs from 513 alcoholics treated in a state hospital. The derived four clusters provided a clinical description of the subjects based on the elevation of certain subscales of the MMPI (profiles). Type I was described as an "emotionally unstable personality," type II was described as having a "neurosis with anxiety reaction or depression," type III alcoholism was associated with a psychopathic personality, while type IV was described as "alcoholism with other drug addictions and paranoid features."

Whitelock et al. (1971) conducted a cluster analysis of the MMPIs from 136 male alcoholic inpatients in a state hospital. Their two types were similar to two of those of Goldstein and Linden. According to the mean MMPI profiles, the two similar clusters were the type I (high elevation of the Pd scale) and the type II (high elevation of D-Sc-Hs-Pd-Pt scales). However, Goldstein and Linden's type III and IV were not found by Whitelock et al.

Several other investigators have also conducted cluster analyses on the MMPI scales (Stein et al., 1971; Skinner et al., 1974; Skinner and Jackson, 1978; Donovan et al., 1978; Conley, 1981). Skinner and Jackson (1978) identified three types of personality characteristics (neurotic, psychotic, and psychopathic) when they examined the association between their classifications and those of Goldstein and Linden's. Their neurotic personality type was moderately correlated with both the type I and type II, while high correlations were found between the psychotic personality type and type II as well as between the sociopathic personality type and type IV. The sociopathic type was also moderately correlated with type I. Conley (1981) found that 48% of individuals with alcohol problems could be classified into one of four types by the addition of classic alcoholism to Skinner and Jackson's types. These four types were examined in terms of alcohol use history and follow-up variables. The "psychopathic" alcoholics tended to develop problem drinking at an early age, but reported the most improvement following treatment.

Blashfield (1984) examined the relationships among clusters developed by several investigators and found that some clusters were highly intercorrelated, i.e., overlapped with each other. Morey and Skinner (1986) have also examined the average MMPI group profiles in studies employing a cluster analysis of alcoholics. Using Goldstein and Linden's typology, they examined the intercorrelation of group profiles among 12 studies. Generally high correlations ranging from .52 to .959 (Q-type correlation) were found between the group profiles and Goldstein and Linden's type I cluster (emotionally unstable personality). However, the correlations were generally lower for the type

II and III clusters (neurosis with anxiety reaction or depression and alcoholism with psychopathic personality) than with those of the other studies.

The statistically derived typology continues to be popular among alcohol researchers (Costello et al., 1978; Donovan et al., 1986; Morey et al., 1987; Alfano et al., 1987; Jackson and Hoffmann, 1987). Some studies have included measures beyond the MMPI to other psychometric measures [cf. prognostic indicators (Gibbs, 1980), and other personality measures (Nerviano, 1976; Nerviano and Gross, 1983)]. Other studies have examined the relevance of empirically derived typologies in relation to treatment outcome (Zivich, 1981; Thurstin and Alfano, 1988) or drinking behaviors (Morey et al., 1984; Kline and Snyder, 1985).

Most investigators, however, have not examined the relationship between statistically derived typologies and etiological (i.e., genetic) factors or other longitudinal data (i.e., outcomes), although there is evidence suggesting that some personality traits might be genetically transmitted (cf. Tarter, 1988; Plomin, 1990). These typologies have been limited to descriptions of the personality features of alcoholics and have not been related to other aspects of alcoholism or its etiology.

The major limitation of most, if not all, statistically derived typological classifications is their lack of comparability across the different studies (Blashfield, 1984). Although numerous typologies have been developed, there has been a failure to produce standard profiles or subtypes. In addition, the studies have utilized a variety of unspecified statistical procedures, computer software packages, and validation methods, all of which make a comparison of the studies impossible (Blashfield, 1984).

Another limitation of most statistical typologies is their focus on only one aspect of the disorder rather than the multidimensional nature of alcoholism, e.g., personality measures. Since the statistically derived typologies have not been examined in relation to external measures, their lack of predictive validity limits their clinical utility. Further, other important factors related to the etiology, course, and consequences of alcoholism, e.g., family history, co-occurrence of psychopathology, alcohol use, and treatment history have not been examined in relationship to empirically derived typologies.

Most empirical typologies have been derived from homogeneous, rather than heterogeneous samples, i.e., studies conducted at VA hospitals using only male samples or at state hospitals. Statistically derived typologies based on samples containing females are rare. Kline and Snyder (1985) studied MMPI subtypes of both men and women and their relationship to drinking behaviors. They found that group profiles of men and women varied somewhat within each subtype. Further, subtypes of women were differentiated according to alcohol use patterns; this was not true among the male subtypes. Their study indicates the importance of including women in studies of alcoholic typologies. With an increase in the number of women seeking treatment for alcoholism, replication of these studies is needed on samples in which females are adequately represented.

Another limitation of typologies based on personality traits is the relative instability of many personality measures, most of which reflect the current state of the individual rather than an underlying personality structure or trait. For example, the MMPI D scale has been criticized for being very sensitive to the respondent's mood at the time of assessment. It is also known that an elevated subscale score does not necessarily indicate the presence of a psychiatric diagnosis. Several studies have found a low concordance between elevated MMPI scores and the presence of a diagnosable condition (cf. Hesselbrock et al., 1983).

Another criticism of the empirically derived typologie is the apparent lack of statistical independence among the identified types. For example, Morey and Skinner's (1986) typology based on the MMPI identified four independent (orthogonal) types. However, both the neurotic and psychotic subtypes were highly correlated with Goldstein and Linden's (1969) type II, while their sociopathic type was highly correlated with both types I and IV. Further, statistically derived typologies (particularly those based on personality measures) might not be specific to only treated alcoholics. For example, Morey and Skinner (1986) have found similar elevations of MMPI scores among driving while intoxicated (DWI) offenders who had not developed alcoholism. These factors, (e.g., lack of consideration of etiological factors, genetic factors, poor predictions of clinical outcome) limit the utility of empirically derived typology for both clinical and research purposes.

Subclassification Based on Childhood Hyperactivity and Conduct Disorder

Problem childhood behavior has served as the basis for other typological studies of alcoholism. Several investigators have found that childhood behavior problems, such as hyperactivity and conduct problems, often developed into alcoholism in adulthood. In a longitudinal study of delinquent boys, McCord and McCord (1960) found that boys who later became alcoholic tended to be more active, aggressive, and sadistic in childhood than their peers. Robins (1966) also found that men who developed alcoholism in adulthood had conduct problems in childhood. These findings were replicated by longitudinal studies of community samples. In the Oakland Growth Study. Jones (1968) identified two types of behavior among boys who developed drinking problems. One is characterized by emotionality, crying easily, anger, and excessive worrying, the second by extrapunitiveness, irritability, and hostility. Similarly, in a retrospective study of problem drinkers drawn from the general population, Cahalan and Room (1974) identified rebelliousness, extroversion, impulsivity, hell-raising, and unhappiness as early predictors of adult drinking problems.

Studies linking childhood behavior problems and alcoholism in adulthood suggest that some alcoholics may have inherited a predisposition for childhood hyperactivity, minimum brain dysfunction (MBD) and conduct disorder (Alterman and Tarter, 1983). An increased risk of hyperactivity, alcoholism, sociopathy, and hysteria has also been found among the relatives of hyperactive children (Morrison and Stewart, 1971; Cantwell, 1972; Tarter, et al., 1985). In the Danish adoption study, male adoptees who became alcoholic as adults had alcoholic biological fathers who were reported to have high rates of hyperactivity and aggressiveness in childhood (Goodwin et al., 1975). Similarly, hyperactive children who were adopted were more likely than nonhyperactive children to have a biological father who was alcoholic (Mendelson et al., 1971;

Wood et al., 1976; Wender et al., 1981; Wood et al., 1983). An association between childhood hyperactivity and alcoholism has also been found in retrospective studies. Many adults who were hospitalized for alcoholism were likely to have suffered from hyperactivity and MBD in their childhood. Tarter et al. (1977) found that a subgroup of primary alcoholics who were characterized by early onset and a severe form of alcoholism reported higher numbers of symptoms of childhood hyperactivity and MBD behavior than secondary alcoholics. Further, primary alcoholism was found to be significantly related to familial alcoholism.

DeObaldia et al. (1983) reported similar findings. Their study found an association between hyperactivity/MBD in childhood, severe symptoms of alcohol dependence, and poor performance on cognitive tests.

While there is evidence suggesting genetic transmission of alcoholism and hyperactivity/MBD in the aforementioned studies, no specific causal mechanism has been described. The relationship between childhood hyperactivity and MBD is further complicated by the vagueness of the concept. The term "hyperactivity/MBD" includes a broad range of behavior problems in children. These behaviors can be classified into three or four categories (e.g., hyperactivity, attention deficit, impulsivity, and conduct problems) to relate the role of specific types of behavior problems to the development of alcoholism. Hesselbrock (1986b) examined childhood behavior problems and antisocial alcoholism in hospitalized alcoholics and found that while the antisocial personality (ASP) alcoholics reported significantly higher numbers of childhood attention deficit, impulsivity, hyperactivity, and conduct problems, conduct problems were the most distinguishing behavior problem between ASP and non-ASP alcoholics.

Stewart et al. (1980) divided hyperactive boys into two groups, unsocialized-aggressive and hyperactive only. Antisocial personality and alcoholism were more frequently found in fathers of the aggressive, antisocial boys than in boys without these characteristics, but the prevalence of these disorders did not distinguish fathers of hyperactive boys from those without hyperactivity. Stewart et. al. cautioned against the argument that hyperactivity is a specific syndrome. Rather, disorders in the parents were related to aggressive conduct disorder in the boys, not hyperactivity alone. Similar findings were reported by August and Stewart (1983). In their study, parents of hyperactive children were divided into family history positive (in which at least one biological parent was diagnosed in the antisocial spectrum) and family history negative (in which neither parent had such a diagnosis). While the two groups of children were similar in terms of inattention and reactivity, family history positive children and their siblings showed conduct problems. These studies suggest that these behaviors (conduct problems, aggressiveness) are of etiologic importance for alcoholism since genetic factors may also be involved.

Zucker and Gomberg (1986), in a review of prospective studies, examined the etiology of alcoholism in terms of a longitudinal developmental framework and found that antisocial behavior and difficulty in achievement-related activity in childhood and adolescence were consistently related to the development of alcoholism in adulthood. For Zucker and Gomberg, antisocial behavior was a specific behavior, such as aggression, sadistic behaviors, antisocial activity, or rebelliousness. The achievement-related variables included poor school performance, low productivity in high school, truancy, and lower educational attainment (i.e., dropping out). These variables were also associated in the high-risk sample with those who did not develop alcoholism, implicating genetic factors. Zucker and Gomberg proposed that the difficulties children experience might be related to biological factors, e.g., neural integrative deficit. This hypothesis contradicts Vaillant (1983a, 1983b), who found, in a longitudinal study of inner-city youths, that antisocial personality disorder was a consequence of alcoholism rather than a risk factor.

Based on his study of Danish adoptees at high and low risk for developing alcoholism, Goodwin (1979) suggested that familial alcoholism be considered a subtype of alcoholism. The familial subtype was characterized by an early onset of alcoholism, a concentration of alcoholism in the biological family members, and severe symptoms requiring treatment at young age, in the absence of other psychopathology. Among males, genetic factors appear to play a pivotal role in the etiology of alcoholism, while developmental and/or environmental factors were associated with the risk for alcoholism in females (Goodwin et al., 1977; Frances et al., 1980; Mirin et al., 1986; Hesselbrock, V. M., 1986). There is, however, evidence questioning aspects of this typology, including the absence of other psychopathology among the biological relatives of family history positive alcoholics (Hesselbrock, V. M., 1986). Further, family history positive alcoholics may experience greater psychosocial and physical consequences of alcohol abuse than alcoholics without a family history of alcoholism (Hesselbrock et al., 1982). However, the presence of antisocial personality in the person affected with alcoholism appears to affect the course of alcoholism to a greater extent than having a positive family history of alcoholism (Hesselbrock et al., 1985).

The relationship between familial alcoholism and childhood behavior problems is complicated by the fact that childhood hyperactivity/MBD is a nonspecific risk since not all children with behavior problems go on to develop either alcoholism or antisocial personality disorder in adulthood. A prospective study of hyperactive children found half of the children diagnosed as hyperactive markedly improved between the ages of 12 and 16. Those children who did not improve displayed a variety of antisocial activities including contact with the police and juvenile court, excessive drinking, and fire setting. Among those children with the most antisocial problems, 22% of their fathers and 4% of their mothers were problem drinkers (Mendelson et al., 1971; Weiss et al., 1979). August et al. (1983) found that hyperactive boys continued to be inattentive and impulsive. However, only those boys who were undersocialized and aggressive as children were aggressive, noncompliant, and antisocial and used alcohol as teenagers at their four-year follow-up evaluation. Robins (Robins, 1978; Robins and Ratcliff, 1979) inferred from several studies that not all children with a conduct disorder problem become antisocial adults, and that violent and aggressive behavior does not appear in adulthood if it has been absent in childhood. While Allen and Frances (1986) proposed that residual symptoms of childhood hyperactivity may persist into adulthood, it appears that only a certain type of childhood behavior (i.e., conduct problem or aggression) is specific in predicting alcoholism and/or antisocial personality disorder. Further, the association between alcoholism and hyperactivity could actually be attributable to the conduct disorder often found in hyperactive children (Alterman and Tarter, 1986).

A review of the literature thus far seems to agree that childhood conduct problems are linked to familial alcoholism and the development of alcoholism, although hyperactivity/MBD without conduct disorder may not be a risk factors for the development of alcoholism. In addition, it is generally agreed that conduct disorder in children is a risk factor for developing alcoholism and antisocial personality disorder in adults. It is not clear, however, how genetics influences the vulnerability between conduct disorder and the development of alcoholism and/or antisocial personality disorder. There are data, however, suggesting that alcoholism and antisocial personality disorder are separate, genetically transmitted disorders (Cloninger and Reich, 1978).

Subclassifications Based on Antisocial Personality Disorder

Investigations of psychiatric comorbidity in clinical and nonclinical samples of alcohol abusers have found a strong association between ASP and alcoholism (cf. Powell et al., 1982; Martin, Cloninger, and Guze, 1982; Hesselbrock et al., 1984; Penick et al., 1984; Hesselbrock et al., 1985; Hesselbrock, 1986b; Lewis et al., 1986; Helzer and Pryzbeck, 1988). By differentiating alcoholics according to the co-occurrence of ASP, investigators found that ASP alcoholics can be characterized as a separate typology. However, it can be difficult to distinguish alcoholism and ASP on the basis of phenomenology alone, leading to diagnostic confusion (Schuckit, 1973; Hesselbrock, V. M., 1986; Meyer, 1986). Persons who are suffering from alcoholism often display a variety of antisocial behaviors (e.g., fights, lying), while persons with antisocial personality disorder often abuse alcohol. The prevalence of ASP (according to the DSM III criteria) among samples of male alcoholics has been reported to approach 50% (Penick et al., 1984; Cadoret et al., 1984; Hesselbrock et al., 1985). Further, it is often difficult to separate antisocial personality disorder from early-onset alcoholism. Alcohol abuse at an early age is a criterion for ASP, while alcoholism may produce behavior problems (Meyer, 1986; Gerstley et al., 1990). ASP alcoholics, compared to non-ASP alcoholics, have an earlier onset of alcoholism followed by a more chronic and severe course. Consequently, they often seek treatment at a much younger age than non-ASP alcoholics. (Lewis et al., 1983; Penick et al., 1984; Hesselbrock et al., 1984; Stabenau, 1984). Hesselbrock et al. (1984) found that hospitalized ASP alcoholics took their first drink and began regular drinking and drunkenness much earlier than their non-ASP counterparts. ASP alcoholics were nearly 10 years younger, on average, than non-ASP alcoholics at the time of hospitalization, but reported having a drinking problem just as long as the older non-ASP alcoholics.

While there is general agreement that ASP alcoholics can be characterized in terms of an early onset and a severe course of alcoholism, there is little agreement regarding their drinking patterns or the severity of the consequences of alcohol abuse they experience. Rimmer et al. (1972) found that ASP alcoholics reported more blackouts, arrests, and driving difficulties than non-ASP alcoholics. Hesselbrock et al. (1984) and Stabenau (1984) found that the social, physical, and psychological problems resulting from alcoholism in the six months prior to hospitalization were similar between ASP and non-ASP alcoholics, despite the young age of the ASP alcoholics. Rimmer et al. (1972) found that ASP alcoholics were not more likely to suffer from withdrawal symptoms or liver cirrhosis than were non-ASP alcoholics, while Hesselbrock et al. (1984) found that ASP alcoholics versus non-ASP alcoholics consumed more alcohol and experienced more symptoms related to withdrawal in the month prior to hospital admission than their non-ASP counter parts. Other investigators have, however, found fewer alcohol-dependence symptoms and medical complications among ASP alcoholics than in non-ASP alcoholics (cf. Virkkunen, 1979). The conflicting findings by different investigators may reflect sample differences (some studies only included men, while others included both men and women), information gathered during different time periods (e.g., 1 month, 6 month before hospitalization, or lifetime), and the retrospective nature of studies. They may also reflect the acute condition of alcoholics at the time of hospitalization.

Findings by Lewis et al. (1983) that ASP alcoholics reported more problems related to loss of control despite fewer years of heavy drinking may indicate a biological vulnerability for alcoholism among ASP alcoholics. That study indicates the importance of examining the lifetime history of alcohol abuse rather than the time period immediately prior to hospitalization when comparing ASP and non-ASP alcoholics.

Penick et al. (1984) found that ASP alcoholics had an early onset of alcoholism, poor psychosocial functioning, more alcohol-related hospitalizations, arrests, alcohol abuse symptoms, and familial psychopathology than non-ASP alcoholics. Similar findings reported by Cadoret et al. (1984) indicate that ASP alcoholics have more alcohol-related problems, including fighting, job problems, arrests, and physical problems. They also found that alcoholism with ASP was associated with other substance abuse problems and a greater number of treatments for alcoholism. Multiple substance abuse probably predispose ASP alcoholics to poor treatment outcomes, especially since poor treatment outcome has in fact been reported for ASP alcoholics (Goodwin et al., 1971). An investigation of psychiatric problems in biological family members of ASP alcoholics has revealed a high prevalence of familial alcoholism among alcoholic probands with the diagnosis of ASP. Hesselbrock et al. (1984; Hesselbrock, 1991a) compared the lifetime prevalence of alcoholism among the father, mother, and siblings of ASP and non-ASP alcoholics, and found that the prevalence of alcoholism in the proband's biological father was higher among ASP alcoholics (both males and females) than non-ASP alcoholic probands. However, the rate of alcoholism in mothers was higher among ASP men than non-ASP men, while non-ASP women alcoholics reported a higher prevalence of alcoholism among their mothers than was found among the mothers of female ASP probands.

While a higher prevalence of sociopathy in the male relatives of alcoholic probands has been compared to the general population (Winokur et al., 1970, 1971), it does appear that alcoholism and ASP are two separately transmitted traits (Hesselbrock, M. N., 1985a). For example, adult, adopted-away sons of Danish alcoholics were found to have an increased prevalence of alcoholism, but not ASP (Goodwin et al., 1973), while Schulsinger (1972) found a high rate of criminality and psychopathy, but not alcoholism, in the offspring of psychopathic parents. Primary alcoholism appears most frequently among the family members of primary alcoholic probands, while primary ASP (but not primary alcoholism) appears mainly in the biological relatives of primary ASP probands (Cloninger et al., 1979). However, the co-occurrence of ASP and alcoholism seems to create a synergistic effect for the transmission of both ASP and alcoholism (Hesselbrock, V. M., 1986; Mirin et al., 1986; Alterman and Tarter, 1986). The relatives of probands with both ASP and alcoholism were found to have an increased risk for both antisocial personality disorder and alcoholism (Reich et al., 1981; Cloninger and Reich, 1983; Lewis et al., 1983; Hesselbrock, V. M., 1986).

Neurobiological-Based Typologies

The studies reviewed thus far have taken a phenomenological approach to the subtyping of alcoholism. More recently, a neurobiological typology that combines antisocial traits and other putative risk for alcoholism has been developed. Cloninger and colleagues have proposed two separate forms of alcoholism based on biological and personality factors thought to be associated with the transmission of alcoholism (Cloninger et al., 1981). One form, thought to be highly heritable and independent of environmental influence, is characterized by moderate alcohol abuse in the probands themselves, and by criminality and severe alcohol use in their fathers. The second form was characterized by either mild or severe alcohol abuse in the probands and no criminality in the fathers. The biological fathers were often mild to moderate alcohol abusers. Both genetic and environmental factors contribute to the development of this form of alcohol abuse (Type 1).

Cloninger et al.'s (1981) typology is based on a study of Swedish men who were adopted away to nonrelatives at an early age. Most were separated from their biological relatives in the first few months of life. The sample included 862 male offspring born between 1930 to 1949 to single women in Stockholm. These men were followed up when they were 23 to 43 years of age. Information about the biological parents and adoptive parents was obtained from hospitals, clinics, and several national health and law enforcement registers that are systematically maintained in Sweden. Information pertinent to the diagnosis of alcohol abuse, age of onset of alcohol abuse, supervision, and treatment of alcohol abuse was obtained through the records of the local Temperance Board register; information regarding criminal convictions came from a criminal register; and information about sick leave, hospitalization, occupational status came from the local office of the National Health Insurance. Through the data from the Temperance Board register, the men were classified into one of four groups of alcohol users: no alcohol abuse; mild alcohol abusers who had been registered with the Temperance Board once but receiving no alcoholism treatment; moderate alcohol abusers who had been registered two or three times but were not treated for alcoholism; and severe alcohol abusers who had been registered four or more times or who received compulsory treatment or psychiatric hospitalization for alcoholism. One-hundred-fifty-one men (17.5%) were classified as alcohol abusers, including 64 mild alcohol abusers (7.4%), 36 moderate abusers (4.1%), and 51 severe alcohol abusers. The three types of alcohol abuse were compared in terms of the biological father's alcohol abuse history, socioeconomic status, and history of maternal alcohol abuse.

Fathers of mild abusers ($N = 64$) were found to have had an adult onset of alcohol abuse, recurrent alcohol abuse, but low criminality and few hospitalizations or treatment for alcohol abuse. The fathers had a relatively high socioeconomic status, while alcohol abuse in the biologic mothers was frequent (Type 1). The biological parents of severe abusers ($N = 51$) were found to be similar to those of mild abusers, except that the fathers had a very low socioeconomic status (Type 1). Alcohol abuse and criminality in the fathers of mild and severe alcohol abusers were similar to those found in the adoptees who were not alcohol abusers (Cloninger et al., 1981).

The biological fathers of moderate abusers ($N = 36$) had a low socioeconomic status, recurrent alcohol abuse, a greater number of hospitalizations or treatments for alcohol abuse, frequent registrations with the Temperance board, and a teenage onset of alcoholism. Criminal convictions dating back to adolescence were also frequent, while no alcohol abuse was seen among the biological mothers of the moderate alcohol abusers (Type 2). Using a discriminant analysis, it was found that mild and severe alcohol abusers shared genetic determinants and several environmental factors. Cloninger et al. (1981) suggest that, while alcohol abuse itself seemed in these cases to be influenced by genetic determinants, environmental factors appeared to determine the level of abuse (i.e., mild and severe alcohol abuse) in the adoptees. On the other hand, moderate abuse was determined by genetic factors alone, and did not seem to be dependent on environmental factors.

To examine the independent contribution of genetic and environmental factors and the interaction between genetic and environmental background, both the biological and adoptive parents of the probands were classified as transmitting high and low risk according to their own alcohol abuse patterns. For adoptees with mild alcohol abuse, both genetic and environmental backgrounds were significant factors, while there was no interaction between these two factors. For adoptees with moderate alcohol abuse, however, a ninefold increase in risk among the genetically predisposed sons was found regardless of their environmental background. No increase in risk was found due to environmental factors alone or to the interaction between genetic and environmental background. With severe alcohol abuse, some increase in risk from genetic background and from environmental factors was noted, but not significantly. These findings differ from those of Goodwin (1979, 1984), who found in the Danish adoption study that alcoholics with a family history of alcoholism tended to have a severe form of alcoholism. The variation in the findings of the two studies could be due to differences in the definition of alcohol abuse. The Swedish adoption study defined types of alcohol abuse in relation to the number of contacts with the Temperance Board or treatment contacts, while Goodwin's (1979, 1984) definition was based on hospitalization records.

Thus, Type 1 (milieu-limited) alcohol abuse is associated with recurrent alcohol abuse without criminality in the biological parents. Both mothers and fathers contribute to the milieu-limited type of alcohol abuse, while Type 2 (male-limited) alcohol abuse is highly heritable from father to son. Mothers of type 2 alcoholics tended to be nonabusers.

In the second part of the study, Bohman et al., (1981) analyzed data on 913 adopted women from the same adoption study. This analysis dichotomized the female adoptees into two categories, abuse and no abuse, instead of dividing them into four categories (probably due to the small number of abusers). Only 31 women (3%) were classified as alcohol abusers, though an increased prevalence of alcohol abuse was found among the daughters whose mothers were alcohol abusers. If both biological parents were alcoholics, the risk for alcohol abuse among the women was also increased. However, there was no increased risk for alcohol abuse among the daughters of alcohol-abusing fathers. As with the male adoptees, a cross-fostering analysis was conducted to determine the risk associated with both genetic and environmental background variables. If the genetic disposition was classified as high, the risk to the adoptee increased threefold over those adoptees with low genetic and environmental background. The presence of both an environmental factor and a high genetic background produced only a slight increment in risk (6.7% for genetic only and 7.7% for both). In the absence of a genetic factor, the environmental factor was related to similar rates of alcohol abuse among daughters who were low in both factors (2.3% for neither and 3.2% for environmental factor only). Thus, the susceptibility to alcoholism was different for adopted men and women. In their analysis, Bohman et al. (1981) found that daughters seemed to inherit alcoholism from their biologic mothers, while the men tended to show the two types of heritability. Maternal alcohol abuse was associated with Type 1 mileu-limited alcohol abuse for male alcoholics, while paternal alcohol abuse was often found in Type 2 male-limited alcohol abuse in male adoptees. Based on these two studies, Bohman et al. (1981) concluded that the pattern of transmission among the adopted daughters was more similar to Type 1 alcoholism.

Several cautions should be applied to the interpretation of the Swedish adoption study data. First, the rates of alcohol abuse among the female sample was very low (N = 31). Because of the small number of women who developed alcohol abuse, Bohman et al. were unable to exactly replicate the analysis done with the adopted men. Similarly, Type 2 alcoholism in the male sample was based on a small number of moderate alcohol abusers (N = 36). Consequently, the relatively small number of cases used in the 2×2 tables for the cross-fostering analysis for adopted sons with moderate alcohol abuse and for women is likely to provide low statistical power. For example, only 5 moderate alcohol-abusing men (Type 2) were from the high genetic and environmental risk group; 12 from the high genetic and low environmental risk group; 8 from the low genetic and high environmental risk group; and 11 from the low genetic and environmental risk group. Similarly, the low congenital and low postnatal group included only 12 women; the low congenital and high postnatal, 7 women, the high congenital, low postnatal, 8 women, and the high congenital and postnatal, 4 women. While the authors offer a caution regarding the findings about environmental factors, the caution should be applied to all of the cross-fostering analyses.

The methods used to classify background into high or low risk are not clearly stated and may limit the generalizability of the findings, making the study difficult to replicate. The criteria are described as "more like average characteristics of adoptees either with no abuse or with any abuse," but the average characteristics are not described.

It should also be noted that the analyses of the men and women samples were not conducted in the same manner. The male alcohol abusers were divided into three groups, while the female abusers were treated as one group. Because of the small number of abusers among the female adoptees, no subdivision was possible. It should not and cannot be assumed however, that female alcoholics are homogeneous in terms of types of alcohol abuse. Also, the variables examined in the two analyses were not identical. For example, criminality in the mothers of male adoptees was not examined in the analysis, while it was considered for the female adoptees. Therefore, the conclusion that alcohol abuse among females is relatively homogeneous and similar to Type 1 alcohol abuse in men may be premature. Despite these limitations, the Swedish adoption study is the first attempt to examine etiologic heterogeneity and the mode of transmission in alcoholic subtypes. The low rates of severe alcohol abuse among the adoptees could be due to the age of the subjects, which range from 23 to 43. Most of the subjects are still at risk for developing alcohol abuse/dependence. Replication of this study 10 to 15 years later may yield different findings.

Cloninger (1986) proposed that "there are biogenetically distinct dimensions underlying personality variation that are moderately heritable and moderately stable across time and situations." He identified three heritable dimensions of personality that influence the behavior patterns of individuals' response to various environmental stimuli: Novelty seeking, defined as a tendency toward frequent exploratory activity and intense excitement in response to novel stimuli; harm avoidance, a tendency to respond intensely to aversive stimuli and to learn to avoid punishment and novelty; reward dependence, defined as a tendency to respond intensely to reward and succorance and to maintain rewarded behavior. According to Cloninger, "these neurobiological dimensions interact to give rise to integrated patterns of differential responses to punishment, reward and novelty." The operational measure of these personality traits, the Tridimensional Personality Questionnaire (TPQ), was based on findings from a longitudinal study of Swedish school children. Cloninger et al. (1988) found that high novelty-seeking, low harm avoidance was highly predictive of alcohol abuse in young adulthood.

Cloninger (1987) combined the genetic transmissibility of alcoholism and these personality traits into the definitions of Type 1 and Type 2 alcoholism. Type 1 alcoholics are described as being dependent on social approval (high reward dependence), cautious (high harm avoidance), and to prefer nonrisk taking situations (low novelty seeking). Type 1 alcoholism, characterized by loss of control, and guilt and fear about alcohol dependence, is associated with "passive-dependent or anxious personality, high reward dependence, high harm avoidance and low novelty seeking."

Type 2s have personality traits opposite to those of Type 1 alcoholics, i.e., low reward dependence, low harm avoidance, and high novelty seeking. Type 2 alcoholism is further characterized by "spontaneous alcohol-seeking behavior or inability to abstain" and is associated with traits of antisocial personality. These traits are opposite those of a passive-dependent personality and feature high novelty seeking, low harm avoidance, and low reward dependence. Cloninger et al. further hypothesize neurophysiological and neurochemical differences in relationship to each personality trait.

Replication Study from the United States

With analytic methods similar to those used in the Swedish study, Gilligan et al. (1987) examined the heritability of alcohol abuse in Caucasian alcoholics hospitalized in the United States. They examined families of 288 alcoholic probands. The mode of transmission in the families of female probands was characterized by a "multifactorial-polygenic model" with no significant evidence of a major gene effect; the analysis of the families of male probands indicated a "transmissible major effect" in addition to a multifactorial-polygenic effect. The male probands were subdivided for further analysis according to the likelihood for the models of male and female families and labeled malelike and femalelike. Using segregation analysis, malelike families were found to have a much higher heritability than the femalelike family. The relatives of malelike alcoholics became alcoholic at an earlier age and had a higher prevalence of antisocial personality according to Feighner criteria (1972) than femalelike male alcoholics and female probands. However, unlike the Swedish sample of adopted women, female probands in this sample had no alcoholism in their mothers.

Gilligan et al. further examined the alcohol-related symptoms (as described in the Feighner (1972) criteria) in the male first-degree relatives of male and female probands. Using discriminant function analysis, male relatives of male probands were characterized by the Type 2 features, i.e., inability to abstain, fights while drinking, reckless driving while drinking, and treatment for alcohol abuse. Male relatives of female probands exhibited Type 1 features, i.e., benders, guilt, onset after 25, loss of control, and cirrhosis and/or liver disease. The examination of subtypes of relatives by transmission liability found that males in female and femalelike families showed a greater number of Type 1 symptoms than malelike males, while female relatives were similar in their symptom picture. Based on these findings, the authors suggested that alcohol abuse in women was more homogeneous than in men.

Gilligan et al. (1987) compared their Type 1 alcoholism to Jellinek's Gamma alcoholism in terms of alcohol-related characteristics. Gamma alcoholism is characterized by loss of control, binges and benders, and feelings of guilt about drinking. On the other hand, the Type 2 style of drinking is associated with Delta alcoholism, and is characterized by the inability to abstain completely and by impulsive behavior when intoxicated. However, Jellinek (1960) emphasized environmental influences on the etiology of alcohol abuse, while Gilligan et al. (1987) found an association between alcohol-related behavior and the mode of transmission.

Gilligan et al. posit an association of alcohol-related symptoms with Jellinek's typology, but their typology was based on a discriminant function analysis done on relatives, not the probands themselves. The only alcohol-related variable from the proband used in Gilligan et al.'s analysis was the age of onset of alcoholism. Therefore, their typology is based on alcohol-related variables found in the proband's relatives. The typology of probands was based only on the likelihood of malelike or femalelike mode of transmission.

Differences in the samples of alcohol abusers between the Swedish study and that of Gilligan et al. (1987) should also be considered. In the first study, alcohol abuse was defined as the number of registered contacts with the Temperance Board or number of hospitalizations recorded, while the U.S. Sample was drawn from persons hospitalized for the treatment of alcoholism. Possible variations in the severity of alcoholism in the probands was not considered. In order to replicate Cloninger and Bohman's typology in a comparable U.S. sample (a community sample), only those who abuse alcohol but are not treated for alcoholism and DWI offenders could be sampled since no system comparable to the Swedish Temperance Board is available in the United States.

Another caution stated by the authors is that the results of the discriminant function analysis did not separate etiologically distinct groups of families with nonoverlapping traits. They suggest that additional variables (e.g., other forms of psychopathology) and quantitative measures of personality are needed to better specify phenotypic patterns of behavior among family members.

Cloninger et al.'s Type 1 and Type 2 classifications have been criticized because of the small sample size ($N = 31$), sample selection methods, indirect measurement of probands' fathers' variables, and other methodological limitations (Vanclay and Raphael, 1990).

Several investigators have attempted to examine Type 1 and Type 2 alcoholism in the United States. For example, Schuckit and Irwin (1989) first raised the issue that the Type 1/Type 2 classification might not apply to U.S. samples of alcoholics. They are concerned that the sample of alcoholics in the Swedish study was too small to make definitive statements about validity. In a study of 171 young men at risk for alcoholism, Irwin et al. (1990) examined the usefulness of novelty seeking, harm avoidance, and reward dependence for predicting alcohol-related problems among young men whose fathers had either severe alcohol-related problems or had no family history of alcoholism. No significant relationship between the personality traits proposed by Cloninger et al. (1987) and either the young men's drinking patterns or their family history of alcoholism was found. Inconsistencies between the Type 1 and Type 2 continuum and personality characteristics among alcoholics have also been reported (von Knorring et al., 1987).

The findings of Schuckit et al. (1990) have been substantiated by Hesselbrock and Hesselbrock (1992) who examined a sample of nonalcoholic young men similar to the subjects in the Schuckit et al. study. While Schuckit et al. examined only one risk factor, a family history of alcoholism, Hesselbrock and Hesselbrock's study examined two risk factors. Antisocial personality disorder and family history of alcoholism were studied in relation to the personality traits proposed by Cloninger (1987) and several additional personality measures: Karolinska Scales of Personality (Schalling and Edman, 1986), Life Orientation Test (Sheirer and Carver, 1985), Rosenberg Self-Esteem Inventory (Rosenberg, 1965), Psychopathic State Inventory (Haertzen et al., 1980), and the Sensation Seeking Scale V (Zuckerman, 1979). The results indicated that ASP, regardless of a family history of alcoholism, is an important factor in describing alcohol use and the personality characteristics among young men at risk of developing serious alcohol abuse. In terms of the subscales of the TPQ, the young men who were at risk for Type 2 alcoholism scored high on the Novelty Seeking scale, but not on the Harm Avoidance or Reward Dependence scales. The young men at risk for Type 1 alcoholism could not be distinguished on these personality scales. ASP men also scored higher than non-ASP men on the Karolinska Scale of Personality, indicating impulsivity, life orientation, psychopathy, and the total sensation-seeking score. A family history of alcoholism was not a significant factor in differentiating young men on most personality measures. These findings indicate that many traits often ascribed to such a family history may in fact be due to ASP.

Schuckit et al (1990) also suggest that the Type 2 alcoholic may represent a separate disorder, i.e., antisocial personality disorder. The findings of Hesselbrock and Hesselbrock (1992) are also consistent with previous findings suggesting that premorbid characteristics and genetic influences due to ASP and a family history of alcoholism are separate (Founds and Hassall, 1969; Cadoret, 1978; Cadoret et al., 1987; Schuckit and Irwin, 1989; Cloninger and Gottesman, 1987; Irwin et al., 1990).

Other investigations have examined Type 1 and Type 2 alcoholism in terms of alcohol-related symptoms. For example, Penick et al. (1990) found that a single criterion, age of onset of alcoholism, was a significant factor in separating the two types of alcoholism. Other alcohol-related symptoms, such as inability to abstain, fights, arrests, loss of control, guilt, and fear of alcohol dependence were frequently reported by both types of alcoholics and did not distinguish Type 1 from Type 2 in their sample. Irwin et al. (1990) also found that the Type 1 and Type 2 criteria were related to the age of onset of alcoholism. Von Knorring et al. (1985) suggest that age of onset rather than any specific symptomatology, is sufficient to classify alcoholics into two discrete subtypes.

The male-limited transmission of Type 2 alcoholism has been examined by Glenn and Nixon (1991). They examined 51 female alcoholics by dividing them into two groups according to the age of onset. They were unable to distinguish these two groups in terms of alcohol-related symptoms, but the early onset group more closely resembled the characteristics of male Type 2 alcoholics, including high familial density and paternal alcoholism. Their finding indicates that Type 2 alcoholism in the United States may not be limited to males. Hesselbrock (1991b) also examined a sample of alcoholic women and men in terms of Type 1 and Type 2 alcoholism. Although the number of women was small, ASP alcoholic women had characteristics resembling Type 2 alcoholism.

Babor et al. (1992) employed an empirical clustering technique to subtype 321 male and female hospitalized alcoholics. Two types of alcoholics were derived from the clustering solution. One type was similar to Cloninger's Type 1 and was characterized by later onset, fewer childhood risk factors, and less psychopathology. The characteristics of the other type resembled Type 2 alcoholism, i.e., high childhood risk factors, familial alcoholism, early onset of alcohol problems, a more chronic treatment history, greater psychopathology, and more life stress. However, several characteristics found in the Babor et al. (1992) study differed from those of Cloninger. For example,

Cloninger et al. found that Type 2, male-limited alcohol abuse was associated with moderate alcohol abuse, while Babor et al.'s subtype was associated with severe and more chronic consequences of alcoholism. Further, Babor et al. found Type 1 and the Type 2 alcoholism in both males and females.

While the Type 1 and Type 2 typology in U.S. samples has not been confirmed, none of the replication studies sampled adoptees. It is difficult to conduct an exact duplication of the Swedish adoptee' study in the United States due to differences in the availability of information about the biological parents of adoptees and the lack of a comparable registering system of the general population (i.e., psychiatric hospitalization and Temperance Board). Further, cultural differences, differences in the variables examined, and differences in the method of the data collection might also contribute to the failure to replicate thus far. Nevertheless, Cloninger and colleagues' typology formulation provides a comprehensive model of genetic vulnerability, personality, and alcohol-related characteristics and their interrelationship. Several studies have replicated aspects of Cloninger et al.'s proposed typology, but further research efforts are needed to clarify the discrepancies.

Summary

This chapter has reviewed several typological classifications of alcoholism and their association with genetic vulnerability. Several issues with respect to alcoholism have been identified. First, alcoholism is indeed a heterogeneous disorder. Like other medical disorders in which subtyping based on a family history of the disorder is often an effective predictor of the severity and natural history of the disorder (e.g., diabetes and cardiovascular disease), similar subtypes of alcoholics may be useful. From the late nineteenth century to the current time, most efforts to develop homogeneous subtypes of alcoholism have been based on phenomenology rather than on etiological considerations or treatment outcome(s). Further research efforts are needed in this area.

Secondly, the heritability of alcoholism seems to be multifaceted. While some typologies have considered the etiology of alcoholism attributable to genetic factors only, others have included environmental factors. Classifications of alcoholism based on phenomenology have considered social, psychological, or physical consequences. A variety of different family constellations and different cultures have also been the focus of study. Variations were also seen in the definition of alcoholism and alcohol abuse, a key element of all typologies. For example, alcohol dependence has been operationalized differently from one study to the other. Some studies include persons with alcohol abuse, while others only sample those with alcohol dependence. Some definitions of a family history of alcoholism included only paternal alcoholism, while in other studies the genetic loading is based on both first- and second-degree relatives.

Despite vast differences in theoretical orientation, key elements of the types of alcoholism defined appear to be similar, i.e., severity of social, psychological, and physical consequences; conduct disorder; delinquencies and crime in childhood and adolescence. All these characteristics seemed to be associated with familial alcoholism, suggesting genetic factors or at least heritable aspects of the transmission of alcoholism.

Another factor is that a type of alcoholism has been consistently associated with ASP. While the labeling has changed over time, the more prominent characteristics describing alcoholism and ASP have remained similar. It is also likely that ASP and alcoholism are transmitted separately. However, the relationship among childhood hyperactivity, conduct problems, and familial alcoholism needs clarification.

Environmental factors also appear to be important in less severe types of alcoholism. These types may represent as much as 20% of alcoholism. While environmental factors may not cause alcoholism, they may well interact with genetic factors. Specific mechanisms, including how this interaction occurs, have yet to be identified.

References

Alfano, A. M., Nerviano, V. J., and Thurstin, A. H. (1987). An MMPI-based clinical typology for inpatient alcoholic males: derivation and interpretation. *J. Clin. Psychol.* **43**:431–437.

Allen, M. H., and Frances, R. J. (1986). Varieties of psychopathology found in patients with addictive disorders: A review. In *Psychopathology and Addictive Disorders,* R. E. Meyer, ed. New York: Guilford Press.

Alterman, A., and Tarter, R. (1983). The transmission of psychological vulnerability: Implications for alcoholism etiology. *J. Nerv. Ment. Dis.* **171**:147–154.

Alterman, A. I., and Tarter, R. E. (1986). An examination of selected typologies: Hyperactivity, familial, and antisocial alcoholism. In *Recent Developments in Alcoholism,* **4**, M. Galanter, ed. New York: Plenum Press.

August, G. J., and Stewart, M. A. (1983). Familial subtypes of childhood hyperactivity. *J. Nerv. Ment. Dis.* **171**:362–368.

August, G. J., Stewart, M. A., and Holmes, C. S. (1983). Four year follow-up of hyperactive boys with and without conduct disorder. *Br. J. Psychiatr.* **143**:192–198.

Babor, T., and Dolinsky, Z. (1988). Alcoholic typologies: Historical evolution and empirical evaluation of some common classification schemes. In *Alcoholism: Origins and Outcome,* R. M. Rose and J. Barett, eds. New York: Raven Press, Ltd.

Babor, T., and Lauerman, R. (1986). Classification and forms of inebriety: Historical antecedents of alcoholic typologies. In *Recent Developments in Alcoholism,* **4**, M. Galanter, ed. New York: Plenum Press, pp. 113–144.

Babor, T. F., Hofmann, M., DelBoca, F. K., Hesselbrock, V. M., Meyer, R. E., Dolinsky, Z. S., and Rounsaville, B. (1992). Types of alcoholics: II. Evidence for an empirically-derived typology based on indicators of vulnerability and severity. *Arch. Gen. Psychiatr.,* **49**, 599–608.

Blashfield, R. K. (1984). *The Classification of Psychopathology.* New York: Plenum Press.

Bohman, M., Sigvardsson, S., and Cloninger, C. (1981). Maternal inheritance of alcohol abuse: Cross-fostering analysis of adopted women. *Arch. Gen. Psychiatr.* **38**:965–969.

Bowman, K., and Jellinek, E. M. (1941). Alcohol addiction and its treatment. *Q. J. Stud. Alcohol* **2**(1):98–176.

Cadoret, R. (1978). Psychopathology in adopted-away offspring of biologic parents with antisocial behavior. *Arch. Gen. Psychiatr.* **35**:176–184.

Cadoret, R., Troughton, E., and Widmer, R. (1984). Clinical differences between antisocial and primary alcoholics. *Compr. Psychiatr.* **25**:1–8.

Cadoret, R., Troughton, E., and O'Gorman, T. (1987). Genetic and environmental factors in alcohol abuse and antisocial personality. *J. Stud. Alcohol* **48**:1–8.

Cahalan, D., and Room, R. (1974). *Problem Drinking Among American Men.* New Brunswick, NJ: Rutgers University Center of Alcoholic Studies.

Cantwell, D. P. (1972). Psychiatric illness in the families of hyperactive children. *Arch. Gen. Psychiatr.* **27:**414–417.

Cloninger, C. R. (1986). A unified biosocial theory of personality and its role in the development of anxiety states. *Psychiatr. Devel.* **3:**167–224.

Cloninger, C. R. (1987). Neurogenetic adaptive mechanisms in alcoholism. *Science* **236:**410–416.

Cloninger, C. R., and Reich, T. (1983). Genetic heterogeneity in alcoholism and sociopathy. In *Genetics of Neurological and Psychiatric Disorders,* S. Ketty, L. Rowland, R. Sidman, and S. Matthysse, eds. New York: Raven Press, pp. 145–166.

Cloninger, C. R., and Gottesman, I. (1987). Genetic and environmental factors in antisocial behavior disorders. In *The Cause of Crime: New Biological Approaches,* S. Mednick, T. Moffitt, and S. Stack, eds. New York: Cambridge University Press.

Cloninger, C. R., Reich, T., and Wetzel, R. (1979). Alcoholism and affective disorders: Familial associations and genetic models. In *Alcoholism and Affective Disorders,* D. Goodwin and C. Erickson, eds. New York: SP Medical & Scientific Books.

Cloninger, C. R., Bohman, M., and Sigvardsson, S. (1981). Inheritance of alcohol abuse: Cross-fostering analysis of adopted men. *Arch. Gen. Psychiatr.* **38:**861–868.

Cloninger, C. R., Sigvardsson, S., and Bohman, M. (1988). Childhood personality predicts alcohol abuse in young adults. *Alcohol.: Clin. Exp. Res.* **12:**494–504.

Conley, J. (1981) An MMPI typology of male alcoholics: Admission, discharge, and outcome comparisons. *J. Pers. Assess.* **45:**33–39.

Costello, R. M., Lawlis, F. L., Manders, K. R., and Celistino, J. F. (1978). Empirical derivation of a partial personality typology of alcoholics. *J. Stud. Alcohol* **39:**1258–1266.

DeObaldia, R., Parsons, O., and Yohman, R. (1983). Minimal brain dysfunction symptoms claimed by primary and secondary alcoholics: Relation to cognitive functioning. *Int. J. Neurosci.* **20:**173–182.

Donovan, D. M., Chaney, E. F., and O'Leary, M. R. (1978). Alcoholic MMPI subtypes: Relationships to drinking styles, benefits and consequences. *J. Nerv. Ment. Dis.* **166:**553–561.

Donovan, D. M., Kivlahan, D. R., and Walker, R. D. (1986). Alcoholic subtypes based on multiple assessment domains, validation against treatment outcome. In *Recent Developments in Alcoholism,* M. Galanter, ed. New York: Plenum Press.

Feighner, J. P., Robins, E., Guze, S. B., Woodruff, A. R., Winokur, G., and Munoz, R. (1972). Diagnostic criteria for use in psychiatric research. *Arch. Gen. Psychiatr.* **26:**57–63.

Fleeson, W., and Gildea, E. F. (1942). A study of the personality of 289 abnormal drinkers. *Q. J. Stud. Alcohol* **3:**409–432.

Foulds, G., and Hassall, C. (1969). The significance of age of onset of excessive drinking in male alcoholics. *Br. J. Psychiat.* **115:**1027–1032.

Frances, R., Timm, S., and Bucky, S. (1980). Studies of familial and nonfamilial alcoholism. 1. Demographic studies. *Arch. Gen. Psychiatr.* **37:**564–566.

Gerstley, L. J., Alterman, A. I., McLellan, A. T., and Woody, G. E. (1990). Antisocial personality disorder in patients with substance abuse disorders: A problematic diagnosis? *Am. J. Psychiatr.* **147:**173–178.

Gibbs, L. E. (1980). A classification of alcoholics relevant to type-specific treatment. *Int. J. Addict.* **15**(4):461–488.

Gilligan, S. B., Reich, T., and Cloninger, C. R. (1987). Etiologic heterogeneity in alcoholism. *Genet. Epidemiol.* **4:**395–414.

Glenn, S. W., and Nixon, S. J. (1991). Applications of Cloninger's subtypes in a female alcoholic sample. *Alcohol. Clin. Exp. Res.* **15:**851–857.

Goldstein, S. G., and Linden, J. D. (1969). Multivariate classification of alcoholics by MMPI. *J. Abnorm. Psychol.* **74:**661–669.

Goodwin, D. W. (1979). Alcoholism and heredity: A review and hypothesis. *Arch. Gen. Psychiatr.* **36:**57–61.

Goodwin, D. W. (1984). Studies of familial alcoholism: A review. *J. Clin. Psychiatr.* **45:**14–17.

Goodwin, D. W., Crane, J. B., and Guze, S. B. (1971). Felons who drink; and eight-year follow-up. *Q. J. Stud. Alcohol* **32:**136–147.

Goodwin, D. W., Schulsinger, F., Hermansen, L., Guze, S., and Winokur, G. (1973). Alcohol problems in adoptees raised apart from alcoholic biological parents. *Arch. Gen. Psychiat.* **28:**238–243.

Goodwin, D., Schulsinger, F., Hermansen, L., Guze, S., and Winokur, G. (1975a). Alcoholism and the hyperactive child syndrome. *J. Nerv. Ment. Dis.* **160:**349–353.

Goodwin, D. W., Schulsinger, F., Knop, J., Mednick, S. and Guze, S. B. (1977). Psychopathology in adopted and nonadopted daughters of Alcoholics. Arch. Gen. Psychiatr. **35:**269–276.

Haertzen, C., Martin, W., Ross, F., and Neidert, G. (1980). Psychopathic State Inventory (PSI): Development of short test for measuring psychopathic states. *Int. J. Addict.* **15:**137–146.

Helzer, J., and Pryzbeck, T. (1988). The co-occurence of alcoholism with other psychiatric disorders in the general population and its impact on treatment. *J. Stud. Alcohol* **49:**219–224.

Hesselbrock, M. N. (1986a). Alcoholic typologies: A review of empirical evaluations of common classification schemes. In *Recent Developments in Alcoholism.* **4**, M. Galanter, ed. New York: Plenum Press.

Hesselbrock, M. N. (1986b). Childhood behavior problems and adult antisocial personality disorder in alcoholism. *Psychopathology and Addictive Disorders,* R. E. Meyer. ed. New York: Guilford Press.

Hesselbrock, V. M. (1986). Family history of psychopathology in alcoholics: A review and issues. In *Psychopathology and Addictive Disorders,* R. E. Meyer, ed. New York: Guilford Press, pp. 41–56.

Hesselbrock, M. N. (1991a). Gender comparison of antisocial personality disorder and depression in alcoholism. *J. Subst. Abuse* **3:**205–219.

Hesselbrock, M. N. (1991b). Dual diagnosis in alcoholism: Gender comparison. Paper presented at the Symposium, Alcoholism in Women: Research Updates. Annual Meeting of the Research Society on Alcoholism, Fort Myers, FL.

Hesselbrock, V. M., Stabenau, J., Hesselbrock, M. N., Meyer, R., and Babor, T. (1982). The nature of alcoholism in patients with different family histories for alcoholism. *Prog. Neuropsychopharmacol. Biol. Psychiatr.* **6:**607–614.

Hesselbrock, M. N., Hesselbrock, V. M., Tennen H., Widenman, M. A., and Meyer, R. E. (1983). Methodological considerations in the assessment of depression of alcoholics. *J. Consult. Clin. Psychol.* **51:**399–405.

Hesselbrock, M. N., Hesselbrock, V. M., Babor, T., Stabenau, J., Meyer, R., and Weidenman, M. (1984). Antisocial behavior, psychopathology and problem drinking in the natural history of alcoholism. In *Longitudinal Research of Alcoholism,* D. Goodwin, K. Van Dusen, and S. Mednick, eds. Boston: Kluwer-Nijhoff Publishing, pp. 197–214.

Hesselbrock, M. N., Meyer, R. E., and Keener, J. (1985a). Psychopathology in hospitalized alcoholics. *Arch. Gen. Psychiatr.* **42:**1050–1055.

Hesselbrock, V. M., Hesselbrock, M. N., and Stabenau, J. (1985b). Alcoholism in men patients subtyped by family history and antisocial personality. *J. Stud. Alcohol* **46**:59–64.

Hesselbrock, M. N., and Hesselbrock, V. M. (1990). Relationship of family history, antisocial personality disorder and personality traits in young men at risk for alcoholism. *J. Stud. Alcohol* **53**:619–625.

Irwin, M., Schuckit, M., and Smith, T. (1990). Clinical importance of age at onset in Type 1 and Type 2 primary alcoholics. *Arch. Gen. Psychiatr.* **47**:320–324.

Jackson, D. N., and Hoffmann, H. (1987). Common dimensions of psychopathology from the MMPI and the basic personality inventory. *J. Clin. Psychol.* **43**:661–669.

Jellinek, E. M. (1945). Heredity of the Alcoholics, Lecture 9. Alcohol, Science and Society; Twenty-nine lectures with discussions as given at the Yale Summer School of Alcohol Studies. *Q. J. Stud. Alcohol* **7**:105–114.

Jellinek, E. M. (1960). *The Disease Concept of Alcoholism.* New Haven: College and University Press.

Jellineck, E. M., and Jolliffe, N. (1940). Effects of alcohol on the individual: Review of the literature of 1939. *Q. J. Stud. Alcohol* **1**:110–181.

Jones, M. (1968). Personality correlates and antecedents of drinking patterns in adult males. *J. Consult. Clin. Psychol.* **32**:2–12.

Jordy, S. (1966). *International Bibliography of Studies of Alcohol. References 1901–1950.* New Brunswick, N.J.: Rutgers Center of Alcohol Studies.

Kline, R. B., and Snyder, D. K. (1985). Replicated MMPI subtypes for alcoholic men and women: Relationship to self-reported drinking behaviors. *J. Consult. Clin. Psychol.* **53**:70–79.

Knight, R. P. (1937). The dynamics and treatment of chronic alcohol addiction. *Bull. Menninger Clin.* **1**:233–249.

Knight, R. P. (1938). Psychoanalytic treatment in a sanatorium of chronic addiction to alcohol. *JAMA* **111**:1443–1448.

Lender, M. E. (1979). Jellinek's typology of alcoholism—some historical antecedents. *J. Stud. Alcohol* **40**(5):361–375.

Levine, H. G. (1978). The discovery of addiction: Changing conceptions of habitual drunkenness in America. *J. Stud. Alcohol* **39**:143–174.

Lewis, C. E., Helzer, J., Cloninger, R., Croughan, J., and Whitman, B. (1986). Psychiatric diagnostic predispositions to alcoholism. *Compr. Psychiatr.* **23**:451–461.

Lewis, C. E., Rice, J., and Helzer, J. (1983). Diagnostic interactions: Alcoholism and antisocial personality. *J. Nerv. Ment. Dis.* **171**:105–113.

Lewis, C. E., Rice, J. P., Andreasen, N., and Endicott, J. (1987). The antisocial and the nonantisocial male alcoholic-II. *Alcohol Alcohol.* **1**:(suppl.)379–383.

McCord, W., and McCord, J. (1960). *Origins of Alcoholism.* Palo Alto, CA: Stanford University Press.

Martin, R., Cloninger, R., and Guze, S. (1982). Alcoholism and female criminality. *J. Clin. Psychiatr.* **43**:400–403.

Marsten, A., Garmanzy, N., Tellegen, A., Pellegrini, D., Larkin, K., and Larsen, A. (1988). Competence and stress in school children: The moderating effects of individual and family qualities. *J. Child Psychol. Psychiatr.* **29**:745–764.

Marston, A., Jacobs, D., Singer, R., Widaman, K., and Little, T. (1988). Adolescents who apparently are invulnerable to drug, alcohol, and nicotine use. *Adolescence* **23**:593–598.

Mendelson, W., Johnson, N., and Stewart, M. (1971). Hyperactive children as teenagers: A follow-up study. *J. Nerv. Ment. Disord.* **153**:273–279.

Meyer, R. E. (1986). How to understand the relationship between psychopathology and addictive disorders: Another example of the chicken and the egg. In *Psychopathology and Addictive Disorders,* R. E. Meyer, ed. New York: Guilford Press.

Meyer, R. E., and Babor, T. F. (1986). Typologies of alcoholics: Overview. In *Recent Developments in Alcoholism,* **4,** M. Galanter, ed. New York: Plenum Press.

Mirin, S. M., Weiss, R. D., and Michael, J. (1986). Family pedigree of psychopathology in substance abusers. In *Psychopathology and Addictive Disorders,* R. E. Meyer, ed. New York: Guilford Press.

Morey, L. C., and Skinner, H. A. (1986). Empirically derived classifications of alcohol-related problems. In *Recent Developments in Alcoholism,* **4,** M. Galanter, ed. New York: Plenum Press.

Morey, L. C., Skinner, H. A., and Blashfield, R. K. (1984). A typology of alcohol abusers: Correlates and implications. *J. Abnorm. Psychol.* **93:**408–417.

Morey, L. C., Roberts, W. R., and Penk, W. (1987). MMPI alcoholic subtypes: Replicability and validity. *J. Abnorm. Psychol.* **96:**164–166.

Morrison, J. R., and Stewart, M. A. (1971). A family study of the hyperactive child syndrome. *Biological Psychiatr.* **3:**189–195.

Nerviano, V. J. (1976). Common personality patterns among alcoholic males: A multivariate study. *J. Consult. Clin. Psychol.* **44:**104–110.

Nerviano, V. J., and Gross, H. W. (1983). Personality types of alcoholics on objective inventories: A review. *J. Stud. Alcohol* **44:**837–851.

Penick, E., Powell, B., Othmer, E., Bingham, S., and Rice, A. (1984). Subtyping alcoholics by coexisting psychiatric syndromes: Course, family history and outcome. In *Longitudinal Research in Alcoholism.* D. Goodwin, K. Van Dusen, and S. Mednick, eds. Boston: Kluwer-Nijhoff.

Penick, E. C., Powell, B. J., Nickel, E. J., Read, M. R., Gabrielli, W. F., and Liskow, B. I. (1990). Examination of Cloninger's Type 1 and Type 2 alcoholism with a sample of men alcoholics in treatment. *Alcohol.: Clin. Exp. Res.* **14:**623–629.

Plomin, R. (1990). The inheritance in behavior. *Science* **248:**183–188.

Powell, B., Penick, E., Othmer, E., Bingham, S., and Rice, A. (1982). Prevalence of additional psychiatric syndromes among male alcoholics. *J. Clin. Psychiatr.* **43:**404–407.

Reich, T., Cloninger, C., Lewis, C., and Rice, J. (1981). Some recent findings in the study of genotype-environment interaction in alcoholism. In *Evaluation of the Alcoholic,* R. Meyer, T. Babor, J. Stabenau, J. O'Brien, and J. Jaffe, eds. NIAAA Research Monograph 5. Washington, D.C.: U.S. Government Printing Office.

Rimmer, J., Reich, T., and Winokur, G. (1972). Alcoholism. V. Diagnosis and clinical variation among alcoholics. *Q. J. Stud. Alcohol* **33,**658–666.

Robins, L. N. (1966). *Deviant Children Grown Up: A Sociological and Psychiatric Study of Sociopathic Personality.* Baltimore: Williams & Wilkins.

Robins, L. N. (1978). Sturdy childhood predictors of adult outcomes: Replications from longitudinal studies. *Psychol. Med.* **8:**611–622.

Robins, L. N., and Ratcliff, K. S. (1979). Risk factors in the continuation of childhood antisocial behavior into adulthood. *Int. J. Ment. Health* **7:**526–530.

Rosenberg, M. (1965). *Society and Adolescent Self Image.* Princeton, NJ: Princeton University Press.

Schalling, D., and Edman, G. (1986). The Karolinska Scales of Personality (KSP): An Inventory for Assessing temperament Dimensions Associated with Vulnerability for Psychosocial Deviance. Unpublished manuscript.

Schuckit, M. A. (1973). Alcoholism and sociopathy-diagnostic confusion. *J. Stud. Alcohol* **34:**157–164.

Schuckit, M. A. (1983). Alcoholism and other psychiatric disorders. *Hosp. Comm. Psychiatr.* **34:**1022–1027.

Schuckit, M. S. (1986). Genetic and clinical implications of alcoholism and affective disorder. *Am. J. Psychiatr.* **143:**140–147.

Schuckit, M., and Irwin, M. (1989). An analysis of the clinical relevance of Type 1 and Type 2 alcoholics. *Br. J. Addict.* **84:**869–876.

Schuckit, M. A., and Morrissey, E. (1976). Alcoholism in women: Some clinical and social perspectives in an emphasis on possible subtypes. In *Alcoholism Problems in Women and Children.* M. Greenblatt and M. Schuckit, eds. New York: Grune and Stratton.

Schuckit, M., Irwin, M., and Mahler, H. (1990). Tridimensional personality questionnaire scores of sons of alcoholic and nonalcoholic fathers. *Am. J. Psychiat.* **147:**481–487.

Schulsinger, F. (1972). Psychopathy, heredity and environment. *Int. Ment. Health* **1:**190–206.

Sheier, M., and Carver, C. (1985). Optimism, coping and health: Assessment and implications of generalized outcome expectancies. *Health Psychol.* **4:**219–247.

Skinner, H. A., and Jackson, D. N. (1978). A model of psychopathology based on an interpretation of MMPI actuarial systems. *J. Consult. Clin. Psychol.* **46:**231–238.

Skinner, H. A., Jackson, D. N., and Hoffman, H. (1974). Alcoholic personality types: Identification and correlates. *J. Abnorm. Psychol.* **83:**658–666.

Stabenau, J. R. (1984). Implications of family history of alcoholism, antisocial personality, and sex differences in alcohol dependence. *Am. J. Psychiatr.* **141:**1178–1182.

Stein, K. B., Rozynko, V., and Pugh, L. A. (1971). The heterogeneity of personality among alcoholics. *Br. J. Soc. Clin. Psychol.* **10:**253–259.

Stewart, M. A., deBlois, G. S., and Cummings, C. (1980). Psychiatric disorder in the parents of hyperactive boys and those with conduct disorder. *J. Child Psychol. Psychiatr.* **21:**283–292.

Tarter, R. (1988). Are there inherited behavioral traits that predispose to substance abuse? *J. Consult. Clin. Psychol.* **56:**189–196.

Tarter, R., McBride, H., Buonpane, N., and Schneider, D. (1977). Differentiation of alcoholics according to childhood history of minimal brain dysfunction, family history, and drinking pattern. *Arch. Gen. Psychiatr.* **34:**761–768.

Tarter, R. E., Hegedus, A. M., and Gavaler, J. S. (1985). Hyperactivity in sons of alcoholics. *J. Stud. Alcohol* **46:**259–261.

Thurstin, A. H., and Alfano, A. M. (1988). The association of alcoholic subtype with treatment outcome: An 18-month follow-up. *Int. J. Addict.* **23:**321–330.

Vaillant, G. E. (1983a). *The Natural History of Alcoholism.* Cambridge, MA: Harvard University Press.

Vaillant, G. E. (1983b). Natural history of male alcoholism. V: Is alcoholism the cart of the horse to sociopathy? *Br. J. Addict.* **78:**317–326.

Vanclay, F. M., and Raphael, B. (1990). Type 1 and Type 2 alcoholics: Schuckit and Irwin's negative findings. *Br. J. Addict.* **85:**683–688.

Virkkunen, M. (1979). Alcoholism and antisocial personality. *Acta Psychiatr. Scand.* **59:**493–501.

von Knorring, L., Palm, U., and Andersson, H. (1985). Relationship between treatment outcome and subtype of alcoholism in men. *J. Stud. Alcohol* **46:**388–391.

von Knorring, L., von Knorring, A-L, Smigan, L., Lindberg, U., and Edholm, M. (1987). Personality traits in subtypes of alcoholics. *J. Stud. Alcohol* **48:**523–527.

Weiss, G., Hechtman, L., Perlman, T., Hopkins, J., and Wender, P. (1979). Hyperactive as young adults: A controlled prospective ten year follow-up of 75 children. *Arch. Gen. Psychiatr.* **36**:675–681.

Wender, P. H., Reimberr, F. W., and Wood, D. R. (1981). Attention deficit disorder (minimal brain dysfunction) in adults. *Arch. Gen. Psychiatr.* **38**:449–456.

Whitelock, P. R., Overall, J. E., and Patrick, J. H. (1971). Personality patterns and alcohol abuse in a state hospital population. *J. Abnorm. Psychol.* **78**:9–16.

Winokur, G., Reich, T., Rimmer, J., and Pitts, F. (1970). Alcoholism. III: Diagnosis of familian psychiatric illness in 259 alcoholic probands. *Arch. Gen. Psychiatr.* **23**:104–111.

Winokur, G., Rimmer, J., and Reich, T. (1971). Alcoholism. IV: Is there more than one type of alcoholism? *Br. J. Psychiatr.* **118**:525–531.

Wood, D. R., Reimberr, F. W., Wender, P. H. (1976). Diagnosis and treatment of minimal brain dysfunction in adults. *Arch. Gen. Psychiatr.* **33**:1453–1460.

Wood, D. R., Wender, P. H., and Reimberr, F. W. (1983). The prevalence of attention deficiency disorder, residual type, or minimal brain dysfunction in a population of male alcoholic patients. *Am. J. Psychiatr.* **140**:95–98.

Zivich, J. M. (1981). Alcoholic subtypes and treatment effectiveness. *J. Consult. Clin. Psychol.* **49**:72–80.

Zucker, R. A., and Gomberg, E. S. (1986). Etiology of alcoholism reconsidered: The case for a biopsychosocial process. *Am. Psychol.* **41**:783–793.

Zuckerman, M. (1979). *Sensation Seeking: Beyond the Optimal Level of Arousal.* Hillsdale, NJ: Lawrence Erlbaum. Inc.

3

Familial Transmission of Psychiatric Disorders Associated with Alcoholism

REMI J. CADORET

Recent developments in the study of alcoholism have both enriched and complicated the role of genetic factors in the etiology of alcohol abuse or dependence. One such development is the increasing recognition in the last decade that alcoholism is a clinically heterogeneous condition in which a number of psychiatric conditions including personality deviations play etiologic roles. In large part this awareness of the heterogeneity of alcoholism has come about because of a revamping of psychiatric diagnostic criteria published in DSM-III (American Psychiatric Association, 1980). In this diagnostic scheme explicit provision was made for multiple diagnoses. Room for multiple diagnoses was made by incorporating them in a multiaxial scheme in which personality disorders were assigned their own axis. Studies of alcoholic patients have consistently revealed the additional presence of psychiatric conditions such as depression and antisocial personality disorder (Fowler et al., 1980; Hesselbrock et al., 1985). As a recent example of such associations, Roy et al. (1991) reported that 81% of 339 alcoholics participating in a research program had other mental disorders. The conditions associated with heavy drinking before age 20 in this study were antisocial traits, drug abuse, bipolar affective disorder, and panic disorder. This correlation of other psychiatric conditions with alcoholism is not just a product of a sampling error, e.g., individuals with two conditions being more likely to be present in a treatment setting. These conditions have also been associated with alcoholism in surveys of the general population.

A Review of Some Pertinent Studies

Studies such as the Environmental Catchment Area (ECA) project have estimated the correlations between alcohol abuse/dependence and other mental illnesses in five different urban sites in the United States. Some of these correlations are shown in Table 3-1, where antisocial personality has the closest relationship with alcohol abuse/dependence. Other conditions such as anxiety and affective disorders show lesser but still significant correlations. These correlations are likely to reflect a variety of factors rather than one underlying cause. Some factors could well be etiologic in that the associated condition would predispose an individual to alcohol abuse/dependency. Other psychiatric conditions might represent consequences of alcohol abuse/dependency. Many of these associated conditions have a genetic component in their etiology.

Considerations based upon developmental timetables would suggest that the correlation between antisocial personality (ASP) and alcoholism develops as part of the socially deviant behaviors that are an early characteristic of ASP. In ASP, drinking generally starts at a young age, so that alcohol abuse/dependency occur at significantly earlier ages in the ASP than in the non-ASP alcoholic (Hesselbrock et al., 1985). Early adolescent drinking and regular drinking that lead to significant alcohol exposure are part of the antisocial lifestyle. Heavy alcohol exposure in turn leads to alcohol abuse/dependence. Antisocials who are admitted for treatment of alcoholism are generally found to have started drinking at an earlier age than primary alcoholics, and their alcohol abuse has been described as commencing anywhere between 7 and 9 years after the onset of overt conduct disorder behaviors (Lewis and Bucholz, 1991). Findings such as these are compatible with a causal effect of deviant behavior leading to alcohol abuse. Later onset of regular drinking in non-ASPs represents a very different lifestyle, one that might have been mediated through different inheritance and/or environmental factors.

Some adoption studies are compatible with the interpretation just offered: that there are at least two kinds of alcoholism. In an analysis of Swedish adoption data Bohman et al. (1982) presented evidence for two types of alcoholism. Type I alcohol abuse involves both severe and mild cases and was called milieu-limited because both genetic diathesis and postnatal environmental factors were necessary for its expression. Type II was defined as male-limited and was increased by a genetic diathesis regardless of the postnatal environment. Type II alcohol abusers have been found to have ear-

Table 3-1 Lifetime Prevalence (%) and Odds Ratios for Alcohol Abuse/Dependence and Mental Disorders

	Antisocial Personality	Schizophrenia	Panic Disorder	Phobia	Bipolar Disorder	Major Unipolar Depression
Alcohol abuse/ dependence prevalence (%) ± standard error	73.6 ± 2.7	33.7 ± 4.4	28.7 ± 3.7	17.3 ± 0.9	43.6 ± 4.3	16.5 ± 1.5
Odds ratio for association with alcohol abuse/ dependence	21.0	3.3	2.6	1.4	5.1	1.3

Source: From Regier et al., 1990, p. 2511.

lier onset of abuse and more social complications and are thought to be similar to antisocial alcoholism (von Knorring et al., 1987), a subdivision of alcoholism first proposed as a subtype by Schuckit et al. (1970). Further genetic support for the concept of
an antisocial alcoholism that is distinct from other types of alcoholism is found in the
adoption studies of Cadoret et al. (1985, 1987).

These data are summarized in Fig. 3-1 where total results from both the 1985 and
1987 reports of two independent adoption studies are presented in a loglinear interaction diagram showing correlations between genetic and environmental factors and
adult adoptee alcoholism and ASP. As can be seen, criminality or delinquency in a biologic parent (which is itself highly correlated with ASP) predicts a significant increase
in adult adoptee ASP, which in turn is highly correlated with adult adoptee alcohol
abuse/dependency. It should be noted that biologic criminality in this best-fitting log-
linear model does not predict directly an increase in adoptee alcohol abuse; nor does
biologic parent alcohol problem predict an increase in adult adoptee ASP. Biologic
parent alcohol problems, however, do predict an increase in adult adoptee alcohol
abuse/dependence. The model is compatible with separate and specific inheritances for
alcohol abuse/dependency and ASP. The time course of onset of drinking in ASP just
discussed suggests that the causal direction shown by the arrow between adult adoptee
alcohol abuse/dependence and ASP is from ASP to alcohol abuse. The third independent pathway to alcohol abuse/dependence shown in this model is an environmental
factor, which increases the possibility of ASP as well as alcohol abuse/dependency.

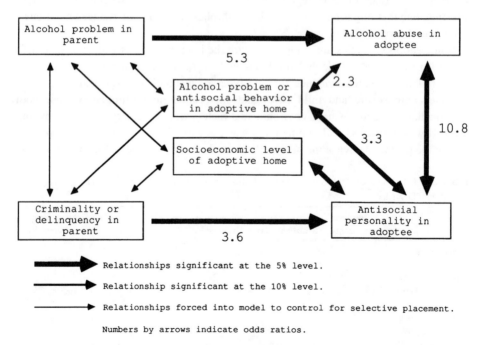

Fig. 3-1 Log-linear model of relationship between adoptee outcomes of antisocial personality and
alcohol abuse and genetic and environmental factors.

This environmental factor involves the presence in the adoptive family of someone (other than the study adoptee) with problem drinking. This individual could be a parent, sibling, or more distant relative such as an uncle or grandparent. The fact that more distant relatives (with whom adoptee contact was limited) had an effect on adoptee drinking suggests that the family drinking problem could have acted as a marker for a common environmental factor that caused the problem for both the adoptee and the adoptive relative. One other environmental factor, in Fig. 3-1, adoptive home socioeconomic states (SES), could also influence alcohol abuse/dependency indirectly through its effect upon ASP. In the presence of a biologic background of criminality, a low SES is associated with an increased incidence of ASP, which in turn leads to an increase in alcohol abuse/dependence. SES did not influence incidence of adoptee ASP when there was no biologic background of criminality. This interactional relationship is shown in Table 3-2 and could explain, in part, the increased alcohol abuse reported in lower SES populations.

In Table 3-1, schizophrenia is seen to be associated with increased alcohol abuse/dependency. Whether alcoholism precedes or succeeds the onset of the schizophrenia is not clear. Evidence from twin and adoption studies is consistent with a genetic etiology of schizophrenia (Rosenthal and Kety, 1968). One adoption study shows that separated-at-birth offspring of schizophrenic mothers tended to have problems with antisocial behavior and alcohol (Heston, 1966). However, in that study it was possible that male ASP/alcoholics were involved in fathering the children, and that the schizophrenic diathesis by itself was not associated with increased alcohol problems in the offspring.

The anxiety disorders, as evidenced in Table 3–1, also seem to be associated with increased alcoholism. Anxiety disorders, including panic and agoraphobia (even including avoidant personality), are more prevalent in alcoholic populations (reviewed in Noyes, 1990). Family studies (Crowe et al., 1983; Noyes et al., 1987) show increased alcoholism in relatives of panic disorder patients and agoraphobic patients.

Table 3-2 Socioeconomic Status of Adoptive Home vs. Antisocial Personality in Adoptee (Interaction with Biologic Parent Criminality or Delinquency)

Biologic Parent Criminal or Delinquent

		Adoptive home SES			
		High	Medium	Low	
Adoptee ASP	Yes	1	9	10	$\chi^2 = 12.02, df = 2$
	No	16	12	4	$P < 0.0025$

Biologic Parent neither Criminal nor Delinquent

		Adoptive home SES			
		High	Medium	Low	
Adoptee ASP	Yes	9	9	8	$\chi^2 = 0.53, df = 2$
	No	73	85	52	$P = NS$

These findings suggest that a genetic factor could be responsible for both alcoholism and anxiety states. However, there are no adoption studies that have tested this hypothesis, as for example, finding more anxiety conditions in adopted-away offspring of alcoholics. If a genetic diathesis for anxiety could also manifest as alcoholism, then examination of adopted-away offspring of alcoholics (some of whom should carry the alcoholism causing anxiety diathesis) should reveal increased anxiety conditions such as panic disorder or agoraphobia.

Apropos of the hypothesis that some psychiatric conditions predispose toward alcoholism is the concept of depressive alcoholism proposed by Winokur et al. (1971). This concept was based on findings from a large consecutively collected series of patients who were admitted for inpatient treatment of alcoholism. A subset of this sample turned out to be individuals who suffered from a depressive illness whose onset clearly *antedated* the development of alcoholic drinking behaviors. These individuals had higher rates of depression in their families when compared to primary alcoholics (that is, alcoholics with no other psychiatric condition) or sociopathic alcoholics (alcoholic ASPs). Almost *all* of these depressive alcoholics were female and had become alcoholic at significantly later ages than primary and sociopathic alcoholics. They had significantly more suicide attempts and fewer driving problems associated with drinking. These data are compatible with a predisposition hypothesis: depression occurring early in life predisposes and leads to alcohol abuse/dependency later in life. It is possible the increase in alcoholism reported with both unipolar and bipolar affective disorder (see Table 3-1) could be due to this type of alcoholism.

Evidence from clinical studies suggests that mania could itself lead to excessive drinking, and some family studies suggest an independent transmission of an alcoholic diathesis. Studies show increased alcohol consumption during manic episodes (Winokur et al. 1969) and high rates of excessive alcohol use in hospitalized bipolars (Reich et al., 1974). Two family studies show increased familial alcoholism in alcoholic bipolars when compared to nonalcoholic bipolars (Morrison, 1975; Dunner et al., 1979), but one study did *not* (Winokur et al., in press). Thus the question of independent transmission of alcoholism in bipolar families is still open.

The Depression Spectrum Hypothesis

Affective disorder's association with alcoholism has been a focus of research attention for a number of years. On the basis of a number of family studies, Winokur postulated two types of depressive illness: depression spectrum disease (DSD) leading to depression in females and alcoholism in males; and familial pure depressive disease (FPDD) with no association with alcoholism (Winokur, 1974). FPDD is defined as family history of depression in a first-degree relative *and* no first-degree relative with alcoholism or antisocial personality. DSD is defined by a family history where at least one first-degree relative has alcoholism or an antisocial personality. Probands for both DSD and FPDD are those with definite depression that is *not* bipolar and not secondary to some other illness (Coryell and Winokur, 1984).

Depression spectrum patients show clinical differences when compared to those with familial pure depressive disease. Spectrum depressives reported more sexual problems, divorce, lifelong irritability, fewer depressive relapses, and hospital admissions (Winokur, 1982). Abnormal dexamethasone suppression tests were fewer in the DSD group than in the FPDD patients (Winokur, 1982; Coryell and Winokur, 1984). One recent family study of depressed patients is supportive of the spectrum hypothesis. Winokur and Coryell (1991) have reported higher rates of alcoholism in the families of depressed women, but not in the families of depressed men in data from the Collaborative Study of Depression. However, not all recent family studies have supported the spectrum hypothesis. Merikangas et al. (1985) found that depressives without a family history of alcoholism did *not* transmit alcoholism, but these authors did not separate results by the sex of the depressed parent as did Winokur and Coryell (1991), and the presence of depressed male parents could have obscured the differences.

The results of two adoption studies are relevant to the depression spectrum hypothesis. The first is Goodwin et al.'s (1979) Danish study of daughters of alcoholics. These investigators reported that daughters who remained in the biologic parent home had higher rates of depression than adopted-away daughters. This result is compatible with an environmental *or* a gene–environment interaction with the biologic home representing a depressogenic environment that in the presence of the biologic background of alcoholism results in increased depression in the females.

The second study was conducted by Cadoret et al. (1985), who found no increase in depression in adopted-away daughters of alcoholics. The study did find, however, that alcohol abuse/dependency in both male and female adoptees was associated with significant increases in major depression, and that environmental factors such as early life loss of a significant figure further increased major depression in females, while alcohol problems in the adoptive home increased both major depression and alcohol abuse/dependence in males. Most of the depressions in the adoptees occurred after the onset of alcohol abuse/dependency. Further analyses of these data indicated that in males, environmental factors such as a rural adoptive home, low adoptive home SES, antisocial behavior in a family member, and later age of placement in the adoptive home resulted in increased affective symptoms (both depression and mania) as adults. The only gene–environment interaction was between affective illness in a biologic parent and later age of adoption: when the biologic background contained an affectively ill parent, then the effect of late adoptee placement (increased depression) was significantly more marked than it was without the affective biologic background (Cadoret et al., 1990). This finding suggested that gene–environment interaction could play a significant role in the etiology of affective disorder.

To relate a genetic diathesis for alcoholism with depression, a multiple regression analysis was done on these data, denoting the number of depressive symptoms as the dependent variable and including an alcohol problem in a first-degree biologic parent as a main effect independent variable. The environmental effects noted previously (rural adoptive home, low adoptive home SES, etc.) were included in the model and crossed with the genetic variable to test for interaction. Results are shown in Table 3-3 for the entire sample of male and female adoptees and demonstrate that the genetic diathesis for alcohol abuse can *interact* in the presence of certain environmental factors

Table 3-3 Multiple Regression Analysis of Genetic and Environmental Contribution to Adult Depressive Symptoms

Source of Variation	Type III Sum of Squares	p
1. Alcohol problem in first-degree biologic relative	0.02	—
2. Year of adoptee birth	15.05	0.07
3. Age of adoption	3.95	0.36
4 Adoptee alcohol abuser/dependent or antisocial	168.26	0.0001
5. Presence of one or more of following: low adoptive home SES rural adoptive home antisocial behavior in family member	60.88	0.0004
6. Interaction terms		
1 × 3	0.02	—
1 × 5	23.94	0.02

(low adoptive home SES, etc.) to produce a higher number of depressive symptoms during adulthood. This interactional effect was similar for both male and female adoptees, a point of variance with the DSD hypothesis, which predicts increased depression for females, though not necessarily for males. Thus the adoption data suggest that DSD might represent an environmental effect or a gene–environment interaction involving the genetic diathesis for alcoholism. Recent genetic linkage studies of DSD and FPDD, however, have reported a linkage between a marker gene for orosomucoid and depression in families with DSD but not in FPDD (Wilson et al., 1989). This finding, if further confirmed, would be excellent evidence for a genetic factor in DSD.

Other Factors in Alcoholism

Psychiatric conditions other than those shown in Table 3-1 have been reported to be associated with increased familial alcoholism. One such condition is Tourette's syndrome. Comings and Comings (1990) report increased alcoholism and/or drug abuse in both first- and second-degree relatives of persons with Tourette's syndrome when compared to relatives of control families (no Tourette's). Obesity was also more frequent among Tourette's syndrome relatives compared to controls. The authors relate their findings to conduct disorder and hyperactivity, which they consider to be a common clinical denominator between alcoholism and Tourette's.

Combinations of comorbid conditions listed in Table 3-1 must also be considered as factors in alcoholism. Liskow et al. (1991) reported that severity of alcoholism was higher in ASPs with depression than in ASPs without depression. The ASP/depression group was further distinguished by higher rates of psychiatric symptoms (other than depression) when compared to nondepressed ASPs. These symptoms were those of anxiety, phobic anxiety, hostility, paranoid ideation, and psychoticism—leading to a higher global psychopathology index.

These findings are compatible with the hypothesis of heterogeneity in antisocial alcoholics proposed by Whitters et al. (1984 and 1987). These authors found evidence for two types of alcoholic ASPs: (1) those with large numbers of psychiatric complaints, such as depression, anxiety, somatic complaints, manic, and psychotic symptoms, and (2) those with very few psychiatric complaints. The authors likened these two groups to previously described breakdowns of ASPs into primary and secondary sociopaths. Contributions to ASP heterogeneity could be made by both genetic and environmental factors, but regardless of etiology the heterogeneity is important in understanding antisocial alcoholism. One analysis of adoption data has examined the question of antisocial heterogeneity (Cadoret et al., 1990) and found that late adoptive home placement was associated with development of higher rates of affective symptoms (both manic and depressive symptoms) in adulthood that were in turn highly correlated with both ASP and substance abuse. Late adoptive home placement involved social disruption during the first year of life, and suggests an environmental contribution that is consistent with the hypotheses of early object-relations investigators (Ainsworth, 1985; Bowlby, 1988), who theorize that disruptions of early life relationships lead to future psychological disturbances, including difficulties in interpersonal relationships.

In addition to the DSM Axis II diagnosis of ASP, other temperament and personality factors that might have genetic roots have been associated with alcoholism. For example, people with borderline personality, which shares some characteristics with ASP, have been reported to have high rates of alcohol and other drug use/abuse (Prasad et al., 1990; Dulit et al., 1990). Many personality traits are transmitted genetically, as evidenced from twin studies (Loehlin and Nichols, 1976; Plomin et al., 1980; Eysenck, 1982) and from adoption studies (Scarr, et al., 1981; Loehlin et al., 1981; Loehlin et al., 1982). There is increased evidence of the importance of within-family environmental factors (especially unique factors) in the genesis of personality traits (Loehlin et al., 1985). There is also evidence that marked changes in personality traits in males during adolescence, especially in individuals with a high-risk profile, could be associated with more intensive substance use (Bates and Pandina, 1991). Tarter et al. (1988) have further developed the relationship between temperament, personality, and alcoholism.

These findings of the genetic transmission of personality traits suggest a number of different etiologies for alcoholism that could involve a variety of such traits. Older studies (Pohlisch, 1933; Bleuler, 1955; Amark, 1951) report large numbers of alcoholic family members with personality disorders. These studies used Schneiderian definitions of personality disorders (Schneider, 1940), which include ASP, obsessive compulsive (anancastic), and other conditions such as dependent, passive-aggressive, and hysterical.

Obviously research needs to be directed toward identifying more specific personality traits or disorders associated with alcoholism. One effort to specify traits is a proposal by Cloninger (1987a, 1987b), who suggested a tridimensional theory of personality based in part on previous dimensional descriptions of personality such as Eysencks (1952). Using this scheme, Cloninger et al. (1988) reported that traits of high novelty seeking and low harm avoidance measured when subjects were an average of

11 years old, predicted alcohol abuse when they reached 27 years of age. A dimensional approach of this type is very relevant to the task of measuring the heterogeneity found within alcoholism, and has occasioned recent attempts at verification of the tridimensional model's validity. Schuckit's group has attempted to identify patient subgroups using the tridimensional description, but reports little success in confirming the presence of specific traits in the two types of alcoholics proposed by Cloninger (Schuckit et al., 1990). In their study, Schuckit et al. concluded that Type 2 alcoholism has as its prototype the antisocial alcoholic, a conclusion echoed by von Knorring et al. (1987), who suggest "that alcoholism accompanied by antisocial behavior . . . be kept separate from alcoholism that is unrelated to antisocial behavior." The fact remains, however, that nonalcoholic sons of alcoholics can be shown to have personality characteristics different from sons of nonalcoholics [for recent examples, see Knowles and Schroeder (1990) and Whipple and Noble (1991)].

The findings in family studies that contrast children of alcoholics with controls are of potential genetic interest, since behaviors or physiologic differences of importance to the development of alcoholism could be genetically mediated. Recent family studies of this type have focused upon psychosocial functioning, and have found that children of alcoholics are characterized by (1) poor verbal ability and impulsive behavior (Schulsinger, et al., 1986); (2) more avoidant responses to stress, characterized by increased drinking, eating, and smoking (Clair and Genest, 1987); (3) higher divorce rate (Parker and Harford, 1987); and (4) more illegal drug use and earlier age of first alcohol intoxication in college age males (McCaul, et al., 1990). Some of these behaviors could obviously lead to substance abuse/dependence; others, such as poor verbal ability, are not as easily conceived as etiologic to alcoholism. These behaviors, however, might serve as markers or predictors of alcoholism and lead to more appropriate interventions.

Summary

This survey of genetically transmitted factors associated with alcoholism suggests that there may be many pathways to alcoholism—temperament, personality traits, deviant personalities, and a number of major psychiatric conditions—all contributing to the heterogeneity found in individual alcoholism. That environmental factors and their interaction with genetic elements are also important is attested to by the examples from adoption studies cited in this chapter. One of the advantages of the adoption paradigm is its ability to detect and measure the importance of both genetic and environmental factors and their interaction, leading to a more balanced assessment of etiologic factors and avoiding one-sided interpretations that can occur when the pendulum swings of the prevailing *zeitgeist* are followed (Vaillant, 1990).

References

Ainsworth, M. D. (1985). Attachments across the life span. *Bull. N.Y. Acad. Med.* **61**:592–812.
Amark, C. (1951). A study in alcoholism: Clinical, social, psychiatric, and genetic investigations. *Acta Psychiatr. Neurol. Scand.* **70**:(suppl.)1–283.

American Psychiatric Association (1980). *Diagnostic and Statistical Manual of Mental Disorders,* 3rd ed. Washington, DC.

Bates, M. C., and Pandina, R. J. (1991). Personality stability and adolescent substance use behavior. *Alcohol.: Clin. Exp. Res.* **15:**471–477.

Bleuler, M. (1955). Family and personal background of chronic alcoholics. In *Etiology of Chronic Alcholism,* O. Diethelm, ed. Springfield, IL: Charles C. Thomas.

Bohman, M., Cloninger, C., Sigvardsson, S., and Von Knorring, A. L. (1982). Predisposition to petty criminality in Swedish adoptees. I. Genetic and environmental heterogeneity. *Arch. Gen. Psychiatr.* **39:**1233–1291.

Bowlby, J. (1988). Developmental psychiatry comes of age. Am. J. Psychiatr. **145:**1–10.

Cadoret, R. J., O'Gorman, T. W., Heywood, E., and Troughton, E. (1985). Genetic and environmental factors in major depression. *J. Affect. Disord.* **9:**155–164.

Cadoret, R. J., Troughton, E., and O'Gorman, T. (1987). Genetic and environmental factors in alcohol abuse and antisocial personality. *J. Stud. Alcohol* **48:**108.

Cadoret, R. J., Troughton, E., Merchant, L. M., and Whitters, A. (1990). Early life psychosocial events and adult affective symptoms. In *Straight and Devious Pathways from Childhood to Adulthood,* M. Rutter, and L. Robins eds. Cambridge, U.K.: Cambridge University Press, chap. 16.

Clair, D., and Genest, M. (1987), Variables associated with the adjustment of offspring of alcoholic fathers. *J. Stud. Alcohol* **48:**345–355.

Cloninger, C. R. (1987a). A systematic method for clinical description and classification of personality varients: A proposal. *Arch. Gen. Psychiatr.* **44:**573–588.

Cloninger, C. R. (1987b). Neurogentic adoptive mechanisms in alcoholism. *Science* **236:**410–436.

Cloninger, C. R., Sigvardsson, S., and Bohman, M. (1988). Childhood personality predicts alcohol abuse in young adults. *Alcohol: Exp. Clin. Res.* **12:**494–505.

Comings, D. E., and Comings, B. G. (1990). A controlled family history study of Jornettes syndrome, II: alcoholism, drug abuse, and obesity. J. Clin. Psychiat. **51:**281–287.

Coryell, W., and Winokur, G. (1984). Depression spectrum disorders: Clinical diagnosis and biological implications. In Neurobiology of Mood Disorders, RM Post and JC Ballenger, eds. Baltimore, MD: Williams & Wilkins, chap. 5.

Crowe, R. R., Noyes, R., Pauls, D., and Slymen, D. (1983). A family study of panic disorder. Arch. Gen. Psychiatr. **40:**1065–1069.

Dulit, R. A., Fyer, M. R., Haas, G. L., Sullivan, T., and Frances, A. J. (1990). Substance use in borderline personality disorder. *Am. J. Psychiatr.* **147:**1002–1007.

Dunner, D., Hensel, B., and Fieve, R. (1979). Bipolar illness: Factors in drinking behavior. *Am. J. Psychiatr.* 136:583–585.

Eysenck, H. J. (1952). The scientific study of personality. New York: Macmillan.

Eysenck, H. J. (1982). *Personality, Genetics, and Behavior.* New York: Praeger.

Fowler, R., Liskow, B., and Tanna, V. (1980). Alcoholism, depression, and life events. *J. Affect. Disord.* **2:**127–135.

Goodwin, D. W., Schulsinger, F., Knop, J., Mednick, S., and Guze, S. B. (1979). Psychopathology in adopted and nonadopted daughters of alcoholics. In *Alcoholism and Affective Disorders, Clinical, Genetic and Biochemical Disorders,* DW Goodwin and CK Erickson, eds. New York: Spectrum.

Hesselbrock, M., Meyer, R., and Kenner, J. (1985). Psychopathology in hospitalized alcoholics. *Arch. Gen. Psychiatr.* **42:**1050–1055.

Heston, L. L. (1966). Psychiatric disorders in foster home reared children of schizophrenic mothers. *Br. J. Psychiatr.* **112:**819–825.

Knowles, E. E., and Schroeder, D. A. (1990). Personality characteristics of sons of alcohol abusers. *J. Stud. Alcohol* **51:**142–147.

Lewis, C. E., and Bucholz, K. K. (1991). Alcoholism, antisocial behavior, and family history. *Br. J. Addict.* **86:**177–194.

Liskow, B., Powell, B. J., and Nichel, E. (1991). Antisocial alcoholics: Are there clinically significant diagnostic subtypes. *J. Stud. Alcohol* **52:**62–69.

Loehlin, J. C., and Nichols, R. C. (1976). *Heredity, Environment and Personality: A Study of 850 Sets of Twins.* Austin: University of Texas Press. 1976.

Loehlin, J. C., Horn, J., and Willerman, L. (1981). Personality resemblance in adoptive families. *Behav. Genet.* **11:**309–330.

Loehlin, J. C., Willerman, L., and Horn, J. M. (1982). Personality resemblance between unwed mothers and their adopted away offspring. *J. Pers. Soc. Psychol.* **42:**1089–1099.

Loehlin, J. C., Willerman, L., and Horn, J. M. (1985). Personality resemblances in adoptive families when the children are late adolescent or adult. *J. Pers. Soc. Psychol.* **48:**376–392.

McCaul, M. E., Turkkan, J. S., Svikis, D. S., Bigelow, G. E., and Cromwell, C. C. (1990). Alcohol and drug use by college males as a function of family alcoholism history. *Alcohol.: Clin. Exp. Res.* **14:**467–471.

Merikangas, K. R., Leckman, J. F., and Prusoff, B. A. (1985). Familial transmission of depression and alcoholism. *Arch. Gen. Psychiatr.* **42:**367–372.

Morrison, J. (1975). The family histories of manic depressive patients with and without alcoholism. *J. Nerv. Ment. Dis.* **160:**227–229.

Noyes, R., Jr. (1990). The psychiatric consequences of anxiety Psychiatr. Med. **8:**41–66.

Noyes, R., Clarkson, C., Crowe, R., Yates, W., and McChesney, C. (1987). A family study of generalized anxiety disorder. *Am. J. Psychiatr.* **144:**1019–1024.

Parker, D. A., and Harford, T. C. (1987). Alcohol-related problems of children of heavy-drinking parents. *J. Stud. Alcohol* **48:**265–268.

Plomin, R., DeFries, J. C., and McClearn, G. E. (1980). *Behavioral Genetics: A Primer.* San Francisco: Freeman.

Pohlisch, K. (1933). *Social and Personliche Bedingungen des Chronischen Alkoholismus.* Leipzig: Georg Thieme Verlag.

Prasad, R. B., Val, E. R., Lakmeyer, H. W., Gavoria, M., Rodgers, P., Weiler, M., and Altman, E. (1990). Associated diagnoses (cormobidity) in patients with borderline personality disorder. *Psychiatr. J. Univ. Ottawa* **15:**22–27.

Reich, T., Davies, R., and Himmelhock, J. (1974). Excessive alcohol use in manic depressive illness. *Am. J. Psychiatr.* **131:**83–86.

Reiger, D. A., Farmer, M. E., Rae, D. S., Loche, B. Z., Keith, S. J., Judd, L. L., and Goodwin, F. K. (1990). Comorbidity of mental disorders with alcohol and other drug abuse: Results from the Epidermiologic Catchment Area (ECA) Study. J. Am. Med. Assoc. **264:**2511.

Rosenthal, D., and Kety, S. S. (1968). *Transmission of Schizophrenia.* Oxford, U.K.: Pergamon Press.

Roy, A., DeJong, J., Lamparski, D., Adinoff, B., George, T., Moore, V., Garnett, D., Kerich, M., and Linnoila, M. (1991). Mental disorders among alcoholics. *Arch. Gen. Psychiatr.* **48:**423–432.

Scarr, S., Webber, P. L., Weinberg, R. A., and Wittig, M. A. (1981). Personality resemblance among adolescents and their parents in biologically related and adoptive families. *J. Pers. Soc. Psychol.* **40:**885–898.

Schneider, K. (1940). Die psychopathischen personlichkeiten. In *Handbook der Psychiatrie,* Vol. 7, G. Aschaffenburg, ed. 5th ed. Vienna: F. Deuticke.

Schuckit, M., Rimmer, J., Reich, T., and Winokur, W. (1970). Alcoholism: Antisocial traits in male alcoholics. *Br. J. Psychiatr.* **117:**575–576.

Schuckit, M. A., Irwin, M., and Mahler, H. M. (1990). Tridimensional personality questionnaire scores of sons of alcoholic and nonalcoholic fathers. *Am. J. Psychiatr.* **147:**481–487.

Schulsinger, F., Knop, J., Goodwin, D. W., Teasdale, T. W., and Mikkelson, V. (1986). A prospective study of young men at high risk for alcoholism: Social and psychological characteristics. *Arch. Gen. Psychiatr.* **43:**755–760.

Tarter, R., Alterman, A., and Edwards, K. (1988). Neurobehavioral theory of alcoholism etiology. In *Theories of Alcoholism,* C Chaudron and D Wilkinson, eds. Toronto: Addiction Research Foundation, pp. 73–93.

Vaillant, G. (1989). The pendulum swings the other way: The role of environment obscured by genes. *Arch. Gen. Psychiatr.* **46:**1151.

von Knorring, L., von Knorring, A. L., and Smegan, L. (1987). Personality traits in subtypes of alcoholics. *J. Stud. Alcohol* **48:**523–527.

Whipple, S. C., and Noble, E. P. (1991). Personality characteristics of alcoholic fathers and their sons. *J. Stud. Alcohol* **52:**331–337.

Whitters, A., Troughton, E., Cadoret, R., and Widmer, R. (1984). Evidence for clinical heterogeneity in antisocial addicts. *Comp. Psychiatr.* **25:**158–164.

Whitters, A., Cadoret, R., and McCaley-Whitters, M. (1987). Further evidence for clinical heterogeneity in antisocial addicts. *Comp. Psychiatr.* **28:**513–519.

Wilson, A. F., Tanna, V. L., Winokur, G., Elston, R. C., and Hill, E. M. (1989). Linkage analysis of depression spectrum disease. *Biol. Psychiatr.* **26:**163–175.

Winokur, G., Clayton, P., and Reich, T. (1969). *Manic Depressive Illness.* St. Louis, MO: Mosby.

Winokur, G., Rimmer, J., and Reich, T. (1971). Alcoholism. IV: Is there more than one type of alcoholism? *Br. J. Psychiatr.* **118:**525–531.

Winokur, G. (1974). The division of depressive illness into depression spectrum disease and pure depressive disease. *Int. Pharmacopsychiatr.* **9:**5–13.

Winokur, G. (1982). The development and validity of familial subtypes in primary unipolar depression. *Pharmacopsychiatr.* **15:**142–146.

Winokur, G., and Coryell, W. (1991). Familial alcoholism in primary unipolar major depressive disorder. *Am. J. Psychiatr.* **148:**184–188.

Winokur, G., Cook, B., Liskow, B., and Fowler, R. (1993). Alcoholism in manic depressive (bipolar) patients. *J. Stud. Alcohol* **54:**574–576.

4

Genetic Influences on Drinking Behavior in Humans

ANDREW C. HEATH

There is an extensive literature on the inheritance of alcohol abuse or dependence (see Chapters 1 and 2). Findings from studies of twin pairs, adoptees, and half-siblings and their families are broadly consistent with an important genetic contribution to risk of alcoholism in males, and though findings for alcoholism in women are more ambiguous (e.g., McGue et al., 1992), the largest study of adult female twin pairs (Kendler et al., 1992) suggests an important genetic contribution to alcoholism risk in females also.

This chapter focuses not on alcohol abuse or dependence, but on variation in patterns of alcohol consumption in general population (and therefore predominantly nonalcoholic) samples. It examines the evidence that differences between individuals in the frequency with which they use alcohol, the average amount that they drink, and the total weekly consumption of alcohol that results, are highly stable over time, and that these stable individual differences in drinking behavior are substantially influenced by genetic factors. For those who consider the importance of genetic factors primarily in the context of the inheritance of diseases, the notion that there might also be a substantial genetic influence on normal variation in drinking patterns in humans may seem strange. However, studies using data from twin pairs (e.g., Eaves et al., 1989, 1992), adoptees and their adoptive and biological relatives (e.g., Scarr et al., 1981; Loehlin et al., 1981, 1985, 1990; Loehlin, 1992; Fulker et al., 1988), and separated twin pairs (e.g., Pedersen et al., 1988; Bouchard et al., 1990) demonstrate a substantial genetic contribution to individual differences in normal patterns of behavior. We shall see that this extends to normal variation in drinking patterns in general population samples.

Why should we consider the role of genetic factors in drinking behavior? A prerequisite for the development of alcoholism is initial exposure to alcohol (Merikangas,

1990). An individual at high genetic risk of alcoholism who remains a lifetime abstainer will not become an alcoholic. It is also possible that a nonabstinent individual at high genetic risk (but without a personal history of alcoholism) who maintains a consistently low level of consumption may have zero risk of alcoholism, though this empirical question has never been rigorously addressed. Thus it is conceivable that genetically determined differences in drinking behavior (the "genetics of exposure to alcohol"; Reich, personal communication) constitute one important route for a genetic contribution to alcoholism risk. It would be a mistake, however, to view the understanding of alcoholism as the sole or even primary goal of research on drinking behavior. Excessive alcohol use, even by those not meeting formal diagnostic criteria for alcohol abuse or dependence, is an important epidemiologic risk factor for a wide range of adverse medical and social conditions (for a recent summary, see Shalala 1993). Understanding the inheritance of the risk factor (drinking behavior) may thus be important for prevention and early intervention efforts.

This chapter reviews the evidence for an important genetic contribution to variation in drinking patterns. Most of this evidence derives from twin and extended twin-family studies. Although adoption studies are most powerful when data from biological parents are available, and while institutional records can be used to identify psychiatric cases who have given up a child for adoption, such records are of no help when we wish to examine normal variation in drinking patterns in biological parents. The comparison of adoptive sibling and adoptive parent–child correlations for drinking behavior with similar correlations estimated from intact nuclear families does provide some information, and as adoptees from prospective adoption studies currently in progress pass through adolescence into early adulthood (e.g., Fulker et al., 1988; Loehlin et al., 1990), we can expect important information to derive from this source.

Data from studies of twin pairs reared together have often been criticized on the grounds that the idiosyncratic early experiences of such pairs must limit the generalizability of findings using twin data. Many of these criticisms, when examined empirically, have proved to be invalid (e.g., Kendler, 1983). Moreover, a wide range of relationships included in the extended twin-family design (Heath et al., 1985)—including cousins related through dizygotic (DZ) twins versus through monozygotic (MZ) twin pairs (MZ half-siblings), uncle/aunt–nephew/niece relationships where the uncle or aunt is an MZ versus DZ cotwin of the parent of the nephew or niece—provide an important additional check on the inference of a genetic contribution to variation in drinking patterns. Findings from the one large-sample twin-family study (Heath et al., unpublished) will therefore be reviewed to provide a test of the validity of inferences from data on twin pairs alone. With rare exceptions (e.g., Partanen et al., 1966), most of the data reviewed derive from studies using self-administered questionnaires. The second part of the chapter deals with the evidence for the validity of these self-report measures which, at least in some studies, is surprisingly strong.

Demonstrating a genetic contribution to variation in drinking patterns is only a starting point in any attempt to understand the determinants of drinking behavior in humans (Heath, 1993). The third and final part of this chapter therefore examines the extent of our knowledge (or ignorance) about such issues as how genetic and social

influences on drinking behavior co-vary (genotype–environment correlation) or interact (genotype $\times$ environment interaction); and how genetic and environmental factors
operate at different stages in the natural history of alcohol use, e.g., to determine initiation of drinking, progression to regular alcohol use, and the development of excessive
drinking. It also considers the question of whether we can identify the mechanisms by
which genetic influences on drinking behavior arise—e.g., identify intervening variables in the causal chain from genotype to drinking behavior—and the moderator variables (vulnerability or protective/resiliency factors) that may exacerbate or diminish
them.

Twin Studies of Alcohol Use

The following review of the literature is quite selective. Sample sizes required for adequate statistical power for resolving genetic and nongenetic hypotheses about the
causes of variation in drinking patterns are large (Martin et al., 1978); small-sample
studies have been excluded. In many early studies, inappropriate data summaries were
used, from which it is not possible to derive estimates of the relative importance of
genetic and environmental factors. In some large-sample studies, although alcohol
consumption patterns were assessed as a potential epidemiologic risk factor, the
assessment was too cursory to be useful for a reanalysis of drinking behavior. Therefore heaviest weight is given to those studies in which I have been directly involved
and still have access to the original raw data. In some studies genetic and environmental models have been fitted to twin data, in which case estimates can be given for the
proportion of the observed variation in alcohol consumption levels that is accounted
for by genetic factors. In other cases, twin pair correlations are reported. Brief summaries of some of the major findings are given here, but we will return to the question
of what can be inferred from these studies in succeeding sections.

　　When interpreting twin correlations reported in these studies, it is helpful to bear in
mind four simple models (e.g., Eaves, 1982): (i) an additive genetic model, whereby
twin pair resemblance for drinking habits is entirely determined by the additive effects
of many genetic loci, a model that predicts that the MZ twin correlations should be
twice the corresponding DZ correlations; (ii) an additive plus nonadditive genetic
model, which also allows for genetic dominance or for epistatic interactions between
genetic loci, and which predicts that the MZ correlations should be greater than twice
the corresponding DZ correlations; (iii) a nongenetic model that predicts that twin pair
resemblance is entirely determined by shared environmental influences (e.g., parental
drinking habits, or schooling, or neighborhood influences), which (in the absence of
any excess environmental correlation between MZ compared to DZ twin pairs) predicts equal MZ and DZ correlations; (iv) a full model allowing for both additive
genetic and shared environmental effects, which predicts that the DZ correlation will
be less than, but greater than one-half, the MZ correlation. All models allow for
within-family environmental effects on drinking behavior, i.e., for differences in experience that lead to even identical twin pairs being imperfectly correlated in their drinking habits. Without data from additional relationships, such as parents of twins, or separated twin pairs, it is not possible to estimate simultaneously both nonadditive genetic

and shared environmental effects from data on twin pairs reared together, unless major environmental variables (e.g. religious affiliation or church attendance) are included as covariates in a multivariate analysis (c.f. Eaves et al., 1990; Truett et al., 1992). Shared environmental effects will mask genetic nonadditivity, or vice versa. In the absence of genetic nonadditivity, approximate estimates of the proportions of the total variance in alcohol consumption levels accounted for by genetic factors (VA) and by shared environmental factors (EC) can be estimated from the observed MZ and DZ twin correlations (r_{MZ}, r_{DZ}) as VA $= 2 \ (r_{MZ} - r_{DZ})$ and EC $= 2 \ r_{DZ} - r_{MZ}$. These estimates aid interpretation of data from those studies in which no model-fitting analyses have been reported.

Assessments of Alcohol Consumption

Compared to the Quantity/Frequency/Variability indices of drinking behavior that have been used in interview-based surveys (e.g., Cahalan et al., 1969), the assessments of drinking behavior in most twin and family studies have been quite limited in scope. Assessments have usually included (i) abstinence, either lifetime (whether the respondent has ever used alcohol) or current (whether the respondent has used alcohol in the preceding 12 months or some other, often undefined, period); (ii) current frequency of alcohol use, assessed as the number of days in a typical week or month that a respondent uses alcohol, sometimes asked separately for beer, wine, spirits, or other beverage types; (iii) current quantity of alcohol taken on days when alcohol is used, usually assessed by asking the respondent to report the number of drinks taken in standard drinks of each beverage type; and (iv) average weekly or monthly total consumption of alcohol, in standard drinks of each beverage type. In most cases, the respondent is given a choice of response categories for reporting frequency of alcohol use, but for quantity or total consumption measures respondents could either be given a range of response categories to select, or asked to fill in the number of drinks. A few studies have obtained additional information about the frequency of heavy drinking (operationalized in different ways in different studies), the frequency of drinking to intoxication, and the frequency of experiencing a hangover. A few studies have obtained additional data on frequency and quantity for that period when the respondent was drinking most heavily. We report in detail the items used to assess alcohol consumption in different studies; in some, the assessment scale used is such that most of the variation in the variable under study is between light and very light drinkers!

Twin correlations for abstinence, frequency, quantity, and heavy drinking measures are summarized in Table 4-1. Twin correlations and estimates of genetic and environmental variance components for total weekly or monthly alcohol consumption are summarized in Table 4-2. Greater detail about the studies on which these tables are based is given in the following sections.

The Finnish Twin Studies

The pioneering survey of Partanen et al. (1966), conducted during 1958–1959, was the first detailed twin study, using reasonably large samples, of the genetic contribution to

Table 4-1 Twin Correlations for Abstinence, Quantity, Frequency and Heavy Drinking Measures: Major Published Twin Studies

Population	Survey	Sex	Birth Dates	Sample Sizes		Abstinence		Frequency		Quantity		Heavy Drinking		Reference
				N_{MZ}	N_{DZ}	r_{MZ}	r_{DZ}	r_{MZ}	r_{DZ}	r_{MZ}	r_{DZ}	r_{MZ}	r_{DZ}	
Finland	1958/1959	Male	1920–1929	198	641	0.92	0.53	0.61	0.32	0.38	0.11	0.62	0.17	Partanen et al. (1966)
Finland	1981	Male	1932–1957	879	1940	—	—	0.41	0.22	—	—	0.44	0.24	Kaprio et al. (1987)
Sweden	1973	Male	1926–1958	2173	3479	—	—	—	—	—	—	0.63	0.48	Medlund et al. (1977)
		Female	1926–1958	2596	3934	—	—	—	—	—	—	0.74	0.53	Medlund et al. (1977)
Australian NH and MRC	1981	Male	1898–1964	567	352	0.85	0.84	0.74	0.52	0.58	0.43	—	—	Heath et al. (1991b)
		Female	1893–1964	1233	751	0.82	0.75	0.66	0.32	0.56	0.32	—	—	Heath et al. (1991b)

Note: See text for further details.

Table 4-2 Twin Correlations, and Variance Component Estimates, for Average Weekly (or Monthly) Consumption of Alcohol: Major Published Twin Studies

Population	Survey	Sex	Birth Dates	Sample Sizes		Correlations		Variance Components (%)		Reference
				N_{MZ}	N_{DZ}	r_{MZ}	r_{DZ}	Additive Genetic (VA)	Shared Environment (EC)	
Finland	1975	Male	1932–1950	1046	2306	—	—	28	—	Kaprio et al. (1991)
			1951–1957	688	1516	—	—	57	—	Kaprio et al. (1991)
		Female	1932–1950	1072	2166	—	—	41	—	Kaprio et al. (1991)
			1951–1957	934	1684	—	—	42	—	Kaprio et al. (191)
	1981	Male	1932–1950	1046	2306	—	—	20	—	Kaprio et al. (1991)
			1951–1957	688	1516	—	—	71	—	Kaprio et al. (1991)
		Female	1932–1950	1072	2166	—	—	17	—	Kaprio et al. (1991)
			1951–1957	934	1684	—	—	72	—	Kaprio et al. (1991)
Sweden	1973	Female	1926–1967	1506	2258	0.75	0.58	34	41	Medlund et al. (1977)
	1973	Male	1926–1967	1674	2503	0.77	0.60	34	43	Medlund et al. (1977)
U.S. Veterans	1967/1970	Male	1917–1927	2390	2571	0.51	0.33	36	15	Carmelli et al. (1990)
Australian NH and MRC	1981	Male	1898–1950	274	206	—	—	—	50	Jardine and Martin (1984)
			1951–1964	293	146	—	—	66	—	Jardine and Martin (1984)
	1981	Female	1893–1950	570	351	—	—	55	—	Jardine and Martin (1984)
			1951–1964	663	400	—	—	58	—	Jardine and Martin (1984)
United Kingdom (Maudsley Register)	1979	Pooled	?–1963	293	266	0.52	0.38	37	—	Clifford et al. (1984)

normal variation in drinking patterns, and remains a landmark study. Male like-sex twin pairs born between 1920 and 1929 were identified from birth records from local birth registers, with a total of 2933 ascertained. A total of 902 twin pairs were interviewed (198 MZ pairs, 641 DZ pairs, and 63 pairs whose zygosity could not be classified). In addition to the twin pairs, male full siblings of twins were also surveyed, so that comparison of the dizygotic and male like-sex sibling correlations would provide a test of the generalizability of findings from the twin data. Assessments of drinking behavior included:

1. Lifetime abstinence;
2. Frequency (called density by the authors): "To which of the groups mentioned below would you say you belong: Those who use alcohol 1) daily, 2) once a week, 3) once a half-year, 4) once a year, 5) less than once a year, 6) don't know";
3. Quantity (amount): "The amount usually consumed 1) very small (strong beverages: 1 drink or not more than 10 cl), 2) small (a couple of drinks or 10-20 cl), 3) moderate (half a bottle or 20–40 cl), 4) large (1 bottle or 40–80 cl), 5) very large (at least two bottles or more than 80 cl)" (with corresponding definitions for each category for wine and beer);
4. Adverse social, occupational, financial, or legal consequences of drinking.

Self-report data on frequency, quantity, and adverse social consequence measures were supplemented by ratings by the respondent's cotwin. The frequency scale groups together in the highest response category all those individuals drinking more regularly than once a week, so that most of the variability in frequency of consumption is between infrequent and very infrequent drinkers.

After the early work of Partanen et al., the Finnish Twin Register was extended to include all same-sex twin pairs in Finland born before 1958, and still alive in 1967 (Kaprio et al., 1981, 1987, 1991, 1992). A questionnaire mailing in 1975, which included assessments of alcohol use (essentially the same assessments as those used in the early Swedish and U.S. NAS/NRC mailings; see below), generated data on 16,269 twin pairs. A further follow-up mailing was conducted in 1981, from which data were reported on 2819 male like-sex twin pairs and 3321 female like-sex pairs (Kaprio et al., 1987, 1991, 1992). Frequency of alcohol use, in days per month, was assessed using separate categorical five-point scales for beer, wine, and spirits, with 16+ days per month forming the highest category, and average monthly consumption was assessed by seven-point categorical scales for each beverage type. Data on drinking habits of a small number of twin pairs separated in early life were reported (Kaprio et al., 1984), but sample sizes for this special group were too small for these data to be useful.

Findings in Brief. From the data summaries reported by Partanen et al. (1966), we have computed intraclass correlations or, in the case of dichotomous variables such as abstinence, tetrachoric correlations (Joreskog and Sorbom, 1988). Substantially higher MZ than DZ male correlations were found for abstinence from alcohol use (0.92 vs. 0.53), frequency of alcohol use (0.61 vs. 0.32), quantity (0.38 vs. 0.11), and presence or absence of heavy drinking, defined as use of at least 7.5 cl of absolute alcohol on the two most recent drinking occasions (0.62 vs. 0.17), raising the possibility of a genetic influence on alcohol consumption patterns. For frequency and quantity measures, but not for heavy use, twin pairs where at least one twin was a lifetime abstainer were excluded by Partanen et al. when computing their summary statistics. For these consumption variables, the MZ correlations are approximately twice as great, or greater than, the corresponding DZ correlations, which is consistent with the hypothesis that shared environmental influences have little influence on differences in drinking patterns, and that twin pair concordance for drinking habits is largely determined by genetic factors. Correlations for reporting of symptoms of alcohol abuse (0.44 vs. 0.41) and arrests for drunkenness (0.55 vs. 0.50), in contrast, did not give much support for a strong genetic contribution to risk of alcohol abuse and suggested that twin pair concordance for abuse was largely determined by shared environmental factors.

From the 1975 survey, reported intraclass correlations for level of alcohol use, defined by factor scores from a factor analysis of frequency and total monthly alcohol consumption items, were 0.54 for male MZ pairs ($n = 1537$ pairs), 0.28 for male DZ pairs ($n = 3507$ pairs), which is again consistent with a genetic contribution to alcohol consumption levels (Kaprio et al., 1981). Pairs in which at least one twin was an abstainer were apparently not deleted from these analyses. In the 1981 survey, male like-sex twin intraclass correlations were 0.41 versus 0.22 for frequency of use of beer, 0.32 versus 0.13 for frequency of use of spirits, and 0.37 versus 0.19 for average monthly consumption of alcohol, again consistent with a genetic contribution to variation in drinking patterns (Kaprio et al., 1987), with comparable results in female like-sex pairs (Kaprio et al., 1991). As in the case of Partanen et al., these twin correlations do not indicate any major influence of shared family environment. An important interaction of genetic effects with age cohort was observed in both males and females, genetic factors accounting for a much higher proportion of the variance in alcohol consumption patterns in those under age 30 than in older respondents (Kaprio et al., 1991). However, interpretation of all these figures is complicated by the fact that although concordant abstainers were excluded from these analyses, data from pairs where one twin was an abstainer were included.

Longitudinal genetic analyses of average monthly consumption and frequency measures from the 1975 and 1981 surveys have also been reported (Kaprio et al., 1992). In interpreting these data, it should be cautioned that the average consumption data were "weight-adjusted," a procedure that may lead to systematic biases to estimates of genetic effects. However, abstainers have been excluded. Stability of drinking patterns was reduced in those aged 18 to 23 at initial assessment, in 1975, compared to older respondents. For the younger twins, longitudinal correlations in men and women were 0.51 and 0.39 for weight-adjusted consumption, 0.30 and 0.32 for frequency of use of beer, and 0.32 and 0.31 for frequency of use of spirits. For the older twins, corresponding correlations were 0.70 and 0.64, 0.53 and 0.52, and 0.43 and 0.49, respectively. Heritability estimates for these measures ranged from 38% to 48% for the older cohort men, 35% to 49% for the older cohort women, 42% to 64% for the younger cohort men, and 45% to 59% for the younger cohort women. From the cross-sectional heritabilities and longitudinal genetic and environmenal correlations reported by Kaprio et al. (1992), I have computed the proportions of the longitudinal stable variance in alcohol consumption that is explained by genetic effects. For the younger cohort, 83% of the longitudinally stable variation in consumption in men, and 70% in women, is attributable to genetic effects; corresponding estimates for the older cohort are 67% for men and 71% for women.

The Swedish Twin Studies

A twin registry consisting of 11,000 like-sex pairs born between 1886 and 1925 (old Swedish twin registry) was compiled in Sweden by researchers at the Department of Environmental Hygiene of the Karolinksa Institute, and was extended, during the period 1971–1975, to include an additional 13,000 twin pairs born between 1926 and 1967 and still living in 1971 (new Swedish twin registry) (Cederlof et al., 1977). Data on drinking habits were obtained from the old registry in a questionnaire mailing conducted in 1967, with complete data returned by 9319 twin pairs. Frequency and quantity measures were obtained separately for beer, wine, and strong liquor, using items that were subsequently translated for use in the NAS/NRC study, which are listed under that study below. In addition, information about registrations with the Swedish Temperance Board (for alcohol-related misdemeanors, drunk driving, etc.) were obtained. Alcohol consumption data were obtained from the new registry twins from 1926–1958 in a questionnaire mailing conducted in 1973, with data obtained from 2733 MZ female, 2292 MZ male, 4170 DZ female, and 3703 DZ male twin pairs. In this latter survey (Medlund et al., 1977), twins were asked whether or not they drank medium-strong or strong beer, wine, or liquor (from which item current or lifetime abstainers were identified), and to report their average monthly consumption of each beverage type, in standard drinks, as well as their monthly consumption at the time they drank the most. To provide an index of heavy drinking, they were also asked to report whether or not they drank at least five bottles of beer (or equivalent) at least once per month. No direct measure of frequency of alcohol use was obtained in the 1973 survey. Detailed assessments of drinking habits have been obtained in a continuing longitudinal study of elderly, separated twin pairs identified from the Swedish Twin Register (Pedersen et al., 1988), with analyses of these data currently in progress (Pedersen, personal communication).

Findings in Brief. Published analyses of alcohol consumption data from the Swedish surveys were quite restricted in scope (Kaprio et al., 1982), and most early publications used inappropriate summary statistics (e.g., Cederlof et al., 1977) from which we cannot derive information about the relative importance of genetic and environmental contributions to variation in drinking patterns. From the paper by Medlund et al. (1977) we have computed twin polychoric correlations for average monthly consumption of alcohol, and tetrachoric correlations for heavy drinking. For average monthly consumption, correlations were MZ male pairs: $N = 1506$, $r = 0.75$; MZ female pairs: $N = 1674$, $r = 0.77$; DZ male pairs: $N = 2258$, $r = 0.58$; DZ female pairs: $N = 2503$, $r = 0.60$), indicating that additive genetic factors are accounting for approximately one-third of the variance in consumption levels, and shared environmental factors as much as 40% of the variance, in both sexes. For heavy drinking (drinking at least five beers on an occasion at least once a month) tetrachoric correlations were MZ male pairs: $N = 2173$, $r = 0.63$; MZ female pairs: $N = 2596$, $r = 0.74$; DZ male pairs: $N = 3479$, $r = 0.48$; DZ female pairs: $N = 3934$, $r = 0.53$, implying that genetic factors are accounting for as much as 42% of the variance in risk of heavy drinking in females, but only 30% in males, and that shared environmental influences are accounting for approximately one-third of the variance in each sex. Abstainers have not been excluded from these analyses.

The U.S. NAS/NRC Twin Studies

Development of the National Academy of Sciences/National Research Council (NAS/NRC) Twin Registry (Jablon et al., 1967; Hrubec and Neel, 1978) was closely coordinated with the early Swedish twin studies, with the early questionnaires used on this panel being essentially translations of the equivalent Swedish twin questionnaires. White male like-sex twin pairs were identified from a search of birth certificates from most states in the United States for the years 1917–1927. Updated address information was obtained by matching to the Veterans Administration Master Index for the period 1958–1959: of the approximately 54,000 multiple births identified in this fashion, some 15,924 twin pairs were identified where both twins served in the Armed Forces, and it was from these pairs that the Twin Registry was formed. Unfortunately, the additional 15,000 pairs where only one twin served in the Armed Forces, and the pairs where neither served, were discarded. There is a potential sampling bias with respect to any health or related problems that might have disqualified a twin from military service. Information about the pairs where only one twin served in the Armed Forces would have provided important information about the areas in which this sampling bias was important. An initial zygosity screening and medical history questionnaire (Q1) was mailed to 27,502 twins, with completed returns received from 20,946 (Hrubec and Neel, 1978). An epidemiologic questionnaire (Q2), based on the questionnaire used in the Swedish twin study, was mailed to 7372 twin pairs who had both returned Q1s, during the period 1967–1970. Completed questionnaires were returned by both members of 4380 twin pairs (Carmelli et al., 1990). A further questionnaire follow-up (Q7) of twin pairs where both twins had returned either Q1 or Q2, was conducted in 1983–1985, with questionnaires returned by both members of 2334 twin pairs. Analyses of these latter data are continuing (Carmelli, personal communication).

Measures of alcohol consumption used in the Q2 survey were:

1. Current abstinence ("Have you at any time during the past year consumed beer, wine, or other alcoholic drinks (liquor)?");
2. Lifetime abstinence ("Have you consumed any alcoholic beverage earlier in your life?");
3. Frequency, estimated separately for beer, wine, and liquor ("How often do you usually drink beer: 1) almost daily; 2) once or twice a week; 3) once or twice a month; 4) once or twice a year; 5) less often; 6) never?");

4. Quantity, estimated separately for beer, wine, and liquor ("On a day when you drink beer, how much do you usually drink: 1) less than one bottle or can (12 oz); 2) one bottle; 3) two bottles; 4) three bottles or more (with equivalent scales for wine and liquor?");

5. Frequency of heavy drinking ("How often do you drink alcoholic beverages in an amount that corresponds to at least one pint of liquor or two bottles of wine or four quarts of beer at one occasion?"), with response categories essentially as in 3;

6. Frequency of drinking to intoxication ("How often do you become really intoxicated: daily/weekly/monthly/less often/never?");

7. Hangover ("How often do you have a hangover?"), with response categories as in 4.

It should be noted that the quantity item will not give good discrimination at high levels of alcohol consumption, having few response categories. With a few changes of response category, similar items were used in the follow-up survey in 1983–1985.

Findings in Brief. Published reports of genetic analyses of alcohol consumption patterns have been quite limited, though the sample is potentially extremely informative about drinking patterns in males in later life. Using data from the Q2 survey, Carmelli et al. (1990) report intraclass correlations for log-transformed average monthly consumption of alcohol, measured in grams of absolute alcohol (as derived from the quantity and frequency questions) of 0.51 in MZ pairs ($N = 2390$ pairs) and 0.33 in DZ pairs ($N = 2571$ pairs), consistent with a genetic influence on level of use. However, pairs where either twin was an abstainer were not excluded from these analyses. Carmelli et al. also report corrected correlations for alcohol use, after adjusting for the impact of sociodemographic variables; however, these latter estimates are technically flawed (e.g. Neale and Cardon, 1992), and have no simple interpretation. Carmelli et al. (1993) have reported fitting longitudinal genetic models to data from the subsample of twin pairs who participated in both Q2 and Q7 surveys, with genetic factors accounting for 82% of the longitudinally stable variance in frequency, 86% of the stable variance in quantity, and 71% of the stable variance in total consumption. Pairs where either twin was an abstainer were excluded from these analyses.

The National Merit Twin Study

Loehlin and Nichols (1976; Loehlin, 1972) report data from the National Merit Twin Study, a survey of 850 high-school junior twin pairs. This study included data on whether or not the respondents had ever used beer, wine, or liquor; had ever done any heavy drinking; had ever used alcohol excessively; had ever become intoxicated; and had ever had a hangover. The sample is socioeconomically advantaged, and the generalizability of findings must therefore be suspect. However, this study is one of the few large-sample studies to report on the genetics of drinking behavior in adolescence (although adolescent twin studies in Australia, Finland, the Netherlands and the United States currently in progress should provide important new information).

Findings in Brief. Loehlin (1972) reports intraclass correlations, though this summary statistic is not strictly appropriate for the dichotomous assessments that were obtained. For use of beer, wine, and spirits, twin correlations were quite comparable for MZ and DZ pairs (0.62 vs. 0.57, 0.59 vs. 0.50, and 0.50 vs. 0.51, respectively); but for heavy drinking (0.46 vs. 0.19), excessive alcohol use (0.24 vs. 0.06), and experiencing a hangover (0.55 vs. 0.24) the much higher MZ than DZ correlations raise the possibility of a genetic contribution to adolescent misuse of alcohol.

The Australian Alcohol Challenge Twin Study

The Australian Alcohol Challenge Twin (AACT) Study (Martin et al., 1985a, 1985b) was designed to assess the genetic contribution to ethanol metabolism and to psychomotor and physiological responses to a challenge dose of alcohol. Its chief importance for this chapter is that it is one of the only studies to address the genetic relationship between normal variation in drinking patterns and reactivity to a challenge dose of alcohol, though other studies still in progress (e.g., Wilson and Plomin, 1985; Nagoshi and Wilson, 1989; see Chapter 5) can be expected to provide important additional data. Small-sample twin studies by Vesell (1972) and Kopun and Propping (1977) have reported a significant genetic influence on the rate of elimination of alcohol, though Propping (1977a, 1977b) has failed to find a genetic contribution to postalcohol deterioration in psychomotor performance. Sample sizes used in these two studies, however, were too small to permit resolution of genetic and nongenetic hypotheses (Martin et al., 1978).

Conducted during the period 1979–1981, the AACT study tested a total of 206 twin pairs (43 MZ female, 42 MZ male, 44 DZ female, 38 DZ female, and 39 DZ opposite-sex twin pairs). All twin pairs were recruited through the Australian NH&MRC volunteer Twin Register, and were aged 18–34. There was no screening to exclude or over-sample twin pairs with a history or family history of alcoholism. Twin pairs were included in the study if both twins were alcohol free at the beginning of testing and both completed the experimental protocol without vomiting or withdrawing from the study for other reasons. Members of a twin pair were tested on the same day, beginning at 9:00 A.M., with multiple twin pairs tested in each session, and no two twins from the same pair tested consecutively (to minimize the possibility of tester effects). Twins completed a questionnaire about their history of alcohol use, which included assessments of the following:

1. Age-of-onset of alcohol use ("At what age did you begin drinking regularly?");
2. Frequency of alcohol use ("Do you drink alcohol 1) every day or most days, 2) a couple of times a week, 3) once every week or so, 4) very rarely?");
3. Average quantity consumed per drinking occasion ("When you drink, how many drinks do you usually have: 1) 9 or more, 2) 6–8, 3) 3–5, 4) 2 or less?");
4. Average weekly consumption of alcohol ("During an average week, how much of the following beverages do you drink 1) beer (middies), 2) cider (glasses), 3) wine (glasses), 4) fortified wine (glasses), 5) spirits (nips)?");

5. Frequency of drinking to intoxication ("Have you ever been drunk 1) often, 2) some-times, 3) never?");
6. Frequency of hangovers ("Have you had a hangover 1) often, 2) sometimes, 3) never?")

From the respondent's age and reported age-of-onset the variable, years of drinking, was computed. For average weekly consumption, the reported numbers of drinks of each type were summed and log-transformed. Average weekly consumption by female subjects was representative of the general population of female drinkers, but male respondents reported slightly lower consumption levels than did the general population of male drinkers (Australian Bureau of Statistics, 1978; Heath and Martin, 1992). Some of these items allow plenty of scope for differences in interpretation by the respondents. As we shall see below, however, they had reasonable validity as assessed by their ability to predict deterioration in psychomotor performance after alcohol chal-lenge.

Baseline assessments of psychomotor performance were also made. The experimen-tal protocol included the following tasks (taken from the test battery of Franks et al., 1976; Belgrave et al., 1979):

1. Subjective intoxication rating: subjects were asked "How drunk do you feel now, on a scale of 1 = completely sober to 10 = the most drunk I have ever been?";
2. Willingness to drive: "Would you drive a car now?" (obtained only during 1980–1981);
3. Body-sway: subjects were asked to stand relaxed and as steadily as possible on a plat-form. A displacement transducer mounted beneath the platform was used to detect for-ward–backward sway. Oscillations were integrated and the time taken in seconds to accumulate a given amount of sway was recorded. Measurements were obtained under two conditions, first with the subject's eyes open, and then with the subject's eyes closed.
4. Motor coordination: the Vienna determination apparatus (VDA) was used to generate a random sequence of visual and auditory stimuli, to which the subject had to give button or foot-pedal responses. One hundred stimuli were presented, and scores were obtained for the number of correct responses, and the number of delayed correct responses (with a response time of greater than 1 second).
5. Eye–hand coordination: a pursuit–rotor task was used, in which subjects attempted to track a light target moving in a clockwise circular motion with a photocell stylus. The number of times off target and the accumulated total time off target were recorded.

In addition, standard visual, auditory, and complex reaction time measures to a white light or tone were obtained.

After baseline assessments, twins ingested a single alcohol dose of 0.75 g ethanol/kg body weight, diluted to 10% (v/v) in sugarless squash, which was consumed over a 20-minute period. After a further 20 minutes, blood alcohol concentration was assessed (see Martin et al., 1985b, for further details of measurement and interpolation proce-dures). Each subject was then retested on the psychomotor battery three times at hourly intervals, with more frequent readings of blood alcohol taken to increase information about the ethanol metabolism curve. A total of 41 twin pairs were retested on a second occasion, to provide information about test–retest correlations for all assessments, at an average test–retest interval of 4.5 months.

Findings in Brief. For measures of alcohol metabolism, a substantial genetic contribution was found for peak blood alcohol concentration (BAC) and for rate of elimination, with genetic factors accounting for, respectively, 62% and 50% of the variance in these variables (Martin et al., 1985b). By fitting structural equation models, Martin et al. (1985a) were able to show that after controlling for genetic differences in baseline performance, there was a substantial genetic contribution to differences in body sway after alcohol challenge (accounting for approximately 44% of the variance in males; 46% of the variance in females), as well as more modest genetic contributions to differences in eye–hand coordination, arithmetic computation, reaction time performance, and perhaps also motor coordination (though for this last variable the twin pair data were equally consistent with a nongenetic model for twin pair concordances for postalcohol performance decrement). An important genetic contribution to differences in postalcohol ratings of intoxication, accounting for 30% of the variance, was also found (Neale and Martin 1989; Heath and Martin, 1992) as well as a genetic contribution to differences in willingness to drive (Martin and Boomsma, 1989). Sizable correlations were noted between reported history of alcohol use, and both postalcohol ratings of intoxication and increase in body sway (Martin et al., 1985a).

The Australian NH&MRC Twin Surveys

During the period 1980–1982 (1981 survey) a 12-page self-report questionnaire was mailed to 5967 adult twin pairs enrolled on the Australian National Health and Medical Research Council (NH&MRC) volunteer twin panel (Jardine and Martin, 1984). The questionnaire included assessments of drinking habits, smoking, exercise, and other health-related habits, as well as basic sociodemographic information and assessments of personality (Eysenck and Eysenck, 1975) and attitudes. Completed questionnaires were returned by both members from 3808 twin pairs (64% pairwise response rate) and by one twin only from 576 pairs (69% individual response rate). During the period 1988–1991 (1989 survey) a similar 12-page follow-up questionnaire was mailed to twins who had both cooperated in the original 1981 survey, with remailings and telephone follow-up of nonrespondents (Heath et al., 1994a). Twins who would not return a mailed questionnaire were given the option of an abbreviated telephone interview. Questionnaire or telephone interview data were obtained from both members of 2997 twin pairs (79% of the pairs who had responded to the 1981 mailing), and to one twin only from 334 pairs (83% individual response rate). Final sample sizes for complete pairs (for 1981 and 1989 surveys, respectively) were MZ females: 1232 and 1021 pairs; MZ males: 567 and 447 pairs; DZ same-sex females: 747 and 602 pairs; DZ same-sex males: 350 and 255 pairs; and DZ opposite-sex pairs: 912 and 672 pairs. Follow-up questionnaires were mailed to 500 male and 500 female twins who returned questionnaires in the 1989 survey, at a retest interval of approximately 2 years, to provide data on short-term test–retest reliability of the questionnaire assessments. Twins who participated in the AACT study were included in the target sample for the original 1981 mailing, so that for a subset of these individuals follow-up data on self-report alcohol consumption levels is available from the 1981 survey, and in some cases from the 1989 survey. Attempts to trace AACT twins who did not participate in the 1981 or 1989 surveys in order to obtain follow-up data on drinking habits are now under way. A survey of the adult relatives—parents, siblings, spouses, and children—of the 1981 survey twins is also currently in progress.

Alcohol consumption measures used in the original 1981 survey are reproduced in Jardine and Martin (1984). We shall make use of a subset of these items:

1. Lifetime abstinence ("Have you *ever* taken alcoholic drinks?");
2. Age-of-onset of alcohol use ("At what age did you start drinking alcohol?");
3. Frequency of alcohol use ("*Over the last year,* about how often have you usually taken any alcoholic drinks: 1) Every day; 2) 3–4 times each week, 3) about twice a week; 4) about once a week, 5) once or twice a month, 6) less often?");
4. Quantity consumed on each day that alcohol is used ("On average, how many *glasses* would you drink on each day that you take some alcohol?"), with separate items for glasses of beer per day, glasses of wine per day, glasses of spirits per day, and glasses of sherry per day, on weekdays and on weekends;
5. Average weekly consumption of alcohol, derived from the quantity question, and separate questions about frequency of alcohol use on weekdays and on weekends;
6. Total weekly consumption by 7-day retrospective diary: respondents were asked to report the number of drinks of beer, wines, spirits, sherry, or other alcoholic beverages taken on each day during the preceding week.

Items similar to those in the 1981 survey were used in the 1989 survey to assess lifetime abstinence, frequency of alcohol use, and weekly consumption by 7-day retrospective diary. These were supplemented by new items to assess:

1. Average weekly consumption ("Write the number which best describes how many drinks (you) *usually* have in a *typical week:* 1) None at all; 2) 1–3; 3) 4–6; 4) 7–12; 5) 13–18; 6) 19–24; 7) 25–42; 8) 43–70; 9) 70+?");
2. Average quantity per drinking day ("On average how many drinks would you have *on each day that you have some alcohol?*"), asked separately for week-days (Monday to Friday) and weekends (Saturday or Sunday), with subjects asked to report the average number of standard drinks;
3. Maximum ever consumed ("What is the greatest number of drinks you have ever had in a single day?"), also asked separately for weekdays and weekends;
4. Maximum consumed within past 12 months ("What is the greatest number [of drinks] you have had in a single day in the past 12 months?").

As in the Finnish survey of Partanen et al. (1966), and the Virginia 30,000 survey (see below), self-report data on lifetime abstinence, frequency of alcohol use, and average weekly consumption were supplemented by ratings on these variables of the respondent's cotwin and also mother, father, and spouse (if any).

Findings in Brief. Genetic analyses of the 1989 survey data, for which data collection was concluded at the end of 1991, are still in progress. In the 1981 survey, for both average weekly consumption and 7-day retrospective diary measures, genetic factors accounted for approximately 55% of the variance in alcohol consumption levels in females and 36% in males (Jardine and Martin, 1984). However, when separate analyses were performed for those twin pairs aged 18–30 and 31+ years old (young and older cohorts), although comparable estimates of the genetic contribution to variation in alcohol consumption levels were obtained in females, in males a substantial heritability estimate was obtained for young males (61%), whereas there was no significant evidence for genetic influences on consumption patterns in older males. Interpretation of these analyses is complicated by the authors' failure to exclude data from lifetime abstainers, though it should be noted that this latter group is rare in Australia, so that serious biases to parameter estimates would not be expected. Separate estimates of the contribution of genetic factors to risk of abstinence, and to quantity and frequency measures for nonabstainers, are given by Heath et al. (1991b; see below). Further analyses of the data on female like-sex pairs, excluding abstainers, indicated an important effect of genotype × environment interaction on alcohol consumption levels in females, with a much stronger genetic contribution to variation in consumption levels (as assessed by 7-day retrospective diary) in those without a marital partner or equivalent (Heath et al., 1989; see below). Preliminary longitudinal analyses of the 1981 and 1989 follow-up data, based on an incomplete dataset, have been reported (Heath and Martin, 1991c), with genetic factors reported to account for approximately 67% of the stable variation in frequency, average weekly consumption, and total consumption by 7-day recall, in females, and for between 27% and 69% of the stable variation (according to measure of consumption) in males.

Analyses of retrospectively reported data on age at onset of alcohol use (Heath and Martin, 1988), focused only on twin pairs aged 20–30 at the time of the 1981 survey (for whom retrospective recall was likely to be more accurate), were consistent with a role of both genetic and shared environmental factors in determining whether or not the respondent had remained an abstainer as a teenager or had become a teenage drinker. Teenage abstinence, however, was too rare a phenomenon to permit a powerful resolution of genetic and nongenetic hypotheses. In those who became adolescent drinkers, early versus late onset in females was influenced by genetic factors, with only a modest effect of shared environment, whereas in males early versus late onset was much more strongly influenced by shared environmental factors, with no evidence for any genetic influence.

The London Twin-Family Survey

Clifford et al. (1981, 1984) report data on alcohol consumption patterns of a small volunteer sample of twin pairs from the Institute of Psychiatry, London (see Eaves et al., 1989, for further discussion of this twin panel), based on a survey conducted in 1979. Data were obtained from twins from 572 families, as well as many parents and siblings of the twins. Alcohol consumption patterns were assessed using a 7-day diary format, with subjects asked to report their total consumption in standard drinks for a typical week.

Findings in Brief. Estimated twin correlations for average weekly consumption, excluding pairs where either twin reported no use of alcohol in a typical week, were 0.52 for MZ pairs and 0.38 for DZ pairs, with no evidence for heterogeneity of twin pair correlations as a function of gender. In a model allowing for cohabitation effects on twin pair resemblance, the maximum-likelihood estimate of the genetic contribution to variation in alcohol consumption levels was 37%.

The Virginia 30,000 Survey

The Virginia 30,000 Survey (Heath et al., unpublished) was a survey of adult twins, ascertained from two sources, and their adult relatives (siblings, parents, spouses, and children), conducted during the period 1985–1991. Twins were ascertained from either the Virginia Twin Register, a birth-certificate confirmed register of twins born in Virginia between 1915 and 1968, or the American Association of Retired Persons (AARP) Twin Panel, a volunteer panel of twins mostly aged 50 years and older. Most of the Virginia Twin Register twins were born after the World War II, so that most of the parents of twins were from the Virginia subsample, whereas most of the adult children of twins were from the AARP subsample. Total sample sizes were approximately 30,000 subjects, including 14,762 twins, 3199 siblings of twins, 132 half-siblings of twins, 2363 parents of twins, 4395 spouses of twins, and 4853 adult offspring of twins, as well as a small number of other relationships. Assessments of alcohol use included both self-report and ratings of cotwin, mother, father, and spouse, for:

1. *Current abstinence* (derived from the frequency-of-use item);
2. *Frequency of use* ("Write in the number which best describes how often the following people have had alcoholic drinks *during the past 12 months:* 1) don't know; 2) more than once a day; 3) every day; 4) 3–4 times/week; 5) 1–2 times/week; 6) 1–2 times/month; 7) less often; 8) not at all.")
3. *Average weekly consumption of alcohol* ("Write in the number which best describes how many drinks the following people *usually* take in a *typical week*"), with response categories the same as in the Australian 1989 survey, except that the highest category was 42 + drinks/week.

These items were supplemented by a retrospective 7-day diary measure of the respondent's alcohol consumption.

Findings in Brief. Figure 4-1 summarizes correlations between male like-sex and female like-sex relative pairs, respectively, for measures of current abstinence and frequency of alcohol consumption. (Correlations for average weekly consumption and total consumption by 7-day diary were broadly consistent in pattern with those for frequency.) If we consider first male like-sex tetrachoric correlations for abstinence, then for the collateral blood relatives we see an ordering consistent with a genetic influence on abstinence, i.e., the ordering of the correlations between relatives is MZ pairs > DZ pairs, sibling pairs > half-sibling, and MZ half-sibling pairs > first cousins, where the coefficient of relationship (i.e., degree of genetic relatedness) for these relationships is, respectively, 100%, 50%, 25%, 12.5%. Likewise for the intergenerational relationships, we observe parent–offspring, MZ uncle–nephew > uncle–nephew. However, these data also indicate either an environmental influence of parental abstinence on offspring abstinence, or an effect of assortative mating, the tendency for abstainers to marry other abstainers: the dizygotic and sibling correlations are greater than one-half the corresponding monozygotic correlations; and the parent–offspring correlation is greater than the MZ uncle–nephew correlation, though in the absence of assortative mating or parent-to-offspring environmental influences, these two correlations are expected to be the same (Heath et al., 1985). Correlations between affine relatives (i.e., relatives by marriage) are very high for abstinence, consistent with a strong effect of assortative mating but, since these are based on measures of current rather than lifetime abstinence, we cannot exclude the possibility of a reciprocal environmental influence of husband's drinking on wife's drinking, and vice versa. Model-fitting analyses would be needed to determine the relative contributions of genetic factors, shared environmental factors, and assortative mating to these correlations between relatives.

For abstinence in females the evidence for an important genetic influence is much weaker, with sibling, half-sibling, and first cousin correlations all approximately equal in magnitude, and the MZ half-sibling correlation actually somewhat lower than might be expected under a simple additive genetic model. The MZ female correlation is only modestly higher than the female like-sex DZ correlation, also consistent with only a modest genetic influence on abstinence by female twins, but the female like-sex sibling correlation is substantially lower than the DZ correlation, indicating an important twin environment effect, i.e., an excess environmental correlation between siblings of the same age growing up together compared to siblings of different ages. As in males, high correlations between affine relatives are observed.

For frequency [and also for average weekly consumption and 7-day diary measures (not shown)], the evidence for a genetic influence on consumption depends largely upon the comparison of correlations between MZ pairs versus DZ and sibling pairs. Correlations for other relationships are all quite similar in magnitude, despite differences in degree of genetic relatedness. Sample sizes are much smaller for many of these relationships than was the case for the analyses of abstinence (because any relationship pair where at least one relative is an abstainer has been excluded), and the standard errors on these correlations correspondingly larger. It is possible that these results arise because much of the genetic influence on alcohol consumption patterns by drinkers is nonadditive (i.e., genetic dominance or epistasis), and therefore makes a relatively modest contribution to correlations between first-degree and more remote relationships. We cannot, however, exclude the possibility of a greater correlation between the environments experienced by MZ twin pairs compared to DZ or sibling pairs.

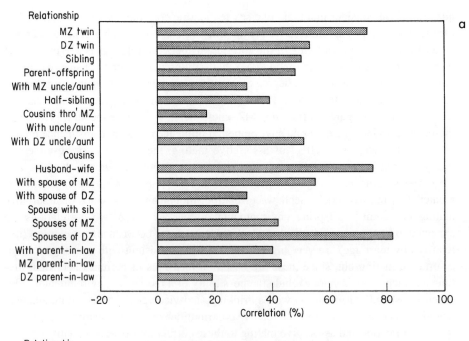

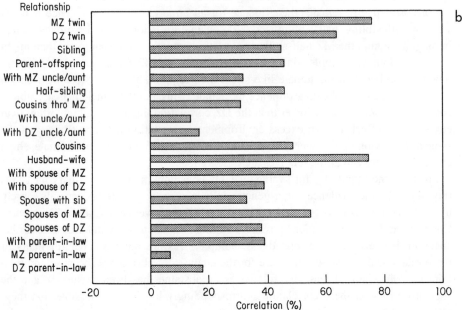

Fig. 4-1 Correlations between twin pairs and their relatives for abstinence and frequency of alcohol use: Virginia 30,000 Survey. (From Heath et al., unpublished.) Correlations are for (a) abstinence in male like-sex relatives, (b) abstinence in female like-sex relatives, (c) frequency in male like-sex relatives, and (d) frequency in female like-sex relatives.

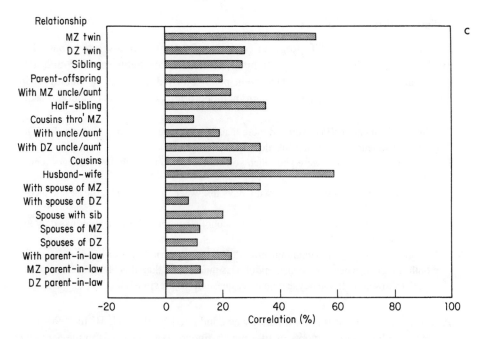

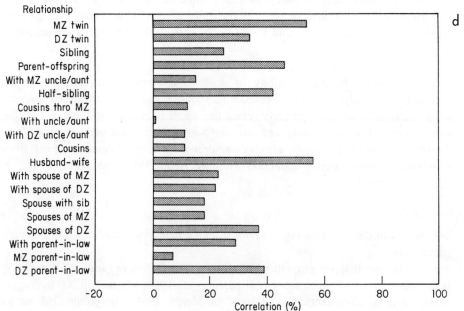

The Vietnam-Era Twin Surveys

The Vietnam-Era Twin (VET) Register comprises 7400 male like-sex twin pairs born 1939–1953, where both twins served in the armed forces between 1965 and 1975 (Eisen et al., 1987). A subset of 4152 twin pairs returned a Survey of Health during 1987–1988 (Goldberg et al., 1990), which included brief assessments of alcohol use:

1. Lifetime abstinence ("Have you had more than 20 alcoholic drinks in your entire life?");
2. Current abstinence ("Do you drink alcoholic beverages now?");
3. Age of onset ("How old were you when you started drinking alcoholic beverages regularly?");
4. Frequency ("On the average, how many days in a week do you drink at least one alcoholic beverage?");
5. Quantity ("On the days when you have an alcoholic beverage, how many drinks do you have on average?");
6., 7. Maximum frequency, maximum quantity ("Was there a period in your life of at least six months in a row when your consumption was much more than this? During that period . . . ," followed by frequency and quantity questions as previously).

A follow-up survey of this twin panel was conducted by the NHLBI in 1990–1991. This survey included assessments of lifetime abstinence (same item as in the Survey of Health); frequency and average quantity questions, separately for each beverage type, for the preceding two weeks; and frequency of heavy drinking during the preceding month.

Findings in Brief. Twin correlations for alcohol consumption patterns have not yet been reported. Analyses of age of onset of alcohol use, based on retrospective reports, suggest a genetic influence on early versus late onset, in contrast to findings for male twins from the Australian study, and raise the possibility that independent factors may determine age at onset in those who become drinkers during adolescence versus those who become drinkers during adulthood (Flick and Heath, 1991, and unpublished).

Conclusions

This review of data on drinking behavior from the major twin studies leads to several conclusions:

1. *Abstinence:* It appears that there is a genetic contribution to variation in the risk of becoming a drinker (Finnish study of Partanen et al., 1966; Virginia 30,000 Survey) or of becoming an adolescent drinker (Heath and Martin, 1988), though the evidence for this in the Virginia 30,000 study is much stronger for males than for females (Heath, et al., unpublished). This apparent genetic influence was an unexpected finding since there is little evidence, at least in the Australian 1981 survey, for a genetic contribution to religious affiliation or church attendance (Eaves et al., 1990), variables that might be expected to be important predictors of abstinence. Reanalysis of the Australian 1981 survey data suggests, however, that there is a subgroup of twins who are abstainers for entirely nongenetic reasons (Heath et al., 1991a, 1991b, and discussed below). In the

National Merit twin sample, the only large-sample study to obtain contemporaneous data on adolescent drinking, there was little evidence for a genetic contribution to probability of use of beer, wine, or spirits; but abstinence from use of all three beverages was not analyzed as a separate variable.

2. *Frequency, quantity, total consumption:* Regardless of which measure is used, data from all the major studies are consistent with a significant and substantial genetic contribution to variation in alcohol consumption levels, though estimates of the magnitude of this effect range between 30% and 60% (if we exclude the unusually low estimates reported for the 1981 Finnish survey). The one exception is the older cohort of Australian male twin pairs aged 30+ at initial assessment in 1981, and even in this group the hypothesis of a genetic influence on alcohol consumption levels cannot be excluded once abstainers are excluded (see Health et al., 1991b, and below). Analyses of longitudinal data on alcohol consumption patterns in the Australian Finnish and U.S. NAS/NRC twin samples suggest that if we consider only that proportion of the variation in alcohol consumption levels that is longitudinally stable (thereby excluding variance due to measurement error and short-term fluctuations in drinking patterns), then a very high proportion of this longitudinally stable component of variation is attributable to genetic factors—as much as two-thirds of the variation in the Australian study, and 70–80% of the variation in the U.S. and Finnish studies.

3. *Heavy drinking:* In the studies that have examined this question—the adolescent sample of Loehlin (1972), the adult male sample of Partanen et al. (1966), and the survey of the new Swedish twin register (Medlund et al., 1977)—a genetic influence on heavy drinking is observed. In the U.S. adolescent data, a genetic influence on reported hangovers is also observed. For symptoms of alcohol abuse, however, Partanen et al. report little excess of the MZ over the DZ correlation. From these studies it is not possible to determine whether the same or different genetic factors are determining excessive or heavy drinking as are determining variation in quantity, frequency, and total consumption measures, i.e., whether or not heavy drinking should be viewed as the extreme point on a continuum of consumption.

4. *Generalizability of findings:* Data from the Virginia 30,000 twin-family study (Heath et al., unpublished) generally support the inference of a genetic influence on abstinence. Evidence for frequency, average weekly consumption, and 7-day diary measures is less consistent, with most of the support for a genetic influence coming from the comparison of MZ pairs versus DZ and sibling pairs. This may be because there are strong nonadditive genetic effects on consumption, or it may suggest that an excess environmental correlation between MZ pairs compared to more remote relatives is causing us to overestimate the importance of genetic factors from twin data.

5. *Sex differences:* In contrast to findings on the inheritance of alcoholism, for which it is widely believed that genetic factors are more important in males than in females (though see, e.g., Kendler et al., 1992), data from the Finnish, Swedish, and Australian samples suggest that genetic influences on alcohol consumption levels are at least as important, and probably more important, in females than in males.

6. *Cohort and cross-cultural differences:* It is apparent that there may be important birth cohort differences in the magnitude of the genetic influence on alcohol consumption patterns. However, these effects appear to be highly culture specific. In Finland,

the importance of genetic factors in both sexes is substantially reduced in older twin pairs, and data from the Swedish separated-twin study of older twins are also consistent with this interpretation (Pedersen, personal communication). In Australia, genetic factors may have a less important genetic influence on alcohol consumption patterns by males born prior to 1951, but still have an important influence on female drinking patterns. In the U.S. NAS/NRC panel of older male twins, in contrast, substantial genetic influence was found. Further analyses of follow-up data from the Australian and Finnish studies may help clarify to what extent this finding reflects a birth cohort difference rather than a developmental phenomenon of middle age.

7. *Shared environmental influences:* Evidence for important shared environmental influences on drinking patterns is less consistent than for genetic effects, and appears to be limited to particular cultures and particular age cohorts. Strong apparent effects of shared environment are observed in the Swedish study, in both sexes, and in the Australian study, in older males, but only weak effects are found in the Finnish study and in Australian females. It should be noted, in addition, that assortative mating for drinking patterns in the parental generation (e.g., if heavy drinkers tend to marry other heavy drinkers) may also lead to a DZ correlation greater than one-half the corresponding like-sex MZ correlation (e.g., Eaves, 1977), so that even in those cases where this pattern of twin correlations is observed, it is not necessarily diagnostic of shared environmental influences on drinking behavior.

8. *Alcohol metabolism and alcohol sensitivity:* From the Australian Alcohol-Challenge Twin Study, a substantial genetic contribution to differences in alcohol metabolism, as assessed by postalcohol peak BAC and rate of elimination, was found. However, these measures showed only weak associations with reported history of alcohol use (Martin et al., 1985b). In contrast, a substantial genetic contribution was found to differences in postalcohol ratings of subjective intoxication and increase in body sway, and performance on these measures did show a strong relationship with reported drinking patterns. This raises the important question of whether some of the genetic variance in alcohol sensitivity, as assessed in the alcohol-challenge paradigm, is determined by the same genetic factors that influence variation in consumption levels, an issue that we address later in this chapter.

Utility of Self-Report Consumption Measures

Lengthy interview assessments have been developed in order to provide detailed information about respondents' patterns of alcohol use (e.g., Cahalan et al., 1969). With the exception of the study of Partanen et al. (1966), most of the data on the inheritance of normal patterns of alcohol use reviewed earlier, in contrast, derive from mailed surveys using short self-report questionnaires. In all studies, assessments of drinking patterns have been quite limited in scope. There is widespread skepticism about the trustworthiness of such self-report measures of consumption which, if justifiable, would undermine any inferences we might make using these data about the genetic contribution to drinking behavior. However, using data from the Australian and Virginia 30,000 studies, we have argued that, at least in the context of general population surveys, this skepticism is unwarranted (Heath et al., 1992b, unpublished). We review some of the evidence to support this assertion here.

Stability of Self-Report Data

While stability of self-report data is no guarantee of the trustworthiness of such data, in the absence of evidence for such stability, any genetic analyses would be of dubious worth. Short-term test–retest correlations, at a retest interval of approximately 5–6 months in the Virginia study and of 2 years in the Australian study, were in the range 0.94–0.99 for abstinence (in both studies), 0.83–0.84 and 0.90–0.93 for frequency (Australian and U.S. data, respectively), 0.76–0.77 for quantity (Australian study only), 0.55–0.61 and 0.9–0.91 for average weekly consumption, and 0.68–0.70 and 0.78 in both genders for total weekly consumption by 7-day retrospective diary, i.e., acceptably high values (Heath et al., 1992b, unpublished). As a measure of quantity, self-report quantity for drinking on weekends was used, since this variable proved much more stable than reported average quantity consumed on weekdays.

In the Australian surveys, long-term 8-year and 10-year test–retest (stability) correlations were also examined (Heath et al., 1992b, unpublished). Important differences in longitudinal stability of drinking patterns were found as a function of age at initial assessment. In those aged at least 26 years at the time of the 1981 survey, there was very little reversion from lifetime abstinence in 1981 to some use of alcohol by 1989 (test–retest tetrachoric correlations of 0.93 in females, 0.97 in males) and considerable stability of measures of frequency of consumption (product–moment correlations of 0.69 in females, 0.71 in males) and reported average weekly consumption (0.60 in females, 0.63 in males).

Comparably high long-term test–retest correlations have been reported for the 15-year follow-up of NAS/NRC male twins [correlations of 0.58 for frequency and 0.55 for total monthly consumption (Carmelli et al., 1993)]; and for the 6-year follow-up of male and female twins from the Finnish twin study who were aged at least 25 at initial assessment [test–retest correlations of 0.57 and 0.56, respectively, for average monthly consumption of alcohol (Kaprio et al., 1991, 1992)]. The quantity measure showed somewhat reduced long-term stability (correlations of 0.41 in females and 0.46 in males), a pattern that has also been noted in the NAS/NRC study (Carmelli et al., 1993), where a somewhat reduced stability correlation of 0.42 is observed for Quantity. Apparently, how much people drink in total and how regularly they use alcohol are highly stable over time, but how many drinks they take when they use alcohol is much more variable from occasion to occasion.

In contrast, considerable changes in drinking patterns were occurring in the youngest Australian cohort, aged 18–25 at initial assessment: those who were more frequent or heavier users of alcohol in 1981 were not necessarily the heaviest drinkers in 1989, and some abstainers had become drinkers. For quantity, frequency, and total consumption measures in both sexes, and for abstinence in males, 8-year stability correlations were all in the range 0.20–0.43, substantially lower than the corresponding correlations for those aged 26 years or higher at initial assessment. A similar tendency for reduced stability of total monthly consumption in early adulthood is noted in the Finnish study, where test–retest correlations of 0.4 for male respondents and 0.32 for female respondents are found for those aged 18–24 at initial assessment (Kaprio et al., 1991). Consistent with other studies (see, e.g., the metanalyses of Fillmore et al., 1991), the period of early adulthood emerges as a period when marked changes in individual drinking patterns occur.

Validity of Self-Report Data

Demonstration that self-report measures of alcohol consumption are highly stable across long assessment intervals need not, of course, imply that these measures have any validity. To provide one check on validity, the early Finnish twin study of Partanen et al. (1966) supplemented self-report data with rating data provided by the respondent's cotwin. For both quantity and frequency measures of consumption, good agreement between self-report and the cotwin's rating was found (correlations of 0.63 and 0.54, respectively). In the Virginia 30,000 and Australian follow-up surveys a similar strategy was used (Heath et al., 1992b, unpublished). In addition to asking respondents to rate the frequency of alcohol use and average weekly consumption of alcohol by their cotwin, however, we also asked for ratings of maternal and paternal alcohol use. In the Australian survey only, twins were also asked to report whether their cotwin had ever used alcohol. Agreement between ratings of parental drinking habits by twins from the same family provides a test of the validity of ratings supplied by an informant. Twins showed very strong agreement in their ratings of how frequently each parent used alcohol, and how much each parent consumed per week, with interrater correlations in the range 0.70–0.86. Agreement between self-report data and rating by an informant (the respondent's cotwin) provides a test of the validity of the self-report data. There was very strong agreement between self-report and rating of alcohol consumption by the respondent's cotwin, with correlations in the range 0.66–0.82 for frequency and average weekly consumption measures, and even higher correlations of 0.85–0.93 in females and 0.87–0.95 in males for abstinence from alcohol use (defined as current abstinence in the Virginia study, but lifetime abstinence in the Australian study). These data suggest that self-report measures of alcohol consumption do have reasonable validity.

Various biochemical markers have also been used to validate self-report assessment of alcohol use. While many of these measures are useful for detecting problem drinking, their ability to discriminate between levels of alcohol use within the normal range is less well established. In the Australian Alcohol Challenge Twin Study, for example, blood levels of gammaglutamyltransferase (GGT), a laboratory marker commonly used to screen for alcohol abuse, showed only a modest though significant association with reported average weekly consumption by male twins (GGT: $r = 0.19$) and no significant association with self-report consumption by female twins ($r = 0.02$). There was a similarly weak though significant association of male self-report alcohol consumption with aspartate aminotransferase (AST: $r = 0.14$) and with alanine aminotransferase levels (ALT: $r = 0.22$), again with no association of either of these plasma enzymes with female self-report consumption levels (AST: $r = -0.02$; ALT: $r = 0.05$) (Whitfield and Martin, 1985a). Mean corpuscular volume (MCV) was likewise correlated with total weekly alcohol consumption reported by male respondents (MCV: $r = 0.30$), but not that reported by female respondents [$r = -0.11$ (Whitfield and Martin, 1985b)].

Data from the Australian Alcohol Challenge Twin Study (Martin et al., 1985a, 1985b; Heath et al., 1992b, unpublished) provide an additional means of validating self-report measures of consumption. In males, certain measures of performance after alcohol challenge showed moderately strong associations with the baseline reports of drinking history and, furthermore, were predictive of future self-report consumption levels in 1981 and 1989 (Heath et al., 1992b, unpublished). Subjective intoxication ratings after alcohol challenge correlated 0.44–0.57 with contemporaneous reports of alcohol use patterns, 0.47–0.6 with self-report data in the subsequent 1981 survey, and 0.26–0.4 with self-report data in the 1989 follow-up survey. Correlations of body sway increase after alcohol challenge (eyes closed condition) were 0.3–0.42 with baseline drinking history, 0.33–0.45 with self-report alcohol use in 1981, and 0.17–0.25 with 1989 self-reports, with only the association with self-report Quantity in 1989 being nonsignificant. Correlations in females were much weaker, perhaps reflecting the reduced variance in drinking habits of the female twins, an interpretation that would also account for the very weak association of self-report consumption data with biochemical measures.

Conclusion

Self-report measures of alcohol consumption, obtained in general population surveys, appear to have good short-term and long-term stability, at least when respondents are aged at least 25 when initially assessed. Despite the skepticism that exists about the utility of self-report measures of alcohol consumption, the agreement observed between self-report and informant rating data, and the association between self-report drinking history and both biochemical measures and postalcohol challenge performance, support the validity of these self-report measures. Indeed, I would argue that the utility of self-report measures of alcohol consumption is much better established for the simple self-administered questionnaire assessments on which most genetic studies have been based than it is for more elaborate interview assessments! This conclusion, however, cannot be generalized to questionnaires completed in other contexts (e.g., applications for life insurance or screening questionnaires administered by primary care physicians).

Unanswered Questions

The demonstration of a significant genetic contribution to variation in drinking patterns in humans should be merely a starting point for research on the determinants of drinking behavior. From there we need to progress to such questions as the following (Heath, 1993).

1. The dimensionality of genetic influences on drinking behavior. Is the same continuum of genetic variability determining abstinence versus moderate use versus heavy use, or are there independent genetic dimensions separating abstainers from moderate users, and moderate users from heavy drinkers? Are these dimensions of genetic variation alcohol specific, or are individuals with an increased genetic risk of heavy drinking also at increased genetic risk of becoming smokers (Madden et al, 1993a,b) or illicit drug users?

2. Genotype–environment correlation. How do genetic and environmental risk factors covary, i.e., are those individuals who are genetically at increased risk of heavy drinking also more likely to be exposed to high-risk environments?

3. Genotype × environment interaction. How do environmental factors moderate (exacerbate or diminish) the genetic influence on alcohol consumption patterns or, conversely, to what extent does genetic predisposition increase vulnerability to environmental risk factors?

4. Mediating/intervening variables. What are the important mediating variables in the inheritance of drinking patterns (c.f. Sher, 1991)? Can we identify personality, biochemical or physiological, or sociodemographic variables that might account for the strong tendency of drinking patterns to aggregate in families, and that might explain some of the genetic (or environmental) influences on alcohol consumption patterns?

5. Moderator variables. Can we identify protective or resiliency factors, or vulnerability factors, which may interact with genetic predisposition to determine drinking behavior (c.f. Sher, 1991)? What are the personality or other behavioral factors that determine whether or not those at high genetic risk progress to become heavy drinkers?

6. Developmental perspectives. How do genetic and environmental influences on drinking behavior unfold during the lifespan? To what extent do the same genetic factors that influence alcohol consumption patterns in early adulthood also affect consumption patterns in middle or old age?

Dimensionality of Genetic Influences

In our literature review, we have seen that different studies have used different definitions of abstinence, and have made different decisions about whether or not to include abstainers in analyses of quantity, frequency, and total consumption measures. We cannot know a priori what is the best approach to take. If the same genetic and environmental factors that determine light versus moderate versus heavy consumption of alcohol also determine nonuse versus use of alcohol (single-dimension model), then exclusion of twins who are abstainers will truncate the distribution of alcohol consumption, leading to biased estimates of genetic and environmental parameters (Heath et al., 1991a). If the genetic and environmental determinants of abstinence versus use of alcohol are independent of the genetic and environmental determinants of level of alcohol use by those who are drinkers (independent-dimensions model), then including abstainers in analyses of consumption level may confound two variables having quite distinct modes of inheritance. In neither case is it appropriate to exclude only those pairs who are concordant for abstinence! Should we consider as an abstainer only someone without any history of exposure to alcohol, or are those who report only very infrequent light use of alcohol also abstainers? If social factors determine strict lifetime abstinence from alcohol use, but genetic differences contribute to the probability that an individual with some initial exposure to alcohol will find that experience aversive and never progress to become a regular drinker, then the exclusion of infrequent drinkers would bias estimates of genetic influences on consumption; whereas, if such genetic influences came into play only once frequency or quantity measures had passed a critical threshold level, exclusion of infrequent drinkers would be appropriate. Fortunately, these different assumptions about the determinants of abstinence versus level of consumption (and about how to define abstinence) lead to different predictions, and hence are testable, in twin data. For example, the single-dimension model predicts that the alcohol consumption levels of nonabstinent twins whose cotwin is an abstainer will be lower than the consumption levels of nonabstinent twins whose cotwin is also a drinker; whereas the independent dimensions model predicts no difference in consumption levels between these two groups (Heath et al., 1991a).

Similar issues of how to define the *phenotype* of drinking behavior arise for measures of frequency, quantity, and total consumption. Some studies have reported twin pair correlations for separate frequency and quantity measures, while others have reported only total weekly or monthly consumption of alcohol. Which data summary is more appropriate will clearly depend upon whether frequency and quantity are independently inherited traits, or whether genetic factors determine only overall level of consumption. Under the latter hypothesis, an identical twin who on average drinks five drinks on two occasions each week is as likely to have a cotwin who drinks two drinks on five days each week as a cotwin with an identical drinking pattern.

Nonmetric multidimensional scaling (MDS) provides one means of exploring such issues in twin or other family data (Heath et al., 1991a; Meyer et al., 1992). Multidimensional scaling uses a matrix of distances between variables, or its inverse, a proximity matrix, to determine the number of dimensions needed to represent the spatial relationships between the variables, and to determine their relative positions in that multidimensional space. Thus, as applied to the matrix of mileages between major U.S. cities it will provide a graphical representation of those cities in a two-dimensional space (Kruskal and Wish, 1978). In twin and other family studies, an initial data summary will often consist of a two-way contingency table, cross-classifying the responses of one relative by that of another, e.g., the average weekly alcohol consumption of first-born MZ female twins by that of their cotwins. While such a two-way table cannot be used directly as a proximity matrix, by adjusting for the marginal frequencies of the table, i.e., the different endorsement frequencies of different response categories, we can create such a similarity matrix. In a reanalysis of data from the 1981 Australian survey, we created a consumption scale with response categories ranging from "Abstinent or drinks less than once a month" to "Drinks at least 3–4 times a week, and takes 7 or more drinks/occasion" (Heath et al., 1991a). Two-way contingency tables were computed, similarity matrices derived, and a nonmetric MDS analysis performed separately for each zygosity group. In each case the best-fitting solution appeared to be one with three dimensions, which yielded separate Abstinence, Frequency, and Quantity dimensions. There was no evidence to support the existence of a fourth dimension separating very heavy drinkers from those with more moderate consumption levels.

Results from the MDS analyses appear to suggest that genetic analyses should be performed separately for abstinence, quantity, and frequency measures. However, MDS uses only distances between variables, which in our application would correspond to differences in drinking behavior within twin pairs. In the case of monozygotic twin pairs, these differences must be determined by within-family environmental effects, i.e., environmental influences that are uncorrelated between twin pairs. Thus on the basis of these analyses, we cannot exclude the possibility that there are independent environmental determinants of abstinence, quantity, and frequency, but a single underlying dimension of genetic variability. To address this issue further, we have developed hierarchical genetic models, an extension of the conventional threshold model used in the genetic analysis of discontinuous data (e.g., Falconer, 1965; Eaves et al., 1978), which allow us to compare the fit of single-dimension and independent-dimension models (Heath, 1990; Heath and Martin, 1993), and have applied these models to abstinence/frequency and abstinence/quantity data from the 1981 survey (Heath et al., 1991b). In each case, we found evidence for the existence of independent Abstinence and Consumption dimensions. Estimates of twin pair correlations on the Abstinence dimension were very high (0.71–0.9) and did not indicate any significant genetic influence. For the Consumption dimension in females, there was no evidence for any influence of shared environment, but a substantial genetic influence was found, accounting for 66% of the variance in the case of frequency of consumption, and 57% in the case of quantity. In males, it appeared that genetic factors accounted for 42% of the variance on the frequency dimension, and 24% of the variance on the quantity dimension, with shared environmental factors accounting for an additional 32% and 35% of the variance, respectively. There was no significant heterogeneity of genetic and environmental parameters as a function of age. The best-fitting model allowed for two routes to abstinence, with some individuals being abstainers because of their position on the nongenetic Abstinence dimension, and others because of their position on the second, heritable consumption dimension. These findings suggest that in order to analyze genetic effects on alcohol consumption level, we need to retain abstinent twin pairs in our analyses, but use a multidimensional model to obtain separate estimates of the genetic and environmental influences on Abstinence and Consumption dimensions. Whether a single underlying genetic dimension is determining both frequency and quantity of alcohol use, however, remains an unanswered question, though the very similar results obtained for quantity and frequency by Heath et al. (1991b) certainly makes this a plausible hypothesis.

Genotype–Environment Correlation

The mechanisms by which genetic risk and environmental risk may come to covary has received exhaustive discussion (e.g., Cattell, 1960; Eaves et al., 1977; Plomin et al., 1977; Scarr and McCartney, 1983). We shall follow the approach of Heath (1992), who distinguishes between three basic mechanisms: (1) genotype–environment (GE) autocorrelation, whereby individuals at high genetic risk also expose themselves to high-risk environments (e.g., individuals at high genetic risk of heavy drinking who live in a neighborhood surrounded by bars), or perceive their environment as being a high-risk environment (e.g., their friends as being heavy drinkers), or simply elicits a high-risk environment from the world at large (e.g., individuals who have inherited physically attractive features may attract many potential drinking partners); (2) primary GE correlation, whereby biologic relatives influence the environment to which an individual is exposed (e.g., sibling influences on drinking behavior, parent-to-offspring transmission, or even possibly offspring-to-parent transmission); and also (3) secondary GE correlation, whereby an assortment process (e.g., assortative mating or assortative friendship, the tendency to select a marital partner, or to select friends, with habits similar to one's own) leads to the selection of individuals who will have an important environmental influence on a subject (spousal or peer influences on drinking behavior). All of these mechanisms might potentially be important determinants of drinking behavior. They will each lead to individuals at high genetic risk also being exposed to high-risk environments.

Behavioral geneticists have made considerable progress in elucidating research strategies that might help to identify examples of GE autocorrelation (e.g., Eaves et al., 1977), primary GE correlation arising through sibling effects (e.g., Eaves, 1976; Carey, 1986) or through parent-to-offspring transmission (Eaves et al., 1978; Fulker, 1982; Heath et al., 1985), and even secondary GE correlation arising through assortment and reciprocal spousal or peer influences on drinking behavior (e.g., Heath and Eaves, 1985; Heath, 1987a). To date, the evidence for correlated genetic and environmental influences on drinking behavior is remarkably weak. As noted in our review of the major twin studies, there is surprisingly little evidence for long-term influences of shared family environment on twin pair resemblance for drinking habits. Results from the London (Clifford et al., 1984) and Finnish (Kaprio et al., 1987) studies, though not the female twin data in the Australian study (Heath et al., 1989), suggest that there may be a cohabitation effect on drinking patterns, i.e., an excess similarity of relatives still living in the same household that is hypothesized to be environmental in origin. Such analyses do not tell us, however, whether such influences arise because of the environmental impact of drinking habits of other household members (i.e., cotwin, parents, or spouse) or because of neighborhood or other effects. Data from the Virginia 30,000 study (Heath et al., 1993, unpublished) are consistent with a strong environmental influence of parental abstinence on offspring abstinence, but do not suggest a major environmental influence of parental frequency or total consumption measures on offspring drinking patterns. Early analyses of data on the drinking habits of twin pairs and their spouses, based on a subsample of the Virginia 30,000 study, were consistent with an important contribution of assortative mating to spousal concordance for drinking patterns, but did not support a major reciprocal environmental influence of husband's drinking on wife's drinking and vice versa (Heath, 1987b). On the basis of the small number of analyses that have been performed, we must conclude that there is remarkably little direct evidence that the drinking habits of those individuals with whom a respondent may have lived for many years, be they parents or spouse, have any lasting influence on the respondent's drinking behavior! It is possible that further analyses will provide evidence for such influences. It is also possible that such analyses will merely confirm that genetic factors play a far more important role in shaping adult drinking patterns, and social environmental influences a far less important one, than has generally been assumed.

Genotype × Environment Interaction

Extensive evidence for the importance of genotype × environment interaction (G × E) in nature has been provided by the carefully controlled experiments of biometrical geneticists working with plants or animals (e.g., Mather and Jinks, 1971). Such research has demonstrated that gene expression may differ under different environmental conditions, that there may be genetic differences in sensitivity to the environment, and that different genes may be involved in the control of environmental sensitivity versus average level of response across a range of environments. While there has been much discussion of how to detect G × E interaction in human populations (e.g., Jinks and Fulker, 1970; Eaves et al., 1977; Plomin et al., 1977; Eaves, 1984), convincing demonstrations of G × E effects have been rare. In order to demonstrate G × E interaction, in the simplest case of a dichotomous or polychotomous measure of environmental exposure, it is necessary to demonstrate differences between environmental conditions in the magnitude of genetic influences on drinking behavior, and to show that such differences cannot be explained by overall variance differences (e.g. Heath et al., 1989; Neale and Cardon, 1992). The birth cohort differences in the genetic influence on alcohol consumption levels observed in male and female twins in the Finnish twin sample (Kaprio et al., 1991) and in male twins in the Australian 1981 survey (Jardine and Martin, 1984) may provide one important example of G × E interaction. However, in these cross-sectional analyses genotype × cohort interaction is confounded with developmental changes in genetic effects, and even should the latter interpretation be excluded by further analyses of the longitudinal data on these two samples, we have little idea about *which* features of the environment are interacting with genetic effects.

The presence or absence of a marital partner, which has been repeatedly found to be an important determinant of the level of alcohol consumption (e.g., Temple et al., 1991), may be an important moderator of genetic influences on drinking patterns. Reanalyzing data on alcohol consumption levels of female Australian twin pairs in the 1981 survey, based on 7-day retrospective diary data, with lifetime abstainers excluded, we found apparent G × E interaction associated with marital status (Heath et al., 1989), with increased genetic influence on consumption levels in those without a marital or other partner. For example, in young adult twins, aged 18–30, genetic differences accounted for only 31% of the variance in consumption levels of married respondents, but for 60% of the variance of unmarried respondents, these figures increasing to 46–59% and 76% of the variance, respectively, in older twins. Eaves (1982), Heath (1993), and others have argued that the most convincing evidence for G × E interaction may be provided by laboratory experiments where the environment can be directly manipulated. From this viewpoint, alcohol challenge studies, in which exposure to a standard dose of alcohol is the experimenter-controlled environmental variable, provide an elegant demonstration of G × E interaction.

Mediating Variables

Given the evidence for a strong genetic influence on drinking patterns, it is natural to ask how this arises, i.e., to attempt to identify potential intervening or mediating variables in the causal chain from genotype to drinking behavior (Sher, 1991). Personality variables (e.g., Eaves et al., 1989; Heath et al., 1992), attitudinal variables (e.g., Eaves et al., 1989), and even such basic sociodemographic variables as educational level (e.g., Vogler and Fulker, 1983) all are influenced by genetic factors, so that it is natural to ask whether these variables can account for the genetic influence on consumption patterns. Carmelli et al. (1990) have attempted to control for the influence of sociodemographic variables, and while their approach is technically flawed (e.g., Neale and Cardon, 1992), their conclusion that there remains substantial unexplained genetic variance in consumption levels is probably correct. Associations between drinking patterns and either personality or attitudinal variables are too weak (e.g., Jardine and Martin, 1984) for the latter to be important mediating variables.

The strong association observed in the Australian Alcohol Challenge Twin (AACT) Study between self-report measures of alcohol consumption and certain measures of postalcohol performance, raises the possibility that inherited differences in alcohol sensitivity might account for much of the genetic influence on drinking patterns. A preliminary factor analysis of the AACT data on drinking history and postalcohol performance decrements yielded two major factors: a drinking-history-sensitive factor, with a high negative loading of average weekly alcohol consumption, high positive loadings of body sway increase, self-rated intoxication, an unwillingness to drive, and only very weak loadings of blood alcohol concentration, and a BAC-sensitive factor, with high positive loadings of deterioration in motor coordination, deterioration in eye–hand coordination and, in females only, increase in body sway (Heath and Martin, 1992). By fitting a multivariate genetic factor model, Heath and Martin (1992) have explored the extent to which the same genetic factors that are influencing psychomotor performance and subjective ratings in the alcohol challenge paradigm are also influencing reported patterns of alcohol use. A two-factor solution was obtained, in which the first genetic factor had a high positive loading on average weekly consumption of alcohol, and high negative loadings on subjective intoxication, willingness to drive, and (in males only) increase in body sway after alcohol challenge. This confirms a substantial overlap of the genetic factors that determine consumption level and the genetic factors that influence performance in the alcohol challenge paradigm (see also Heath and Martin, 1991a).

This initial finding is open to several alternative explanations. It is possible that differences in experience with alcohol were influencing performance in the alcohol challenge paradigm, i.e., that the primary direction of causation was from drinking history to alcohol sensitivity (consumption → sensitivity). Alternatively, it could be the case that inherited differences in alcohol sensitivity were influencing alcohol consumption, with increased sensitivity leading to decreased consumption (sensitivity → consumption). Both processes might be operating, i.e., inherited differences in alcohol sensitivity might indeed restrict consumption, but in those with low sensitivity heavy drinking might further reduce sensitivity (reciprocal causation). Fortunately, twin, adoption, or other family data can, under certain circumstances, provide a very powerful test of such hypotheses about direction of causation (Heath et al., 1989; Heath et al., 1993c). In brief, this is possible whenever two correlated traits have rather different modes of inheritance, e.g., one but not the other is strongly influenced by nonadditive genetic factors, or by shared environmental factors. As a didactic example, we might consider the hypothetical case where alcohol sensitivity and consumption are both influenced by additive genetic effects, but alcohol sensitivity is also strongly influenced by nonadditive genetic effects, whereas alcohol consumption is also strongly influenced by shared environmental effects (except for any such effects on sensitivity mediated through the causal influence of consumption on nonadditivity, or any nonadditive genetic effects on consumption mediated through the causal influence of sensitivity on consumption, respectively). It can be shown for this hypothetical example, by considering the implied structural equations, that the two unidirectional causal hypotheses lead to different predictions for the cross-correlations between twin pairs, with the DZ cross-correlation predicted to be greater than one-half the MZ cross-correlation if the direction of causation is consumption → sensitivity, but predicted to be less than one-half if the direction of causation is sensitivity → consumption. If both traits are influenced by both additive and nonadditive genetic effects, or both additive genetic and shared environmental effects, but the ratios of these effects differ between traits, the same rationale will apply, though in practice there will be considerable loss of resolving power (Heath et al., 1993c).

We have tested such direction-of-causation models using the AACT data in separate ånalyses of the relationship between alcohol consumption and self-report intoxication (Heath and Martin, 1991a) and between alcohol consumption and increase in body sway (Heath and Martin, 1991b). In females, there was insufficient statistical power for resolving alternative causal hypotheses, a finding that may be explained by the much weaker association between alcohol consumption patterns and the alcohol challenge variables. In males, however, our initial analyses in each case indicated that the direction of causation was from consumption to sensitivity, i.e., differences in experience with alcohol were having a major effect on performance in the alcohol challenge paradigm. Further theoretical analysis of direction-of-causation models (Heath et al., 1993c) has convinced us that these models are quite sensitive to differences in measurement error between variables, a complication that we had neglected in the initial analyses. Once measurement error is allowed for, results for alcohol consumption and self-report intoxication in males do not change (Neale and Cardon, 1992), but we are no longer able to resolve direction of causation in the case of body sway, even in males (Heath and Martin, unpublished data). Alcohol sensitivity, as measured by postalcohol intoxication ratings, certainly does not function as a mediating variable in the causal pathway from genotype to consumption in males, but for females, and for other measures of alcohol consumption in males, more data are needed to clarify this issue.

Moderator Variables

In principle, twin and other family data provide a powerful means by which to detect moderator variables, i.e., resiliency or protective factors that might determine which individuals who are genetically at high risk progress to become heavy drinkers (c.f. Sher, 1991). It might be hypothesized, for example, that personality differences would interact with inherited differences in alcohol reactivity to determine risk of becoming a heavy drinker. Surprisingly, this question does not appear to have been addressed in any detail.

Life-Span Developmental Questions

Most of the analyses that we have reported have used cross-sectional data, and most have used adult subjects. Many unanswered questions remain about how genetic factors influence experimentation with alcohol and the emergence of drinking patterns during the period of adolescence and early adulthood. In this area, as in many others, advances in the formulation of developmental genetic models—including autoregressive (Eaves et al., 1986), growth curve (Goldsmith et al., 1989), and survival models (Meyer and Eaves, 1988; Meyer et al., 1991)—have not yet been matched by the collection of the longitudinal data on drinking patterns that are needed to test such models. Beyond the period of early adulthood, longitudinal analyses of data from the Finnish, Australian, and U.S. NAS/NRC studies indicate substantial longitudinal stability of drinking patterns, and model-fitting analyses of these datasets indicate that a substantial proportion of the longitudinally stable variation in drinking patterns is explained by genetic influences. From these studies alone we cannot necessarily infer that the same genetic factors are influencing consumption levels through ages 25–65 and beyond, though continuing analyses of data from the adult offspring of twins in the Australian and Virginia 30,000 studies should help clarify this question.

Summary

The evidence for a genetic contribution to normal variation in drinking patterns in humans has been reviewed. Although this evidence is largely based on studies using self-administered questionnaire measures of drinking behavior, such measures have good validity, as assessed by the strength of the agreement between self-report and informant rating data and by the strength of the association between self-report consumption and subjective ratings and objective performance measures after alcohol challenge. Twin studies from Scandinavia (Finland and Sweden), the United Kingdom, the United States, and Australia provide evidence consistent with the hypothesis that there is a substantial genetic contribution to variation in levels of alcohol intake. Much higher MZ than DZ twin correlations are observed whether these are based on measures of the frequency with which alcohol is used, the average quantity of alcohol consumed on each day that alcohol is taken, or the total weekly consumption of alcohol. Correlations between the relatives of twins in the Virginia 30,000 study suggest that this finding cannot be explained simply by a higher correlation between the environments experienced by MZ versus DZ twin pairs. Beyond the period of early adulthood, from age 25 onward, alcohol consumption patterns exhibit substantial long-term stability. Genetic factors may account for as much as 67–80% of the longitudinally stable proportion of variation in drinking patterns. Differences in body sway and in ratings of intoxication after a challenge dose of alcohol appear to be strongly influenced by genetic factors, and these measures of alcohol sensitivity are strongly correlated with alcohol consumption pattern. It does not appear, however, that genetically determined differences in sensitivity to alcohol can explain the genetic influence on consumption patterns. Quite basic questions about the dimensionality of genetic influences on drinking behavior and the intervening variables that might account for these genetic influences remain unanswered. Comparatively little is known about how genetic influences on drinking behavior co-vary with, or are modified by, environmental factors, or about how these genetic and environmental influences unfold across the life span.

Acknowledgments: Preparation of this manuscript was supported in part by ADAMHA grants AA03539, AA07535, AA07728, DA05588, MH31302, and MH40828.

References

Australian Bureau of Statistics (1978). Alcohol and tobacco consumption patterns. Catalogue No. 4312.0.

Belgrave, B. E., Bird, K. D., Chesher, G. B., (1979). The effect of tetrahydrocannabinol alone and in combination with ethanol on human performance. *Psychopharmacol.* **62**:53–60.

Bouchard, T. J., Lykken, D. T., McGue, M., Segal, N. L., and Tellegen, A. (1990). Sources of human psychological differences: The Minnesota study of twins reared apart. *Science* **250**:223–228.

Cahalan, D., Cisin, I. H., and Crossley, H. M. (1969). *American Drinking Practices: A National Study of Drinking Behavior and Attitudes.* New Brunswick, NJ: Rutgers Center of Alcohol Studies, Monograph No. 6.

Carey, G. (1986), Sibling imitation and contrast effects. *Behav. Genet.* **16**:319–341.

Carmelli, D., Swan, G. E., Robinette, D., and Fabsitz, R. R. (1990). Heritability of substance use in the NAS-NRC twin registry. *Acta Genet. Med. Gemellol.* **39**:91–98.

Carmelli, D., Heath, A. C., and Robinette, D. (1993). Genetic analysis of drinking behavior in World War II veteran twins. *Genet. Epidemiol* **10**:201–213.

Cattell, R. B. (1960). The multiple abstract variance analysis equations and solutions: For nature-nurture research on continuous variables. *Psychol. Rev.* **67**:353–372.

Cederlof, R., Friberg, L., and Lundman, T. (1977). The interactions of smoking, environment and heredity and their implications for disease aetiology: A report of epidemiological studies on the Swedish twin registries. *Acta Med. Scand.* **612**(suppl.):1–128.

Clifford, C. A., Fulker, D. W., Gurling, H. M. D., and Murray, R. M. (1981). Preliminary findings from a twin study of alcohol use. In *Twin Research. 3: Epidemiological and Clinical Studies,* L. Gedda, P. Parisi, and W. E. Nance, eds. New York: Alan R. Liss, pp. 47–52.

Clifford, C. A., Hopper, J. L., Fulker, D. W., and Murray, R. M. (1984). A genetic and environmental analysis of a twin family study of alcohol use, anxiety, and depression. *Genet. Epidemiol.* **1**:63–79.

Eaves, L. J. (1976). A model of sibling effects in man. *Heredity* **36**:205–214.

Eaves, L. J. (1977). Inferring the causes of human variation. *J. Roy. Stat. Soc.* **140B**:324–355.

Eaves, L. J. (1982). The utility of twins. In *Genetic Basis of the Epilepsies,* V. E., Anderson, W. A. Hauser, J. K, Penry, and C. J. Sing, eds. New York: Raven Press.

Eaves, L. J. (1984). The resolution of genotype × environment interaction in segregation analysis of nuclear families. *Genet. Epidemiol.* **1**:215–228.

Eaves, L. J., Last, K. A., Martin, N. G., and Jinks, J. L. (1977). A progressive approach to non-additivity and genotype-environmental covariance in the analysis of human differences. *Br. J. Math. Stat. Psychol.* **30**:1–42.

Eaves, L. J., Last, K., Young, P. A., and Martin, N. G. (1978). Model-fitting approaches to the analysis of human behavior. *Heredity* **41**:249–320.

Eaves, L. J., Long, J., and Heath, A. C. (1986). A theory of developmental change in quantitative phenotypes applied to cognitive development. *Behav. Genet.* **16**:143–162.

Eaves, L. J., Eysenck, H. J., and Martin, N. G. (1989). *Genes, Culture, and Personality: An Empirical Approach.* London: Academic Press.

Eaves, L. J., Martin, N. G., Heath, A. C. (1990). Religious affiliation in twins and their parents: Testing a model of cultural inheritance. *Behav. Genet.* **20**:1–22.

Eaves, L. J., Heath, A. C., Neale, M. C., Hewitt, J. K., and Martin, N. G. (1992). Sex Differences and Non-additivity in the Effects of Genes on Personality. Unpublished manuscript.

Eisen, S., True, W., Goldberg, J., Henderson, W., and Robinette, C. D. (1987). The Vietnam era twin (VET) registry: Method of construction. *Acta Genet. Med. Gemellol.* **36**:61–67.

Eysenck, H. J., and Eysenck, S. B. G. (1975). *Manual of the Eysenck Personality Questionnaire.* London: Hodder & Stoughton.

Falconer, D. S. (1965). The inheritance of liability to certain diseases estimated from the incidence among relatives. *Ann. Hum. Genet.* **29**:51–75.

Fillmore, K. M., Hartka, E., Johnstone, B. M., Leino, E. V., Motoyoshi, M., and Temple, M. T. (1991). A meta-analysis of life course variation in drinking. *Br. J. Addict.* **86**:1221–1268.

Flick, L. H., and Heath, A. C. (1991). Genetic influences on adolescent vs. adult onset of regular alcohol use. *Behav. Genet.* **21**:571A.

Flick, L. H., Heath, A. C., Eiser, S. A., True, W. R., and Goldberg, J. (1994). Onset of regular drinking: different genetic and enviromental risk-profiles during adolescence and adulthood among veteran twins. Unpublished manuscript.

Franks, H. M., Hensley, V. R., Hensley, W. J., Starmer, G. A., and Teo, R. K. C. (1976). The relationship between alcohol dosage and performance decrement in humans. *J. Stud. Alcohol* **37**:284–297.

Fulker, D. W. (1982). Extensions of the classical twin method. In *Human Genetics. Part A: The Unfolding Genome.* B. Bonne-Tamir, T. Cohen, and R. M. Goodman, eds. New York: Alan R. Liss.

Fulker, D. W., DeFries, J. C., and Plomin, R. (1988). Genetic influence on general mental ability increases between infancy and middle childhood. *Nature* **336**:767–769.

Goldberg, J., Eisen, S. A., True, W. R., and Henderson, W. G. (1990). A twin study of the effects of the Vietnam conflict on alcohol drinking patterns. *Am. J. Public Health* **80**:570–574.

Goldsmith, H. H., McArdle, J. J., and Thompson, B. (1989). Longitudinal twin analyses of childhood temperament. *Behav. Genet.* **19**:759–760A.

Heath, A. C., (1987a). The analysis of marital interaction in cross-sectional twin data. *Acta Genet. Med. Gemmelol.* **36**:41–49.

Heath, A. C. (1987b). Marital concordance for alcohol consumption: Contributions of spousal selection and marital interaction. *Behav. Genet.* **17**:625–626. (abstract).

Heath, A. C. (1990). Persist or quit? Testing for a genetic contribution to smoking persistence. *Acta Genet. Med. Gemellol.* **39**:447–458.

Heath, A. C. (1992). What can we learn about the determinants of psychopathology and substance abuse from studies of normal twins.

Heath, A. C., and Eaves, L. J. (1985). Resolving the effects of phenotype and social background on mate selection. *Behav. Genet.* **15**:15–30.

Heath, A. C., and Martin, N. G. (1988). Teenage alcohol use in the Australian twin register: Genetic and social determinants of starting to drink. *Alcohol.: Clin. Exp. Res.* **12**:735–741.

Heath, A. C., and Martin, N. G. (1991a). The inheritance of alcohol sensitivity and of patterns of alcohol use. *Alcohol Alcohol.* **1**(suppl.):141–145.

Heath, A. C., and Martin, N. G. (1991b). Intoxication after an acute dose of alcohol: An assessment of its association with alcohol consumption patterns by using twin data. *Alcohol.: Clin. Exp. Res.* **15**:122–128.

Heath, A. C., and Martin, N. G. (1991c). Persistence and Change in Drinking Habits. Paper presented at the Research Society on Alcoholism, Marco Island, FL.

Heath, A. C., and Martin, N. G. (1992). Genetic differences in psychomotor performance decrement after alcohol: A multivariate analysis. *J. Stud. Alcohol* **53**:262–271.

Heath, A. C., and Martin, N. G. (1993). Genetic models for the natural history of smoking: Evidence for a genetic influence on smoking persistence. *Addictive Behaviors* **18**:11–34.

Heath, A. C., Kendler, K. S., Eaves, L. J., and Markell, D. (1985). The resolution of cultural and biological inheritance: Informativeness of different relationships. *Behav. Genet.* **15**:439–465.

Heath, A. C., Jardine, R., and Martin, N. G. (1989). Interactive effects of genotype and social environment on alcohol consumption in female twins. *J. Stud. Alcohol* **50**:38–48.

Heath, A. C., Meyer, J., Eaves, L. J., and Martin, N. G. (1991a). The inheritance of alcohol consumption patterns in a general population twin sample: I. Multidimensional scaling of quantity/frequency data. *J. Stud. Alcohol* **52**:345–352.

Heath, A. C., Meyer, J., Jardine, R., and Martin, N. G. (199b). The inheritance of alcohol consumption patterns in a general population twin sample: II. Determinants of consumption frequency and quantity consumed. *J. Stud. Alcohol.* **52**:425–433.

Heath, A. C., Cloninger, C. R., and Martin, N. G. (1992a). Testing a Model for the Genetic Structure of Personality. JPSP in press.

Heath, A. C., Eaves, L. J., and Martin, N. G. (1992b). Stability and Validity of Self-report Measures of Alcohol Consumption in General Population Surveys. Unpublished manuscript.

Heath, A. C., Eaves, L. J. Hewitt, J. K. Neale, M. C., and Martin, N. G. (1993). Twin-family correlations for alcohol consumption patterns. Unpublished manuscript.

Heath, A. C., Kessler, R. C., Neale, M. C., Hewitt, J. K., Eaves, L. J., Kendler, K. S. (1993). Testing Hypotheses About Direction of Causation Using Cross-sectional Family Data. *Behavior Genetics* **23**:39–50.

Hrubec, Z., and Neel, J. V. (1978). The National Academy of Sciences—National Research Council twin registry: Ten years of operation. In WE Nance, ed. *Twin Research. Part B: Biology and Epidemiology,* New York: Alan R. Liss, pp. 154–172.

Jablon, S., Neel, J. V., Gershowitz, H., and Atkinson, G. F. (1967). The NAS-NRC Twin Panel: Methods of construction of the panel, zygosity diagnosis, and proposed use. *Am. J. Hum. Genet.* **19**:133–161.

Jardine, R., and Martin, N. G. (1984). Causes of variation in drinking habits in a large twin sample. *Acta Genet. Med. Gemellol.* **33**:435–450.

Jinks, J. L., and Fulker, D. W. (1970). A comparison of the biometrical genetical, MAVA and classical approaches to the analysis of human behavior. *Psychol. Bull.* **73**:311–349.

Joreskog, K., and Sorbom, D. (1988). PRELIS: A preprocessor for LISREL. Mooresville, IN: Scientific Software.

Kaprio, J., Koskenvuo, M., and Sarna, S. (1981). Cigarette smoking, use of alcohol, and leisure-time physical activity among same-sexed adult twins. In *Twin Research. 3: Epidemiological and Clinical Studies* (Progress in Clinical and Biological Research, Vol. 69C), L. Gedda, P. Parisi, and W. E. Nance, eds. New York: Alan R. Liss.

Kaprio, J., Hammar, N., Koskenvuo, M., Floderus-Myrhed, B., Langinvainio, H., and Sarna, S. (1982). Cigarette smoking and alcohol use in Finland and Sweden: A cross-national twin study. *Int. J. Epidemiol.* **11**:378–386.

Kaprio, J., Koskenvuo, M., and Langinvainio, H. (1984). Finnish twins reared apart. IV: Smoking and drinking habits. A preliminary analysis of the effect of heredity and environment. *Acta Genet. Med. Gemellol.* **33**:425–433.

Kaprio, J., Koskenvuo, M. D., Langinvainio, H., Romanov, K., Sarna, S., and Rose, R. J. (1987). Genetic influences on use and abuse of alcohol: A study of 5638 adult Finnish brothers. *Alcohol.: Clin. Exp. Res.* **11**:349–356.

Kaprio, J., Rose, R. J., Romanov, K., and Koskenvuo, M. (1991). Genetic and environmental determinants of use and abuse of alcohol: The Finnish twin cohort studies. *Alcohol Alcohol.* **1**(suppl.):131–136.

Kaprio, J., Viken, R., Koskenvuo, M., Romanov, K., and Rose, R. J. (1992). Consistency and change in patterns of social drinking: 6-year follow-up of the Finnish twin cohort. *Alcohol.: Clin. Exper. Res.* **16**:234–240.

Kendler, K. S. (1983). Overview: A current perspective on twin studies of schizophrenia. *Am. J. Psychiatr.* **140**:1413–1425.

Kendler, K. S., Heath, A. C., Neale, M. C., Kessler, R. C., and Eaves, L. J. (1992). A Population-based Twin Study of Alcoholism in Women. *JAMA* 268 1877–1882.

Kopun, M., and Propping, P. (1977). The kinetics of ethanol absorption and elimination in twins and supplementary repetitive experiments in singleton subjects. *Eur. J. Clin. Pharmacol.* **11**:337–344.

Kruskal, J. B., and Wish, M. (1978). Multidimensional scaling. In *Sage University Paper Series on Quantitative Applications in the Social Sciences,* Beverly Hills, CA: Sage Publications, Series No. 07-011.

Loehlin, J. C. (1972). An analysis of alcohol-related questionnaire items from the national merit twin study. *Ann. N.Y. Acad. Sci.* **197**:117–120.

Loehlin, J. C. (1992). *Genes and Environment in Personality Development* Newbury Park CA: Sage Public Press.

Loehlin, J. C., and Nichols, R. C. (1976). *Heredity, Environment, and Personality: A Study of 850 Sets of Twins.* Austin: University of Texas Press.

Loehlin, J. C., Horn, J. M., and Willerman, L. (1981). Personality resemblance in adoptive families. *Behav. Genet.* **11**:309–330.

Loehlin, J. C., Willerman, L., and Horn, J. M. (1985). Personality resemblances in adoptive families when the children are late-adolescent or adult. *J. Pers. Soc. Psychol.* **48**:376–392.

Loehlin, J. C., Horn, J. M., and Willerman, L. (1990). Heredity, environment, and personality change: Evidence from the Texas Adoption Project. *J. Pers.* **58**:221–243.

McGue, M., Pickens, R. W., and Svikis, D. S., (1992). Sex and age effects on the inheritance of alcohol problems: A twin study. *J. Abnorm. Psychol.* **101**:3–17.

Madden, P.A.F., Heath, A. C., Bucholz, K. K., Dinwiddee, S. H., Dunne, M. P. and Martin, N. G. (1993a). The genetic relationship between problems related to alcohol use, smoking initiation and personality. Paper presented at the annual meeting of the Research Society on Alcoholism, San Antonio, Texas, June 19–20.

Madden, P.A.F., Heath, A. C., Bucholz, K. K., Dinwiddee, S. H., Dunne, M. P. and Martin, N.

G. (1993b). Novelty-seeking and the genetic determinants of smoking initiation and problems related to alcohol use in female twins. Paper presented at the 23rd annual meeting of the Behavior Genetics Association, Sydney, Australia, July 13–16.

Martin, N. G., and Boomsma, D. I., (1989). Willingness to drive when drunk and personality: A twin study. *Behav. Genet.* **19**:97–111.

Martin, N. G., Eaves, L. J., Kearsey, M. J., and Davies, P. (1978). The power of the classical twin study. *Heredity* **40**:97–116.

Martin, N. G., Oakeshott, J. G., Gibson, J. B., Starmer, G. A., Perl, J., and Wilks, A. V. (1985a). A twin study of psychomotor and physiological responses to an acute dose of alcohol. *Behav. Genet.* **15**:305–347.

Martin, N. G., Perl, J., Oakeshott, J. G., Gibson, J. B., Starmer, G. A., and Wilks, A. V. (1985b). A twin study of ethanol metabolism. *Behav. Genet.* **15**:93–109.

Mather, K., and Jinks, J. L. (1971). *Biometrical Genetics: The Study of Continuous Variation.* London: Chapman and Hall Ltd.

Medlund, P., Cederlof, R., Floderus-Myrhed, B., Friberg, L., and Sorensen, S. (1977). A new Swedish twin registry. *Acta Med. Scand.* Suppl. 600:1–111.

Merikangas, K. R. (1990). The genetic epidemiology of alcoholism. Psychol. Med. 20:11–22.

Meyer, J. M., and Eaves, L. J. (1988). Estimating genetic parameters of survival distributions: A multifactorial model. *Genet. Epidemiol.* **5**:265–276.

Meyer, J. M., Eaves, L. J., Heath, A. C., and Martin, N. G. (1991). Estimating genetic influences on the age-at-menarche: A survival analysis approach. *Am. J. Med. Genet.* **39**:148–154.

Meyer, J. M., Heath, A. C., and Eaves, L. J. (1992). Using multidimensional scaling on data from pairs of relatives to explore the dimensionality of categorical multifactorial traits. *Genet. Epidemiol.* 9:87–107.

Nagoshi, C. T., and Wilson, J. R. (1989). Long-term repeatability of human alcohol metabolism, sensitivity and acute tolerance. *J. Stud. Alcohol* **50**:162–169.

Neale, M. C., and Martin, N. G. (1989). The effects of age, sex, and genotype on self-report drunkenness following a challenge dose of alcohol. *Behav. Genet.* **19**:63–78.

Neale, M. C., and Cardon, L. R. (1992). *Methodology for Genetic Studies of Twins and Families,* NATO ASI Series Dordrecht. Kluwer.

Partanen, J., Bruun, K., and Markkanen, T. (1966). Inheritance of drinking behavior: A study on intelligence, personality, and use of alcohol of adult twins. In *Alcohol Research in the Northern Countries.* The Finnish Foundation for Alcohol Studies, Vol. 14. Stockholm: Amquist & Wiksell.

Pedersen, N. L., Plomin, R., McClearn, G. E., and Friberg, L. (1988). Neuroticism, extraversion, and related traits in adult twins reared apart and reared together. *J. Pers. Soc. Psychol.* **55**:950–957.

Plomin, R., DeFries, J. C., and Loehlin, J. L. (1977). Genotype-environment interaction and correlation in the analysis of human variation. *Psychol. Bull.* **84**:309–322.

Propping, P. (1977a). Genetic control of ethanol action on the central nervous system: An EEG study in twins. *Hum. Genet.* **35**:309–334.

Propping, P. (1977b). Psychophysiologic test performance in normal twins and in a pair of identical twins with essential tremor that is suppressed by alcohol. *Hum. Genet.* **36**:321–325.

Scarr, S., and McCartney, K. (1983). How people make their own environments: A theory of genotype → environment effects. *Child Dev.* **54**:424–435.

Scarr, S., Webber, P. L., Weinberg, R. A., and Wittig, M. A. (1981). Personality resemblance among adolescents and their parents in biologically related and adoptive families. *J. Pers. Soc. Psychol.* **40**:885–898.

Sher, K. J. (1991). *Children of Alcoholics. A Critical Appraisal of Theory and Research.* Chicago: University of Chicago Press.

Shalula, D. E. (1993). Eighth Special Report to the U.S. Congress on Alcohol and Health. Rockville, MD: U.S. Dept. of Health and Human Services, Public Health Service.

Temple, M. T., Fillmore, K. M., Hartka, E., Johnstone, B., Leino, E. V., and Motoyoshi, M. (1991). A meta-analysis of change in marital and employment status as predictors of alcohol consumption on a typical occasion. *Br. J. Addict.* **86**:1269–1281.

Truett, K. R., Eaves, L. J., Meyer, J. M., Heath, A. C., and Martin, N. G. (1992). Religion and education as mediators of attitudes: A multivariate analysis. *Behav. Genet.* **22**:43–62.

Vesell, E. S. (1972). Ethanol metabolism: Regulation by genetic factors in normal volunteers under a controlled environment and the effect of chronic ethanol administration. *Ann. N.Y. Acad. Sci.* **197**:79–88.

Vogler, G. P., and Fulker, D. W. (1983). Familial resemblance for educational attainment. *Behav. Genet.* **13**:341–354.

Whitfield, J. B., and Martin, N. G. (1985a). Genetic and environmental influences on the size and number of cells in the blood. *Genet. Epidemiol.* **2**:133–144.

Whitfield, J. B., and Martin, N. G. (1985b) Individual differences in plasma ALT, AST and GST: Contributions of genetic and environmental factors, including alcohol consumption. *Enzyme* **33**:61–69.

Wilson, J. R., and Plomin, R. (1985). Individual differences in sensitivity and tolerance to alcohol. *Soc. Biol.* **32**:162–184.

5

Alcohol Metabolism, Sensitivity, and Tolerance: Testing for Genetic Influences

JAMES R. WILSON AND
ELIZABETH LAFFAN

Familial aggregation of alcohol abuse has been noted for a long time, and has led to the belief that the tendency to abuse alcohol is heritable. But the two major sources of familial resemblance—shared genes and shared environment—are difficult to disentangle in data from cohabiting family members. A number of behavioral genetic strategies have been developed to estimate the relative influence of genes and environment on individual differences in behavioral phenotypes, and many of these have been applied to studies of alcohol abuse and/or alcoholism. Some of these methods are outlined below, as an introduction to findings from research utilizing behavioral genetic methods.

Animal Studies

Though misuse of ethyl alcohol is exclusively or almost exclusively a human problem, significant advances in understanding the effects of alcohol have been made with animal models. One of the most powerful behavioral genetic techniques is that of selective breeding, in which lines of animals are developed whose members exhibit a high amount of a desired phenotype. We are all familiar with the successes of this technique, for example, in increasing butterfat production in dairy cows, running speed in race horses, or desired behavioral characteristics in dogs. Many selection studies of alcohol-relevant phenotypes have been conducted to develop animal models that will help illuminate some of the actions of ethyl alcohol. Among these valuable selection studies are the alcohol preferring/alcohol nonpreferring (AP/ANP) rat lines (Erikkson, 1981), the alcohol accepting/nonaccepting (AA/ANA) rats lines (Li et al., 1981), the withdrawal seizure prone/resistant (WSP/WSR) mouse lines (Crabbe et al, 1983), the long sleep/short sleep (LS/SS) mouse lines developed by McClearn and Kakihana (1973) for differential time of loss of the righting reflex (the sleep time) to an anesthetic dose of ethyl alcohol, and others—see Chapters 6–8. The LS/SS lines have been studied extensively as an animal model of alcohol *sensitivity* and are, of course, proof positive that this type of sensitivity has a significant additive genetic component in this species, otherwise selection would not have succeeded. The success of this model was a principal impetus for the Colorado Alcohol Research on Twins and Adoptees studies of alcohol sensitivity in humans discussed later.

Human Behavioral Genetic Methodologies

Ethical, legal, and practical considerations appropriately limit the kinds of experimentation done with animals, and the constraints are greater for human research. We would not, for example, undertake a selective breeding study with humans, despite Plato's early advice to the contrary (Plato, 1980). Yet there remain many human behavioral genetic methodologies that are widely seen as acceptable and valuable. Many of these methods take advantage of existing human family relationships, special genetic relationships, such as those enjoyed by monozygotic twins, or special rearing arrangements, such as those experienced by adoptees. In essence, researchers do not manipulate human population structure or rearing, but glean information by focusing on existing subgroups. These methods include family studies—often of parent-offspring resemblance, but including studies of resemblance among siblings and other family members—studies of twins in which the phenotypic resemblance of monozygotic twins is contrasted with that of dizygotic twins; and adoption studies in which an adopted child is compared to its adoptive parents and to its birth parents. In some cases additional power is gained by combining methods or groups in the same study.

Family Studies

Comment on apparent familial aspects of alcohol abuse has been made since earliest times. And it has been well documented that some families do have a disproportionate amount of alcohol abuse (e.g., Goedde and Agarwahl, 1987; Cotton, 1979). But from studies of intact nuclear families it is extremely difficult to ascribe familial alcohol abuse to genes or to common environment or, stated more accurately, to determine what proportion of the individual differences in alcohol abuse is traceable to genes and what proportion to environment. Since the parents furnish all the genes and a large portion of the rearing environment, genetic and environmental influences are confounded in most family studies.

A familial methodology of considerable current interest involves the selection and aggregation of families into two contrasting groups, family history positive (FHP) and family history negative (FHN), for a phenotype. For example, families could be assigned to FHP on the basis of diagnosed alcoholism in one or both parents (usually the father), or to FHN if neither parent was alcoholic. Interest, then, is focused on contrasting FHP/FHN *offspring* characteristics, the idea being that if the offspring differ by group, something has been transmitted genetically. This idea is not formally correct. Note that if a (mixed) group of Breton and English parents were grouped as FHP for speaking French and FHN for English, a test of the offspring would argue that the language spoken is genetic. The difficulty obviously is that genes and environment are still confounded. Yet from another view, reliable FHP/FHN differences can be thought-provoking, especially if the difference is not on the phenotype itself, but rather on a system that could be propaedeutic or logically related. For example, if FHP offspring show cognitive, personality, or physiological differences than FHN when the groups are young and have not drunk (or not much) alcohol. A replicable FHP/FHN difference would be of interest whether it was transmitted genetically *or* environmentally since it could help illuminate the pathway from use to abuse. Provocative FHP/FHN differences have been reported by Schuckit (e.g., 1984, 1985), Begleiter et al. (1984); Tarter et al. (1984), Workman-Daniels and Hesselbrock (1987), and others (see Chapters 1, 2, and 11).

Adoptee Studies

A powerful method of distinguishing genetic from environmental influences is to compare adoptees with their adoptive parents (environmental path) and, if possible, with their birth parents (genetic path). The method is not without difficulties. Many persons are not aware that they were adopted, and cannot be included. Late adoption allows for both genetic and environmental transmission from birth parents. Birth parents may have reasons for declining to participate. Selective placement may have occurred; that is, a child may have been adopted into the home of a relative or by adoptive parents who resemble the birth parents in important ways, thereby inflating both the genetic and environmental transmission estimates. In practice, however, these difficulties can be overcome, and adoption studies offer convincing evidence that the risk of alcohol abuse and/or alcoholism is influenced by genes (Goodwin et al., 1973; Cloninger et al., 1981). At present, the risk estimate is useful for groups; the predictive power for individuals is weak. For example, the finding by Goodwin et al. (1973) that 24% of sons of (Danish) alcoholics adopted into nonalcoholic homes themselves become alcoholic garners attention, and is certainly important. It is difficult to conceive of anything but genes linking the adopted-away son with his birth father. But one sees from the same figure that 76% of the adopted-away sons of alcoholic fathers don't become alcoholics.

Monozygotic/Dizygotic Comparisons

Since Merriman's (1924) explication of the method, geneticists have used the naturally occurring difference in the genetic resemblance of monozygotic (MZ) and dizygotic (DZ) twins. This difference is simply that MZ twins arise from an early splitting of a single fertilized egg, and thus have all the same genes, while DZ twins arise from two, separate fertilized eggs, and share an average of 50% of the same genes just as do non-twin siblings. Thus, for any gene-influenced trait, we expect to find the intraclass correlation, t, of MZ twins to be roughly twice as great as that of DZ twins. Conversely, if the trait is not influenced by genes, it should be essentially a random matter which t is larger. Symbolically, using V_A for additive genetic variance, V_D for dominance (genetic) variance, V_E for environmental variance common to both types of twins, and V_P for the total phenotypic variation of the trait:

$$t_{MZ} = 100\% \frac{V_A}{V_P} + 100\% \frac{V_D}{V_P} + 100\% \frac{V_E}{V_P} \tag{5–1}$$

$$t_{DZ} = 50\% \frac{V_A}{V_P} + 25\% \frac{V_D}{V_P} + 100\% \frac{V_E}{V_P} \tag{5–2}$$

Subtracting the second equation from the first, we get

$$(t_{MZ} - t_{DZ}) = 50\% \frac{V_A}{V_P} + 75\% \frac{V_D}{V_P} \tag{5–3}$$

And, attempting to obtain an estimate of broad-sense heritability,

$$h^2 = \frac{V_G}{V_P} = \frac{V_A}{V_P} + \frac{V_D}{V_P} \tag{5–4}$$

we continue to follow Falconer's (1989) method and double the difference between the MZ and DZ intraclass correlations, we obtain

$$2(t_{MZ} - t_{DZ}) = 100\% \frac{V_A}{V_P} + 150\% \frac{V_D}{V_P} \tag{5–5}$$

which is an approximate but useful solution for broad-sense heritability despite the inflation of V_D, since V_D is usually small. A useful way to visualize the variance components derived from twin analyses is with a box diagram. In Fig. 5-1, E_1 represents within-family environmental factors, while E_2 represents common environment, the same as V_E previously, which makes twins and other family members more similar. The results of doubling the difference between the MZ and DZ intraclass correlations can be seen in the middle section where the genetic components are labeled. Common environment E_2 can also be estimated from the resemblance of adoptees to their adoptive parents.

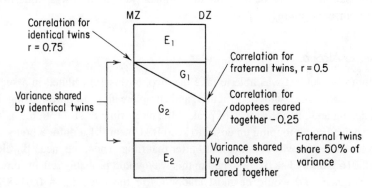

Fig. 5-1 Diagram of components of variance.

This method (and its extensions) has been used extensively to learn whether a phenotype of interest is influenced by genes. It has been used several times (including Partanen et al., 1966; McGue et al., 1991; see also Chapters 1 and 4, to look for genetic influence on rates of alcoholism or alcohol abuse. To our knowledge, however, it has been used only once to look for genetic influence on alcohol *sensitivity* (see Wilson and Plomin, 1985).

Twin/Adoptee (Combined) Studies

In the Colorado Alcohol Research on Twins and Adoptees (CARTA) study conducted between 1981 and 1987, we attempted to use the strengths and counterbalance the weaknesses of the twin and adoption methods by combining them into one study. We also added a group of nontwin sibling pairs, to serve as a further comparison group, a group of placebo controls whose dose of alcohol was minuscule, a group of singletons who repeated all tests and procedures one month after initial testing, and a group of singletons who repeated after one year.

Colorado Alcohol Research on Twins and Adoptees

The design of the CARTA study is described more fully in Wilson and Plomin (1985). Briefly we set out to test 50 pairs each of MZ twins, DZ twins, unrelated adoptee pairs, and pairs of nontwin siblings on a variety of psychomotor, cognitive, and mood tasks before and after dosing with 0.8 g/kg ethyl alcohol. Blood alcohol concentration (BAC) was monitored via breath alcohol readings from an (Omicron Systems) intoxylizer. For *sensitivity* to alcohol, we use the residual from regression of each measure, taken near peak 1 BAC, on the baseline (sober) score for that measure (Nagoshi et al., 1986). For acute behavioral *tolerance,* we use the residual from regression of a score 3 hours after dosing (while BAC has been maintained at about 0.1 g/dl via topping up doses) on the peak 1 score. Subjects were tested individually, a testing day spanning the period 0800 (8.00 A.M.) to 1800 or 1900 hours (6:00 or 7:00 P.M.), and a subject was released when their BAC had fallen to 0.02 g/kg or lower. Subjects were paid for their participation and are being paid to complete annual follow-up questionnaires about their current drinking.

Responses to Alcohol

Practically every subject was able to take the alcohol dose(s) (diluted in a sugar- and caffeine-free soft drink) without difficulty, and complete all procedures. Using the time between dosing and the occurrence of peak 1, the mean time of absorption was 40 minutes. As we used small topping up doses to keep BAC near 0.1 g/dl for 3 hours, no estimate of clearance rate was obtained until after that time. Then, the mean β_{60} clearance rate was 0.016 g/dl/hr. The β_{60} obtained in this way would probably reflect some dispositional tolerance, and would be most analogous to the rate ($\beta_{60} = 0.0178$ g/dl/hr) obtained by Wilson et al. (1984a) for clearance of a second dose of alcohol given after each subject had cleared one-half the original dose.

For essentially every function measured, *sensitivity* was seen as a mean change (usually a decrement) in performance after dosing. The variation in sensitivity was large, however, with a few individuals showing little or no performance deficit after dosing. Further analyses of the variation in sensitivity are given below. Acute behavioral *tolerance* was also seen, on average, for most of the measures taken. In most cases, mean performance after 3 hours with a BAC near 0.1 g/dl was improved from that seen at peak 1, and approached sober performance. Again, individual differences in tolerance were large, and are discussed later. It should be noted that this acquisition of acute tolerance is likely to be a factor in driving while intoxicated (DWI) cases, since a person may well "monitor" their BAC by walking ability, etc., after a few hours of drinking, and may yet have a BAC well in excess of legal limits for driving.

Individual Differences in Response

Within Populations

There are individual differences in ethanol metabolism. For example, Vesell et al. (1970) describe intrasubject differences in ethanol elimination and ethanol metabolism. Wagner (1973) and Martin et al. (1985b) report considerable variation on all ethanol metabolism variables between individual subjects. The CARTA study also found individual differences on many metabolic parameters. For example, peak blood alcohol level (BAL) ranged from 70 to 130 mg/dl, despite the fact that dosages were calculated (taking body weight into account) to produce a BAL of 100 mg/dl.

Sensitivity and tolerance to alcohol also vary widely between individuals. In the CARTA study (Wilson, 1988) some individuals showed decrement, some no change, and some improvement for tasks in which a decrement was expected after alcohol dosing. The variability in sensitivity and acute behavioral tolerance among individuals is far greater than any average effect. Thus an individual's response is poorly predicted by the average effect.

Many studies have focused on the average effects of a certain dose of alcohol, and current legal limits on BAL are based on the assumption that most people will respond similarly at the same BAL. There is, however, increasing evidence to indicate that BAL is a poor predictor of individual performance. In addition, Martin (1987) reports that BAC is a poor predictor of psychomotor sensitivity.

Short-Term Stability of Response

Beyond the intersubject variability, there is a growing body of evidence that suggests there is considerable intrasubject variability. Martin et al. (1985b) retested subjects and found metabolic parameters were only low to moderately repeatable. Wagner (1973) reported larger intra- than intersubject variability for ethanol metabolism when he reanalyzed Vesell's data. Wagner and Patel (1972) report wide variation in Km (the alcohol concentration at $V_{M+X}/2$) and Vm (V_{M+X} = theoretical maximum decay rate) in the same subject from one time to another. The study of short-term (one month) stability of response in the CARTA study (Wilson and Nagoshi, 1987) showed considerable day-to-day variation in metabolic parameters in agreement with the studies just cited.

This lack of repeatability carried over into the repeatability of sensitivity and tolerance. While the baseline measurements are highly repeatable on the tests used, the measures of sensitivity and acute tolerance have only low to moderate repeatability. This general lack of repeatability is probably due to undetermined environmental factors.

Long-Term Stability of Response

The CARTA study also looked at stability of response after a longer time (3 to 39 months) in order to determine the extent of the intrasubject variability (Nagoshi and Wilson, 1989). The repeatability of alcohol clearance rate was zero and the other metabolic parameters were low to moderate (time to peak 0.36, peak BAL 0.50). Sensitivity had a near zero repeatability for this longer term stability, and acute tolerance was low at about 0.10. The rank order of subjects should remain the same from one test session to the next if the measure is repeatable. This would mean that intersubject variability exceeded intrasubject variability. CARTA data indicate that intrasubject variability equals or exceeds intersubject variability.

Group Differences

The large and pervasive individual differences in response to alcohol arise from a variety of sources. One source of variation may be membership in a particular subset of a population. Groups in a population defined by gender, age, or ethnic background may respond differently to alcohol and explain some of the variation observed between individuals.

Gender

Historically, the majority of alcohol research was done on college-age white males because of the ease of recruiting this group and the lack of fluctuating hormonal levels that create complications in females. However, recent research has focused more on the potential differences between men's and women's response to, use of, and dependence on alcohol. Gender differences in ethanol metabolism, sensitivity, and tolerance may help explain the gender differences in the development of alcoholism.

The CARTA study tested a large number of males and females for a wide variety of responses to alcohol. Wilson and Plomin (1985) report few gender differences in sensitivity or tolerance on an early small sample of subjects. As the dataset increased, some interesting gender effects emerged. While sensitivity measures never showed any significant gender effects, many metabolic and acute tolerance measures showed significant differences between males and females (Wilson and Nagoshi, 1988).

Gender had significant effects on most metabolic parameters measured in the CARTA study. Females took significantly longer to reach their peak BAC, which indicates a slower absorption of ethanol. Martin et al. (1985b) also found a longer time to peak for females in a large sample. Some studies with smaller sample size report no significant differences in time to peak between males and females (Sutker et al., 1983; Nicholson et al., personal communication; Marshall et al., 1983). The difference in time to peak may be very slight and require a larger sample size, or it may be extremely variable and depend on other environmental factors.

In agreement with most studies, the CARTA data indicate that women reach a higher peak BAC, given a similar dose of alcohol per kilogram (e.g., Martin et al., 1985b). Many investigators have attributed this difference to the difference in body composition between males and females. Females have more body fat and less total body water than males, and thus have a smaller volume of distribution for ethanol (Batt, 1989). CARTA data show a significantly lower Widmark r for females, indicating a smaller volume of distribution. Some recent work by Frezza et al. (1990) on gastric alcohol dehydrogenase activity suggests that women have less gastric alcohol dehydrogenase activity than men, and thus a significantly lower first-pass metabolism. They propose that both differences in the volume of distribution and the lower dehydrogenase activity lead to the differences in peak BAC between men and women. Whitfield's et al. (1990) results from the Australian twin study support this hypothesis. More research in this area is needed to partial out the various factors affecting peak BAC.

In the CARTA study, the rate of alcohol clearance was estimated with β_{60} values, and a significantly faster clearance rate in females was found (Cole-Harding and Wilson, 1987). Testosterone suppression of ethanol elimination in men may be responsible for this difference. It should be noted that the β_{60} values were calculated after the subjects had been maintained at high BAL for 3 hours, and thus were probably affected by an acute metabolic tolerance to ethanol. A recent study by Mishra et al. (1989) also found higher elimination rates in females. However, other investigators have not found these differences in clearance rates (e.g., Whitfield et al., 1990), perhaps because of the wide variety of ethanol dosing procedures and subject population characteristics.

Another factor that may affect the metabolism of ethanol in women is the fluctuating hormonal levels created by the menstrual cycle and birth control pills. Although Cole-Harding and Wilson (1987) found no evidence that either the phase of the menstrual cycle or taking birth control pills influenced ethanol metabolism in females, the results of other investigators are mixed. Jones and Jones (1976) reported variation in peak BAC due to menstrual cycle phase and effects of birth control pills on metabolism. Sutker et al. (1987) found no differences in peak BAC or absorption, but faster elimination rates with increased levels of progesterone. Hay et al. (1984) found no metabolic differences between women on and not on birth control pills, and no phase differences in either group. The wide variety of results may be due to the differences in alcohol administration, variation and inaccuracies of cycle reporting, and differences in testing days during the cycle.

The effects of gender on acute tolerance in the CARTA study were most apparent in the motor coordination and reaction-time behavioral tasks. Females are less tolerant than males on these tasks, even after average alcohol consumption is partialed out (Wilson and Nagoshi, 1988). The metabolic differences just described probably contribute to these differences in acute tolerance. The higher peak BAC and faster clearance rate observed in females may affect acute tolerance. It is also possible that body composition, drinking history, or stress levels affect the development of acute tolerance.

Age

In the large Australian study of twins, Jardine and Martin (1984) found age-dependent differences in genetic and environmental contributions to drinking habits. There was a small positive correlation between age and BAC that Martin et al. (1985b) speculate is due to habit reinforcement or a decline in general health. The metabolic differences due to age in the CARTA study agree with the Australian study and show older groups with higher BACs at peak. There were no strong effects of age on acute tolerance, but a wide variety of measurements showed sensitivity scores that were affected by age even after partialing out the effect of average alcohol consumption (Wilson and Nagoshi, 1988).

Few studies have considered age effects on alcohol response parameters, so further investigation in this area would provide valuable information. For example, the changing response to alcohol might indicate certain ages at which people are more susceptible to alcohol effects on motor coordination or mood, and could possibly influence a persons susceptibility to alcoholism. Due to the large individual variation in alcohol response, however, longitudinal research would be preferable.

Ethnicity

The CARTA study did not have any ethnic exclusion criteria, but due to the ethnic makeup of the Boulder area and the tendency for volunteers to be mostly Caucasian, very few non-Caucasian subjects were tested. Previous work by Wilson et al. (1984a) in Hawaii addressed the question of ethnic variation in responses to alcohol. The Hawaii study found that men of Oriental ancestry had a faster clearance rate than men of either Caucasian or Polynesian ancestry. Differences between those of Oriental ancestry and those of Caucasian ancestry have been well documented. Increased metabolic rate has also been observed in North American Indians (Reed, 1985). Both Oriental and some American Indians show a flushing response to alcohol in much higher percentages than other ethnic groups. This flushing difference may be due to an atypical alcohol and/or acetaldehyde dehydrogenase (ADH, ALDH) (see Chan, 1986, Reed, 1985; Chapter 8) found in those populations. Agarwal et al. (1985) have proposed an autosomal codominant inheritance pattern for ALDH alleles. While these differences are interesting and may help identify some of the genes contributing to alcohol responses, it should be remembered that most of the variation seen in alcohol responses is within racial groups, not between them.

Genetic Contributions

Evidence from Other Studies

Most genetic studies of alcohol in humans have focused on the genetic influences on alcohol abuse and alcoholism. Genetic etiologies for various forms of alcoholism (e.g., Type I and Type II), as well as factors affecting alcoholism, have been proposed (e.g., Cloninger, 1987; McGue et al., 1991) There is general agreement that alcohol abuse demonstrates familial aggregation, but its sources are still being debated (Searles, 1988). Response to alcohol would be expected to influence the development of alcohol abuse. Thus alcohol metabolism, tolerance, and sensitivity would be expected to demonstrate familial aggregation also. A limited number of studies in humans have focused on these alcohol response variables.

Vesell et al. (1970) attributed ethanol metabolism almost entirely to genetic factors. This finding has never been replicated, but the study did inspire more extensive investigations. One of the largest genetic studies of alcohol response has been the Australian twin study (Martin, 1987). This study estimated moderate heritabilities for peak BAC and rate of elimination and almost no heritability for time to peak. Martin mentioned problems with repeatability and extensive environmental influences that are difficult to detect in a short-term laboratory experiment. He and his colleagues also found genetic variation in response to alcohol on some psychomotor tasks beyond the baseline genetic variation that exists before alcohol dosing. In this study, psychomotor response to alcohol was poorly predicted by BAC. The Hawaii study (Wilson et al, 1984b) found some familiality for both motor coordination and writing (clerical skill) sensitivity to alcohol, as well as significant familiarlity for behavioral tolerance on one motor task (hand steadiness). These results were promising enough to inspire the CARTA study.

CARTA Results

Analysis of the extensive CARTA dataset has revealed some indication of genetic influences on specific aspects of alcohol-related behavior. Gabrielli and Plomin (1985a, 1985b) showed genetic influence on anticipation of alcohol sensitivity for physical symptoms and coordination, but not for mood or driving ability. They also report genetic influence on the amount and rate of alcohol drinking, but not on the maximum amount. However, the majority of the analyses on metabolism, sensitivity, and tolerance have shown no significant genetic influences. The magnitude of the individual differences coupled with the lack of stability of an individual's response across time have overwhelmed whatever genetic influences exist. An analysis of FHP and FHN subjects from the CARTA sample found no significant differences between the groups on response variables (Wilson and Nagoshi, 1988). Searles (1988) has argued that attention to the influences of environment and genetic–environment interactions and correlations has been lacking. The CARTA data would appear to support environmental variation, which creates the fluctuation within individuals across time. The CARTA data also suggest that large studies of genetically informative individuals may need to be conducted in a repeated testing design instead of a single testing session design.

The yearly follow-up questionnaires filled out by the CARTA study participants allow analysis of the predictive power of sensitivity on later alcohol use and abuse. The theory that more sensitive individuals who experience negative effects when drinking alcohol will subsequently be less likely to drink and develop alcohol abuse problems can be tested with these data. Rodriguez et al. (1992) conducted such an analysis using latent variable modeling. They report that when the effects of previous drinking are controlled for, sensitivity (as measured by the CARTA psychomotor battery) is not predictive of later alcohol use or abuse. This does not necessarily rule out the theory that sensitivity affects subsequent use. The authors suggest that our definition of sensitivity may be too restrictive in this case. Consumption reported at the time of testing does predict later reports of consumption and alcohol problems in the yearly follow-up questionnaires.

Future Research

Human response to alcohol is a complex puzzle that will require carefully designed research to untangle. Future research would be greatly aided by standardized testing procedures. Past studies used a wide variety of alcohol dosing, behavioral testing, and variable definition. The results have been interesting but often conflicting and/or difficult to compare. The difficult problems of repeatability and environmental influences on human response to alcohol need to be addressed in an organized manner. A laboratory consortium between the alcohol research centers might help improve the standardization of testing methods. A clearer picture of the nature of human response to alcohol will help address the problems of treating and predicting individuals with actual or potential alcohol abuse problems.

Summary

Following the success of genetic selection for sensitivity to ethyl alcohol in laboratory mice (long-sleep/short-sleep lines), a group of investigators at the Colorado Alcohol Research Center decided to test for genetic influences on alcohol sensitivity in humans. Within an extended twin/adoptee/sibling genetic design, over 500 men and women were tested individually for their sensitivity and acute behavioral tolerance to a dose of ethanol that brought their BAC to about 0.1 g/dl. All those who were tested were invited to complete an annual questionnaire that inquires about alcohol consumption and any current problems stemming from their alcohol use. Two related hypotheses are being tested: (1) Does relative sensitivity (or acute behavioral tolerance) predict future alcohol use? That is, are those more insensitive to alcohol more at risk for increased consumption and/or related problems? (2) To what extent are individual differences in measured sensitivity influenced by genetic variation? Though maximum likelihood, model-fitting alternatives are still being worked on, it is clear that, while earlier alcohol consumption predicts later consumption (and problems), relative sensitivity either does not or has a minor influence. It also appears that the antecedents of adult individual differences in measured sensitivity are largely nongenetic. A potentially important aspect revealed by analyses of the responses of people who repeated all tests, one month or one year later, was that the *stability* of sensitivity response is low: rank order on sensitivity is quite different a month or a year after initial testing, despite acceptable psychometric reliability of the tests and instruments. Given this fluctuation, it is not surprising that MZ twin resemblance is not high on many tests, since the correlations for individuals across occasions is not high. It may be that single-occasion measurements of sensitivity and tolerance are not adequate, given the large short-term and intermediate-term fluctuations in individual sensitivity.

Acknowledgments: The partial support of NIAAA Grant AA-03527 for the CARTA study reported herein, NIAAA Grant AA-08118 for current analyses, and NIDA Grant DA-05464 (Fellowship to Dr. Laffan) is gratefully acknowledged, as are the contributions to CARTA and its follow-up studies of S. A. Rhea, A. K. Watson, Dr. C. T. Nagoshi, L. A. Rodriguez, Michael Roberts, and the many other students and staff members who have helped significantly with this work.

References

Agarwal, D. P., Harada, S., and Goedde, H. W. (1981). Racial differences in biological sensitivity to ethanol: The role of alcohol dehydrogenase and aldehyde dehydrogenase isozymes. *Alcohol.: Clin. Exp. Res.* **5**:12–16.

Batt, R. D. (1989). Absorption, distribution, and elimination of alcohol. In *Human Metabolism of Alcohol, Vol. I,* K. E. Crow and R. D. Batt, eds. Boca Raton, FL: CRC Press, pp. 3–8.

Begleiter, H., Porjesz, B., and Kissin, B. (1984). Event-related brain potentials in boys at risk for alcoholism. *Science* **225**:1493–1496.

Chan, A. W. K. (1986). Racial differences in alcohol sensitivity. *Alcohol Alcohol.* **21**:93–104.

Cloninger, C. R. (1987). Neurogenetic adaptive mechanisms in alcoholism. *Science* **236**:410–416.

Cloninger, C. R., Bohman, M., and Sigvardsson, S. (1981). Inheritance of alcohol abuse: Cross-fostering analysis of adopted men. *Arch. Gen. Psychiatr.* **38**:861–868.

Cole-Harding, S., and Wilson, J. R. (1987). Ethanol metabolism in men and women. *J. Stud. Alcohol* **48**:380–387.

Cotton, N. S. (1979). The familial incidence of alcoholism: A review. *J. Stud. Alcohol* **40**:89–116.

Crabbe, J. C., Rosebud, A., and Young, E. R. (1983). Genetic selection for withdrawal severity: Differences in replicate mouse lines. *Life Sci.* **33**:955–962.

Eriksson, C. J. P. (1981). Finnish selection studies of alcoholism and alcohol actions: Factors regulating voluntary alcohol consumption. In *The Development of Animal Models as Pharmacogenetic Tools,* G. E. McClearn, R. A. Deitrich, and V. G. Erwin, eds. Washington, DC: U.S. Government Printing Office (DHHS publ. no. (ADM) 81–1133).

Falconer, D. S. (1989). *Introduction to Quantitative Genetics.* New York: Wiley.

Frezza, M., Di Padova, C., Pozzato, G., Terpin, M., Baraona, E., and Lieber, C. S. (1990). High blood alcohol levels in women. *New Engl. J. Med.* **322**:95–99.

Gabrielli, W. F., and Plomin, R. (1985a). Individual differences in anticipation of alcohol sensitivity. *J. Nerv. Ment. Dis.* **173**:111–114.

Gabrielli, W. F., and Plomin, R. (1985b). Drinking behavior in the Colorado adoptee and twin sample. *J. Stud. Alcohol* **46**:24–31.

Goedde, H. W., and Agarwal, D. P. (1987). *Genetics and Alcoholism.* New York: A. R. Liss.

Goodwin, D. W., Schulsinger, F., Hermanson, L., Guze, S. B., and Winokur, G. (1973). Alcohol problems in adoptees raised apart from alcoholic biological parents. *Arch. Gen. Psychiatr.* **28**:238–243.

Hay, W. M., Nathan, P. E., Heermans, H. W., and Frankenstein, W. (1984). Menstrual cycle, tolerance and blood alcohol level discrimination ability. *Addict. Behav.* **9**:67–77.

Jardine, R., and Martin, N. G. (1984). Causes of variation in drinking habits in a large twin sample. *Acta Genet. Med. Gemellol.* **33**:435–450.

Jones, B. M., and Jones, M. K. (1976). Women and alcohol: Intoxication, metabolism, and the menstrual cycle. In *Alcoholism Problems in Women and Children,* M. Greenblatt and M. A. Schuckit, eds. New York: Grune & Stratton, pp. 103–136.

Li, T.-K., Lumeng, L., McBride, W. J., and Waller, M. B. (1981). Indiana selection studies on alcohol-related behaviors. In *Development of Animal Models as Pharmacogenetic Tools,* G. E. McClearn, R. A. Deitrich, and V. G. Erwin, eds. Washington, DC: National Institute of Alcohol Abuse and Alcoholism, Research Monograph No. 6 (DHHS publ. no. (ADM) 81-1133), pp. 171–191.

Marshall, A. W., Kingston, D., Boss, M., and Morgan, M. Y. (1983). Ethanol elimination in males and females: Relationship to menstrual cycle and body composition. *Hepatology* **3**:701–706.

Martin, N. G. (1987). Genetic differences in drinking habits, alcohol metabolism and sensitivity in unselected samples of twins. In *Genetics and Alcoholism,* H. W. Goedde, and D. P. Agarwal, eds. New York: Alan R. Liss, pp. 109–119.

Martin, N. G., Perl, J., Oakeshott, J. G., Gibson, J. B., Starmer, G. A., and Wilks, A. V. (1985b). A twin study of ethanol metabolism. *Behav. Genet.* **15**:93–109.

McClearn, G. E., and Kakihana, R. (1973). Selective breeding for ethanol sensitivity. *Behav. Genet.* **3**:409–410.

McGue, M., Pickens, R. W., and Svikis, D. S. (1992). Sex and age effects on the inheritance of alcohol problems: A twin study. *J. Abnorm. Psychol.* **102**:3–18.

Merriman, A. N. (1924). The intellectual resemblance of twins. *Psychol. Monogr.* **33**:1–58.

Mishra, L., Sharma, S., Potter, J. J., and Mezey, E. (1989). More rapid elimination of alcohol in women as compared to their male siblings. *Alcohol.: Clin. Exp. Res.* **13**:752–754.

Nagoshi, C. T., and Wilson, J. R. (1989). Long-term repeatability of human alcohol metabolism, sensitivity and acute tolerance. *J. Stud. Alcohol* **50**:162–169.

Nagoshi, C. T., Wilson, J. R., and Plomin, R. (1986). Use of regression residuals to quantify individual differences in acute sensitivity and tolerance to alcohol. *Alcohol.: Clin. Exp. Res.* **10**:343–349.

Partanen, J., Bruun, M., and Markkanen, T. (1966). *Inheritance of Drinking Behaviors. A Study of Intelligence, Personality, and Use of Alcohol of Adult Twins.* Helsinki: The Finnish Foundation for Alcohol Studies.

Plato. *The Republic.* (1980). B. Jowett (trans.). Norwalk: The Easton Press, p. 252ff.

Reed, T. E. (1985). Ethnic differences in alcohol use, abuse, and sensitivity: A review with genetic interpretation. *Soc. Biol.* **32**:195–209.

Rodriguez, L. A., Wilson, J. R., and Nagoshi, C. T. (1993). Does psychomotor sensitivity to alcohol predict subsequent alcohol abuse? *Alcohol.: Clin. Exp. Res.* **17**, 155–161.

Schuckit, M. A. (1984). Subjective responses to alcohol in sons of alcoholics and control subjects. *Arch. Gen. Psychiatr.* **41**:879–884.

Schuckit, M. A. (1985). Ethanol-induced changes in body sway in men at high alcoholism risk. *Arch. Gen. Psychiatr.* **42**:375–379.

Searles, J. S. (1988). The role of genetics in the pathogenesis of alcoholism. *J. Abnorm. Psychol.* **97**:153–167.

Sutker, P. B., Goist, K. C., and King, A. R. (1987). Acute alcohol intoxication in women: Relationship to dose and menstrual cycle phase. *Alcohol.: Clin. Exp. Res.* **11**:74–79.

Sutker, P. B., Tabakoff, B., Goist, K. C., and Randal, C. L. (1983). Acute alcohol intoxication, mood states and alcohol metabolism in women and men. *Pharmacol. Biochem. Behav.* **18**:349–354.

Tarter, R. E., Hegedus, A. M., Goldstein, G., Shelly, C., and Alterman, A. I. (1984). Adolescent sons of alcoholics: Neuropsychologic and personality characteristics. *Alcohol.: Clin. Exp. Res.* **8**:216–222.

Vesell, E. S., Page, J. G., and Passananti, G. T. (1970). Genetic and environmental factors affecting ethanol metabolism in man. *Clin. Pharmacol. Ther.* **12**:192–201.

Wagner, J. G. (1973). Intrasubject variation in elimination half-lives of drugs which are appreciably metabolized. *J. Pharmacokinet. Biopharm.* **1**:165–173.

Wagner, J. G., and Patel, J. A. (1972). Variations in absorption and elimination rates of ethyl alcohol in a single subject. *Res. Commun. Chem. Pathol. Pharmacol.* **4**:61–76.

Whitfield, J. B., Starmer, G. A., and Martin, N. G. (1990). Alcohol metabolism in men and women. *Alcohol.: Clin. Exp. Res.* **14**:785–786.

Wilson, J. R. (1988). Individual differences in drug response. In *Biological Vulnerability to Drug Abuse,* R. W. Pickens and D. S. Svikis, eds. Rockville, MD: U.S. Department of Health and Human Services, pp. 93–107.

Wilson, J. R., and Nagoshi, C. T. (1987). One-month repeatability of alcohol metabolism, sensitivity and acute tolerance. *J. Stud. Alcohol* **48**:437–442.

Wilson, J. R., and Plomin, R. (1985). Individual differences in sensitivity and tolerance to alcohol. *Social Biol.* **32**:162–184.

Wilson, J. R., and Nagoshi, C. T. (1988). Adult children of alcoholics: Cognitive and psychomotor characteristics. *Br. J. Addict.* **83**:809–820.

Wilson, J. R., Erwin, V. G., and McClearn, G. E. (1984a). Effects of ethanol: I. Acute metabolic tolerance and ethnic differences. *Alcohol.: Clin. Exp. Res.* **8**:226–232.

Wilson, J. R., Erwin, V. G., DeFries, J. C., Petersen, D. R., and Cole-Harding, S. (1984b). Ethanol dependence in mice: Direct and correlated responses to ten generations of selective breeding. *Behav. Genet.* **14**:235–256.

Workman-Daniels, K. L., and Hesselbrock, V. M. (1987). Childhood problem behavior and neuropsychological functioning in persons at risk for alcoholism. *J. Stud. Alcohol* **48**:187–193.

Selective Breeding Studies

II

6

Genetic Influences on Alcohol Metabolism and Sensitivity to Alcohol in Animals

RICHARD A. DEITRICH AND
RODNEY C. BAKER

It has been recognized for millenia that there are individual differences in the reaction of humans to ethanol. Some people are "able to hold their liquor" while others "pass out with a whiff of the cork." That such individual variability exists in lower animals is a more recent observation that forms the basis for the work reviewed in this chapter.

Assuming equal access of ethanol to the blood stream and brain in two individuals or groups of individuals, there are several ways that individual variability in initial sensitivity to ethanol can arise. One possibility is that the central nervous system itself is differentially sensitive to the effects of ethanol. A second possibility is that one individual or group may simply get rid of the ethanol faster. Both of these possibilities have subleties associated with them that may not be readily apparent.

The central nervous system may have a resistance or sensitivity to the initial depressant effects of ethanol that is genetically determined. A complication often encountered in humans is the development of tolerance after long-term exposure to ethanol. This tolerance can be controlled in animal studies. However, there is also the problem of rapidly developing acute tolerance, that is, tolerance that develops within the period of effect of a single dose of ethanol. Genetic influences are just as likely to be exerted on this phenomenon as on initial sensitivity, but unless recognized, they will appear as initial sensitivity.

In a similar way, chronic tolerance to ethanol can develop because of increased metabolic activity, a factor that can be controlled in animals but not in human studies. Moreover, several metabolic pathways capable of metabolizing ethanol exist, and genetic influences on any of them are possible.

Methodology

The interacting effects of the three different modes of response to alcohol—initial sensitivity, the development of acute tolerance, and increased metabolic activity—all of which show similar clinical manifestations, make differentiation among them difficult. Toward that end, complex batteries of tests have been developed to establish independent measures for each parameter. The tests for initial sensitivity are most direct since they are based on the administration of a single dose of ethanol to a naive animal population. Those for the development of acute tolerance are more complex because they involve a test–retest situation after the administration of a single large dose or the sequential administration of two smaller doses. Rates of ethanol metabolism are routinely determined through blood alcohol levels.

Methods for Determining Initial Sensitivity to Ethanol

The battery for testing initial sensitivity to ethanol is necessarily complex because many different systemic responses are studied. A few, such as sleep time and hypothermic effect, are essentially physiological in nature and are most appropriate for testing the effects of large doses of alcohol. Most of the other tests are behavioral, involving more subtle distinctions in performance and as a result, are more effective in differentiating among the effects of smaller doses of ethanol.

The *sleep-time test* consists of determining the sleep time, that is, the time during which an animal is devoid of the righting response (Kakihana et al., 1966). The ethanol is given intraperitoneally, orally, by inhalation, or occasionally intravenously or subcutaneously. The time from administration of the dose, or from the loss of righting response, to the time of regaining the response is measured. Normally the criterion for this response is turning completely over three times within 30 or 60 seconds. Blood ethanol levels should be measured when the animals regain the righting response. With subcutaneous or oral administration that allows for slower absorption, both the time to loss of the righting response and the blood ethanol level at the point can be accurately determined. The sleep-time method will normally yield the highest blood ethanol levels at the point of regaining function since even after regaining the righting response, animals might not be able to accomplish any of the more demanding tasks discussed below.

The *aerial righting response* is carried out in the same way as the sleep time test, except that the righting response used as an end point, is the ability of the animal to right itself when dropped from a specified height onto a cushioned surface (Grant et al., 1989). Alternatively, the height from which the animal must be dropped in order for it to turn over is measured.

The *moving belt test* is used extensively by the Addiction Research Foundation in Toronto (see Campanelli et al., 1988, for an example). Rats are trained to walk on the moving belt and then injected with ethanol. The measure of ataxia is the time the animal spends off the moving belt. The advantage of this type of test is that it is a more sensitive measure of ataxia than either of the righting response tests; the disadvantage is that it requires an apparatus and training of the animals to a criterion level before the experiment.

The *inclined plane test* was used in a Finnish study to select rats for initial sensitivity differences (Eriksson and Rusi, 1981). In this task the rat is placed on a board one end of which is slowly raised. The angle is measured at which the animal begins to slide from the board. The difference between the angle of sliding before and after ethanol dosing is determined. Again an apparatus is required, but prior training is not necessary. In both of these tests, the blood ethanol is measured when the animals reach the control level of time on the belt or the control sliding angle.

The *roto-rod task* measures the ability of animals to maintain themselves on a rotating rod for a specified period of time. This task measures even lower levels of impairment than the preceding tests. A variant of this is the stationary *dowel,* wherein the animal is required to maintain itself on a small wooden dowel for a certain length of time (Gallaher et al., 1982). These tasks also require that the animal be trained beforehand, but it usually takes only a few trials to achieve a criterion level of performance (30 to 60 seconds on the roto-rod or dowel).

A somewhat different measure of ataxia is one that allows an animal to run down an enclosed corridor with a floor made of hardware cloth (Belknap, 1975). Under the hardware cloth is a detector of some type, usually a simple balance. Ethanol produces ataxia so that the animal can no longer keep its feet on the screen and the feet slip through to make contact with the balance surface. The number of slips is counted for a single trip through the corridor.

Both the roto-rod and dowel tasks have been used to measure acute tolerance because low doses can be administered and recovery of the ability occurs relatively rapidly.

At even lower doses of ethanol both mice (Crabbe, 1986) and to some extent rats (Brick et al., 1984; Lewis and June, 1990) show increased locomotor activity. Various tasks to detect this activation have been devised. The simplest is activity in a checkerboard arena where crossing of squares is counted. Several automated procedures are also available to detect increased activity. Animals are also being selectively bred for this trait, e.g., the Fast and Slow mice (Crabbe et al., 1990).

The *hypothermic effect* is another measure of acute sensitivity. Ethanol causes animals to lose body temperature, and the magnitude of the loss of heat following a dose of ethanol is genetically controlled. This effect has been used to selectively breed mice as well (Crabbe et al., 1990). The temperature drop is measured at times following the dose of ethanol and the area under the curve calculated.

Methods for Testing Acute Tolerance

The recognition that animals develop acute tolerance to the effects of ethanol came from a study by Mellanby (1919), who found that tasks capable of being performed at a certain point on a rising phase of the blood ethanol curve could be performed at a higher blood ethanol level on the falling phase of the curve. Any of the measures described earlier can be used to detect acute tolerance. Since they all involve different amounts of time to accomplish, however, the definition of *acute* becomes a problem. At first glance it is relatively simple: it is the tolerance that developes within the time frame of the effect of a single dose of ethanol. For large doses of ethanol, this period may be several hours, and the distinction between acute and chronic becomes somewhat fuzzy. Gallaher et al. (1982) demonstrated that tolerance could be measured using the dowel technique by first giving a low dose of ethanol and waiting until the ability to stay on the rod was regained. A second dose, half the amount of the first, was then given and the ability to remain on the dowel again measured. The difference in blood ethanol levels at time 1 and time 2 represent the amount of acute tolerance that has developed. Here two doses were given, but often several doses can be given before a plateau in the blood ethanol at regain-of-response is reached.

Nearly all of the measures of initial sensitivity can be contaminated by the presence of acute tolerance. Indeed, if acute tolerance develops within the time period of the measurement of initial sensitivity, it will simply be lost in that time. How short must the measure of acute tolerance be? Looking at the development of tolerance in the effect of ethanol on Purkinje cells, Sorensen et al. (1980) found that some of the cells from short-sleep (SS) mice developed acute tolerance within minutes. A similar finding was made by Palmer with Purkinje cells in the cerebellum of Low Alcohol Sensitive (LAS) rats (Palmer et al., 1991). Since we do not have a behavioral measure of initial sensitivity that can work in this time frame, we must try to devise a method to separate acute tolerance from initial sensitivity.

One way to separate the two is to trace a dose response curve using various doses of ethanol, and to determine the blood ethanol level at the time when the response in question is regained. Different doses of ethanol result in different periods before recovery of the response. The blood ethanol levels at regaining the response are plotted as a function of the time to regain that function. If there is a positive slope, it is a measure of the amount of acute tolerance that developed; the extrapolated intercept is the blood ethanol level at zero time to regain the response, i.e., ED_{100} for that response in units of blood level of ethanol. If no acute tolerance develops during the time that the response is absent, there will be no slope to the response; in fact, a negative slope would indicate sensitization, not tolerance. Such a procedure has been carried out for very young SS and long-sleep (LS) mice (Keir and Deitrich, 1990) where the response was sleep time.

A complicating factor has come to light as a result of such studies. This complication apparently arises because the dose response curve for the development of acute tolerance in mice is to the left of the dose response curve for sleep-time response. This is illustrated by theoretical curves in Fig. 6-1. It is possible that the failure to observe acute tolerance to sleep time in adult mice is due to the fact that the dose necessary to cause loss of the righting response is sufficient to produce all of the acute tolerance possible. The reason that acute tolerance is more easily observed in young mice is that the anesthetic dose is much smaller and in the range of the dose required to produce acute tolerance.

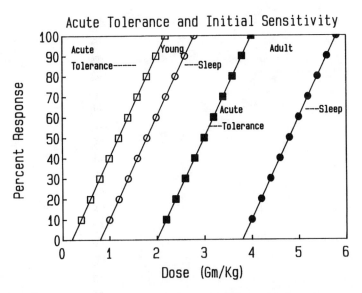

Fig. 6-1 Theoretical curves for dose–response relationships for sleep time and acute tolerance in very young and adult mice.

Blood Alcohol Measurement

Another complicating factor in acute tolerance studies is the measurement of blood ethanol. The most accurate procedure is to measure brain ethanol, but since this requires sacrifice of the animal it is not practical. We need an ethanol concentration determination both at the loss and at the regain of the response in many of the methods; blood ethanol must therefore be taken at these two time points. The conclusions then are based on the assumption that there is an equilibrium between brain and blood ethanol. This equilibrium requires considerable time if the blood is obtained from the tail (Goldstein, 1983); however, if it is obtained from the retroorbital sinus, blood and brain blood ethanol content comes to equilibrium within a few minutes (Fig. 6-2).

Genetic Strategies for Mechanistic Studies of the Initial Sensitivity to Alcohol

General Considerations

There are a number of procedures for analyzing the mechanisms by which genes influence initial sensitivity to ethanol. It should be realized, however, that not all behavioral responses to ethanol will show demonstrable genetic differences in any given animal model. Nor will genetic differences found in one animal model necessarily be discovered in another. This extends, of course, to humans as well. Likewise, the fact that we discover a genetic heterogeneity in behavioral responses to ethanol in one animal model does not mean that it must exist in any other animals nor in humans. If this is so, why then would one wish to study the genetics of a behavioral response in mice, for example, if it has not been shown that a similar polymorphism also exists in humans? The answer, of course, is that such a genetic heterogeneity in animals gives us a pow-

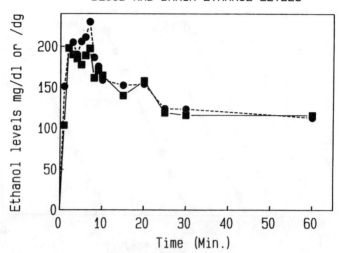

Fig. 6-2 Blood ■ and brain ● ethanol levels in mice following 1.75 g/kg ethanol injected intraperitoneally.

erful tool to understand how ethanol affects behavior in another animal, even if there is little or no genetic variability in that other species with regard to the effect. In practical terms, another consideration is that the discovery of the location of a gene on the mouse chromosome gives us a starting place to look for a similar gene on the corresponding human chromosome because of the synteny between the human and mouse chromosomes.

What are the genetic tools that have been used in such studies? The usual studies involved the investigation of differences between inbred strains of animals to see how their initial sensitivity to ethanol differed. While inbred strain comparisons are an excellent place to start, there are a number of drawbacks to such studies. The most often quoted disadvantage is the fact that all the genes in an inbred strain are fixed randomly and thus give rise to fortuitous associations that may have nothing to do with the mechanism under study. If a sufficient number of inbred strains are investigated, then one can learn something about the mechanism by carrying out linkage studies.

There is, however, another method by which to discover meaningful associations between behavior and mechanism. This is the process of selective breeding, which has been widely used in the alcohol field. In this process a genetically heterogenous population of animals (preferably one made up by crossing several inbred strains, usually eight) is used. The selection of the inbred strains to go into the base population is made on the basis of differences between the strains in the behavioral trait to be selected for and the independent genetic history of the strains. This base population is tested by one of the methods mentioned earlier and the low responders and the high responders identified. These animals are then bred within each group, always selecting the extreme animals to be the parents of the next generation. This process has a number of different ways in which separation of behavioral traits can be accomplished: the number of breeding pairs per generation, whether within-family or mass selection is used, and the amount of selection pressure that is applied, to name but three. All these variables will influence the speed and extent to which differences between selected lines can be achieved. These differences are discussed in detail elsewhere (DeFries, 1981).

The process of selection on a polygenic behavioral trait is made on the basis of slowly gathering all the alleles that contribute to the upward direction in one line and all the alleles that contribute to the downward direction in the other. The more important genetic factors, i.e., those that contribute more strongly to the trait, will be present in those animals that are higher or lower in that trait to begin with, and thus will be pulled into the parents for the next generation at earlier time points in the selection. This is why it is important to test suspected mechanisms throughout the selection process, even when there may be no statistical difference in the behavior between lines. By the time that the selection is complete, even very minor players on the genetic stage will have been selected and it is more difficult at that point to tell the bit players from the leading actors when they take their curtain bows together. If we pay attention earlier, the leading actors take their bows alone.

The process of selective breeding is a constant but losing battle against the random fixation of genes. The larger the selection population, the longer it takes. But given a finite population, eventually some genes that have nothing to do with behavioral sensitivity are going to be fixed in the high or low lines. Paradoxically, until that occurs, the animals are extremely valuable, primarily for ruling *out* possible mechanisms. If the animals differ behaviorally but do not differ in some physiological or biochemical function, that function cannot be involved in the genetic differences between lines. This is not to say that the mechanism might not be important for the actions of ethanol; it is just that there is no *discernable* genetic heterogeneity in the system in that particular group of animals. A corollary to this line of reasoning involves the use of inbred strains where all genes have been fixed at random. Comparison of any two strains can *only rule out* mechanisms if the behavioral response is different and the biochemical measures are not different. Otherwise, the only useful information provided is of the nature of preliminary experiments that need to be carried out in a number of other inbred strains or with individual animals of a heterogenous stock.

For example, there is the study of Durkin et al. (1982) in which they used C56Bl/6 and Balb/c mice to study the effect of ethanol on choline acetyltransferase and the kinetics of choline uptake into the P2 fraction of the striatum and hippocampus. They found that acute treatment of the mice with ethanol produced rapid inhibition of the V_{max} of high-affinity choline uptake only in the striatum of the C57 mice. In the hippocampus, inhibition of high-affinity choline uptake V_{max} *was found for both strains.* Thus the only firm conclusion that can be drawn concerning the differences in the many behavioral response differences to ethanol in these two strains is that the choline uptake in the hippocampus is *not* involved in these behavioral differences. We have no idea whether or not the differences in high-affinity choline uptake in the striatum is correlated with ethanol's behavioral actions, because this difference may have been fixed randomly and be completely unrelated to the behavioral differences in responses to ethanol.

Table 6-1 Quantitative Genetic Correlations between Ethanol Responses in Rats and Mice

	1	2	3	4	5	6	7	8
1. Sleep time	1	−.76[a][a] −.22[b]	−.51[a] −.35[b]	.03[c]	−.2[c] −.38[g][a]	−.89[d][a] −.79[e][a]	.9[h][a]	
2. Preference		1	.71[a][a] .47[b][a]					
3. Acute tolerance			1					
4. Hypothermia				1	−.15c			.5[f][a]
5. Locomotor activation					1			
6. Cerebellar Purkinje cell sensitivity						1		
7. Convulsive sensitivity							1	
8. Ataxia								1

(a) Spuhler and Deitrich (1984): Inbred rats
(b) Erwin et al. (1980): HS mice
(c) Erwin et al. (1990): RI LSXSS
(d) Spuhler et al. (1982): Inbred mice
(e) Palmer et al. (1987): HAS, LAS rats
(f) Crabbe (1983): Inbred mice
(g) Erwin, personal communication, RI LSXSS
(h) Peris et al. (1989): RI LSXSS

[a]p < .05 at least.

If a difference between lines or strains is found, it must be confirmed in some other genetic model to avoid the possibility that it is the product of random fixation of genes for that system differentially in the two lines. The existence of replicate control lines and replicate selection lines for selective breeding is the preferred procedure. Inbred strains can be used, or if recombinant strains between two lines or strains exist, they can be used to great advantage. Perhaps even more convincing is evidence of the existence of the identified difference in another species altogether (see Table 6-1).

High-Dose Sensitivity

One of the oldest selection studies is that of SS and LS mice begun by McClearn and Kakihana in the 1960s (Kakihana et al., 1966; McClearn and Kakihana, 1981). Observations of these animals have advanced our knowledge not only about the reasons for the behavioral differences but also about how alcohol depresses the central nervous system. The results from the use of these animals have been reviewed in detail recently, so only the highlights will be covered here (Deitrich, 1990).

The marked difference in sleep time present at generation 16 of the selection between SS and LS mice was initially postulated to be due to a difference in metabolic rates. Early experiments apparently dispelled this possibility (Heston et al., 1974). Subsequently, following further selection and a different dose for selection of SS and LS mice, some differences in metabolism of ethanol were found (Smolen et al., 1986). This result is probably due to two factors: a difference in volume of distribution between the lines, and a lower body temperature in the alcohol-treated LS mice, which in turn slows the rate of ethanol metabolism (Romm and Collins, 1987). The measure of blood ethanol at the time of regain of the righting response is a way to avoid the problem of differential metabolic rates. This measure also shows that there is a marked difference in the brain sensitivity to ethanol between these two lines (Erwin et al., 1976).

A number of observations have been made with regard to neurotransmitter receptor system differences between the lines and in other selectively bred lines, as well as in inbred and outbred animal models. The most interesting differences have to do with the GABA, adenosine, nicotinic, and adrenergic receptor systems. While a great deal of information is available concerning neurotransmitter systems (Deitrich, 1990), the discussion here is confined to those aspects that appear to have the best chance of explaining some of the central nervous system depressant effects of ethanol.

Genetics of the GABA System. The GABA system is generally regarded as the major inhibitory neurotransmitter system in the brain. If ethanol were to interact with such a system, it would presumably augment the effects of GABA agonists and GABA antagonists counteract the effects of ethanol. This reasoning led to early tests of this thesis, which amply confirmed it. Although there were earlier studies on the interactions of GABA active drugs and ethanol (Hakkinen and Kulonen, 1976), the first use of genetic models was in the demonstration by Martz et al. (1983) that LS mice were more affected by THIP (4,5,6,7-tetrahydroisoxazole (5,4-*c*) pyridin (3-*ol*) and baclofen (a GABAb agonist) than were SS mice.

With the advent of studies of radioactive chloride uptake into synaptoneurosomes (Allan and Harris, 1986; Suzdak, et al., 1986), it became possible to study the actions of ethanol on the GABA system in an in vitro system. These investigators confirmed the idea that ethanol potentiated GABA actions, but at a more fundamental level. Allan and Harris (1986) found that mice selected for ethanol sensitivity also had differences in the in vitro sensitivity to the effects of ethanol on chloride uptake. A convincing confirmation came in the finding that rats bred in a similar protocol to be sensitive or resistant to ethanol (High Alcohol Sensitive [HAS] and Low Alcohol Sensitive [LAS] rats) were likewise differentially sensitive to the in vitro effects of ethanol on the GABA chloride channel (Allan et al., 1991). Even mice from an unselected population of heterogenous mice (HS) used to develop the LS and SS lines had differential responses to the effects of ethanol on the GABA system when they were chosen from the extremes of a population distribution of mice sensitive or resistant to the actions of ethanol (Allan et al., 1988a). Interestingly, genetic selection for benzodiazepine ataxia results in functional changes in the chloride channel as well (Allan et al., 1988b).

The availability of the frog oocyte expression system afforded an elegant technique by which these results could be further pursued. It was found that when mRNA from LS mouse brain was injected into frog oocytes there was an increased sensitivity to ethanol-facilitated GABA responses, but there was an inhibition of this response in eggs injected with mRNA from SS mouse brain (Wafford et al., 1990). Interestingly, there was no difference in the responses of these oocytes to barbiturates or GABA itself.

Simultaneously studies were being carried out on the genes that code for the various components of the GABA receptor; this was done on the assumption that such marked functional differences could well be due to alterations in the structural genes coding for one or more of the subunits of the GABA receptor. The first attempts at demonstrating this were disappointing since there was no difference between SS and LS mice in the sequence of the gene coding for the alpha-1 subunit of the GABA receptor (Keir et al., 1991). Subsequent studies, however, clearly demonstrated that the gamma subunit conferred ethanol sensitivity on oocytes injected with mRNA from LS mouse brain. This was first demonstrated by the use of antisense sequences to various subunits. It was found that only the antisense sequence to the gamma subunit abolished the sensitivity to ethanol augmentation of GABA-mediated chloride currents in these oocytes (Wafford et al., 1991). Subsequently this fact was demonstrated directly by injecting oocytes with sequences coded for the alpha, beta, and gamma subunits. A major discovery was made when it was found that the gamma subunit came in two forms, due to alternate splicing. One form, the long form (gamma 2L), had an extra eight amino acids on the putative intracellular loop of the receptor. Only when the gamma 2L form of the cRNA was injected into oocytes along with alpha-1 and beta-1 subunit cRNA was ethanol sensitivity found. When the short form of the gamma 2 subunit, lacking this sequence was used, no ethanol sensitivity was present. Expression of either gamma 2 short (25) *or* gamma 2L along with alpha-1 and beta-1 cRNA resulted in GABA responses enhanced by both diazepam and pentobarbital. More importantly the gamma 2L subunit contains a consensus sequence for protein kinase C phosphorylation. It is not known whether or not protein kinase C will, in fact, phosphorylate this site in vivo. It is known that mutation of the serine in the sequence to an alanine abolishes ethanol sensitivity (Wafford and Whiting, 1992).

The obvious question now is whether the SS and LS mice differ in the gamma 2S and gamma 2L subunit. Preliminary data suggest that this may not be the case since both LS and SS mice contain mRNA for the gamma 2L in the cortex and cerebellum. A firm conclusion on this point must await analysis of the protein from gamma 2L and gamma 2S mRNA in the brains of these mice (Wafford et al., 1991).

Another interesting series of experiments that implicate phosphorylation in the sensitivity of GABA receptors to ethanol have been carried out by Lin and co-workers (1991, 1993a, 1993b). In these experiments, cerebellar Purkinje cell firing was recorded from rats. GABA application slowed the rate of firing, and application of isoproterenol somewhat augmented the GABA-mediated firing rate depression. Addition of ethanol in the presence of isoproterenol greatly potentiated the depression of firing rates, while addition of ethanol in the absence of isoproterenol had no effect on the GABA-mediated depression of firing rate. One explanation of these effects is that activation of the beta-adrenergic receptors and subsequent activation of protein kinase A are somehow involved in the interaction between GABA and ethanol.

Similarly, Liu et al. (1992) found that the dopamine D2 receptor subtypes D2long and D2short were differentially sensitive to phosphorylation by protein kinase C. Given the putative role of the dopamine D2 receptor in alcoholism (Pato et al., 1993), these results take on significance for the actions of ethanol.

It is possible that, at least for some receptors, we will find that ethanol has little if any direct effect on the receptor, but brings about its effects by acting on protein kinases, phosphatases, or other posttranslational events. Thus we may find an "ethanol cascade" effect. As a consequence of this possibility, Quantative Trait Loci (QTL) studies may show a marked association of the actions of ethanol with the gene for one of these enzymes rather than with the gene for the receptor itself.

GABA Studies with Other Anesthetics. As a corollary to the effects of ethanol, the effects of other anesthetic agents including the barbiturates have been evaluated by using genetically selected lines of animals. Since the barbiturates also affect the GABA system, it was logical to assume that reactions to them would be in the same direction as reactions to ethanol in the selected lines of animals. Initial experiments indicated that this was not the case; in fact, the reverse was true, i.e., LS mice were less sensitive to pentobarbital than were SS mice (Erwin et al., 1976). This view was later challenged (Alpern and McIntyre, 1985). An early explanation for the differences in reactions of SS and LS mice to the barbiturates was that the two lines had different rates of metabolism for barbiturates but that the brain barbiturate levels upon awakening were similar (O'Connor et al., 1982). The matter was finally put to rest by Howerton et al. (1984), who demonstrated that pentobarbital- and ethanol-induced sleep time sensitivities segregated differently in the F2 cross between SS and LS mice. Later Allan and Harris (1989) got similar results in the HS mice, showing that sensitivities to ethanol and pentobarbital did not cosegregate. Finally, the fact that oocytes expressing GABA subunits adequate for augmentation of GABA responses to pentobarbital, but not ethanol, argues against the idea that pentobarbital sensitivity is genetically related to ethanol sensitivity in these mice (Wafford et al., 1991).

The question of whether or not the gaseous anesthetics have the same mechanism of action as ethanol has also been investigated using selectively bred lines of mice. Initially it was found that the SS and LS mice were equally sensitive to ether (Erwin et al., 1976). Since ether is a relatively slow acting anesthetic and requires a long period to come to equilibrium, the experiment was repeated with the more potent halothane. Again it was found that the SS and LS mice did not differ in response to this anesthetic (Baker et al., 1980). A somewhat different conclusion was reached by Koblin and Deady (1981), who found that there was a 34% and a 20% greater requirement respectively, for nitrous oxide and enflurane concentration for the loss of righting response in SS than in LS mice. Marley et al. (1986) carried out a large study on the sensitivity of SS and LS mice to various hypnotics, and found that there was a good correlation between the difference in sensitivity of SS and LS mice and the oil/water solubility quotient. The more water soluble the agent, the greater the difference in sleep time between the two lines. This series did not include any of the gaseous anesthetics, however.

More recently, two studies have been completed with gaseous anesthetics. In both cases brain levels of the anesthetics at regain of the righting response were measured. The HAS and LAS rats were found to be differentially sensitive to enflurane, isoflurane, and halothane (Deitrich et al., 1994). A similar study carried out with SS and LS mice (Simpson, personal communication) found that the lines were differentially sensitive to isoflurane, but confirming earlier studies of Baker et al (1980) they are not differentially sensitive to halothane.

Other Studies in the GABA System. Many of the mechanisms as to why SS and LS mice might differ in their response to ethanol in the GABA system have been explored. Some of these have been investigated, but the studies have either found no difference between the lines or they have not been followed up vigorously. For example, the binding of flunitrazepam does not differ in brain membranes from SS and LS mice (Harris and Allan, 1989) even though there are marked differences between the sensitivity of these membranes to the augmentation of mucimol-stimulated-chloride flux. This discovery led to the suggestion that there is a difference in the two lines of mice in the coupling of the receptors to the chloride channel.

Another finding is that there are physical differences between the GABA and benzodiazepine receptors in SS and LS mice. Marley et al. (1988) found that GABA protected benzodiazepine receptors from heat inactivation more effectively in LS than in SS mice, although again there was no difference in the flunitrazepam binding to these receptors. Similarly, McIntyre et al. (1988) found that benzodiazepine receptors from LS mice were more rapidly heat inactivated, but that GABA was *less,* rather than more, effective in LS membranes in protecting against heat inactivation. Both Marley and Wehner (1986) and McIntyre et al. (1988) found that GABA enhancement of flunitrazepam binding was greater in SS than in LS mouse brain cortex.

Other areas of investigation are the release and uptake of GABA from neurons as well as turnover of GABA (Hellevuo and Kiianmaa, 1989). Howerton and Collins (1984) found that ethanol inhibited K^+-stimulated GABA release at a lower concentration in LS than in SS cortical slices, though spontaneous release was the same in LS and SS cortical slices. While ethanol inhibited GABA uptake into cortical and cerebellar slices, it did so equally in SS and LS brain slices (Howerton et al., 1982).

In rats selectively bred for ethanol-induced ataxia, the alcohol tolerant (AT) and alcohol nontolerant (ANT) lines, the ANT rats had a higher concentration of GABA in the striatum and a higher rate of GABA turnover than the AT rats. However, ethanol suppressed the turnover of GABA to a greater degree in the AT than in the ANT rats (Hellevuo and Kiianmaa, 1989). This is in contrast to the results of Howerton and Collins (1984) (see above), who found that while ethanol suppressed the release of GABA from slices, it did so equally in SS and LS mouse brains. The AT and ANT rats also showed differential behavioral effects to barbital (Hellevuo et al., 1989). Rats selected for high and low ethanol sleep times differ in response to pentobarbital as well (Draski et al., 1991; Deitrich et al., 1994), which would indicate a fundamental difference between mice and rats in the structure and function of the GABA receptor. In mice the barbiturate site would be uncoupled from the ethanol site, but in rats the opposite would be true.

Recently an extensive comparison between selectively bred rat and mouse lines with regard to cerebellar GABAa receptors has been carried out by Uusi-Oukari and Korpi (1991). They found that AT rats had more high affinity muscimol binding sites in the cerebellum than did ANT rats, and that Ro15-4513 was displaced from its binding sites by benzodiazepine agonists at lower concentrations in ANT than AT rats. However, these results were confined to the AT and ANT rats and were not found in the LS/SS, HAS/LAS rats, Hot/Cold mice, Fast/Slow mice, nor in the AA/ANA rats.

Since, of this group of selectively bred animals, the AT and ANT rats are the only ones selected for low levels of ataxia, these results may be a consequence of the selection process. Confirmation would await a correlative study between the potency of ethanol in causing ataxia and the in vitro binding data in an F2 cross of the AT and ANT rats or in *individual* rats from the mixed (M) line from which the AT and ANT rats were derived.

The AT and ANT rats also do not differ in ethanol sleep times or in hypothermic reaction to ethanol. This would indicate that these traits did not cosegregate with ethanol ataxia in this selection process (Kiianmaa et al., 1988). The HAS and LAS rats do not differ in hypothermic reactions to low doses of ethanol (Draski et al., 1991), but do differ at higher doses of ethanol (deFiebre et al., 1991).

Low-Dose Sensitivity

This selective breeding protocol was started in order to develop two lines of mice that differed markedly in the activating effects of low-dose ethanol (Crabbe et al., 1990). The procedure is to inject a mouse with a dose of saline (control) or, on another day, a dose of 2 g/kg of ethanol. The number of line crossings in an open arena are counted. The difference between the activity recorded after saline injection and that after ethanol injection is the score for that animal. The base stock was the HS population from the Institute of Behavioral Genetics. The lines do not differ in response to saline injections. This is an important facet of the selection since it is possible to select for open field activity by itself (DeFries, 1981). While separation between the lines has been accomplished, it was largely obtained in the first generation when the order of testing was saline followed by ethanol. When the order of testing was the opposite, i.e., ethanol followed by saline, there was an increase in activity in all lines and a greater separation between the lines. The animal response to correlated ethanol-invoked measures of depression usually show that the Fast mice are relatively more impaired than the Slow mice. Responses to pentobarbital, diazepam, and d-amphetamine were variable between the two selections. There was no difference in ethanol-induced hypothermia between the lines (Crabbe et al., 1990).

This same group has selectively bred mice, again from the HS stock, for hypothermic response to ethanol (Crabbe et al., 1990). In this case a dose of 3g/kg ethanol was used as the selection dose and was temperature measured at 30 and 60 minutes. Animals that reacted with a marked decrease in temperature were termed the Cold lines, and those that reacted with a more modest or with no temperature drop were designated the Hot lines. It appears that the selection is primarily in the cold direction since the control mice nearly parallel the Hot mice. A differences in rates of metabolism is an important complication since Romm and Collins et al. (1987) have shown that the greater hypothermic effect in LS mice can account for a considerable amount of the difference in ethanol metabolism between the LS and SS mice. In the case of the Cold and Hot mice, it was found that the Hot mice did metabolize ethanol somewhat faster, but only at higher doses of ethanol (Crabbe et al., 1990). Other central nervous system depressants also elicited a difference in the hypothermic response between these two lines. Several straight-chain alcohols, pentobarbital, phenobarbital, methyprylon, ethchlorvynol, and diazepam all elicited a differential effect on body temperature in the Hot and Cold mice. There was a difference to hydralazine after 12 but not after 7 selected generations (Feller and Crabbe, 1991).

Sensitivity to Convulsions

Early studies by Sanders and Sharpless (1978) and Greer and Alpern (1978) using the convulsant gaseous agent, flurothyl, found that SS mice were more susceptible to clonus than were LS mice. Similar findings with the convulsant bicuculline have been found by two groups. One, Peris et al. (1989), found that LS mice were less sensitive than SS mice. There was a significant negative correlation between time to bicuculline-induced clonus and B_{max} for TBPS binding in the colliculi of SS and LS mice and five of the LSXSS recombinant strains. That is, there is an increased binding of TBPS in those mice (SS and SS-like RI strains) that are *more* sensitive to bicuculline seizures. The other, Phillips et al. (1989), obtained similar results in their stock of SS and LS mice with bicuculline and picrotoxin. There was no correlation between TBPS binding and ethanol-induced sleep time in these same lines and strains of mice (Peris et al., 1989). There appears to be a significant correlation ($p < .005$) between sleep time and time to bicuculline-induced clonus in this study (data recalculated from Peris et al., 1989). Susceptibility to bicuculline seizures was increased in both LS and SS mice after adrenalectomy (Bowers et al., 1990).

On the other hand, Tuominen et al. (1990) using the ANT and AT lines of rats found that the ANT rats (corresponding to the LS mice) were *more* rather than less susceptible to seizures induced by 3-mercaptopropionate, which depletes the brain of GABA. The difference was in the final seizure score at a dose of 50 g/kg of 3-mercaptopropionate and not in the latency for a score of 1 or 2.

It is difficult to conclude that the seizure susceptibilities of rats and mice, both selected for initial sensitivity to ethanol, are different since different convulsive agents were used. In the case of 3-mercaptopropionate, brain levels of GABA are decreased, and presumably all GABA receptors are deprived of the endogenous agonist. In the case of bicuculline, its binding is probably to only one receptor subunit type. The other aspect to be considered is that there may indeed be a qualitative difference in the GABA receptor function between mice and rats.

Genetic Correlations in Sensitivity Studies

Crabbe (1983) did not find any significant genetic correlation between duration of the loss of the righting reflex (sleep time) and open field activity, loss of balance, locomotor ataxia, home cage activity, home cage ataxia after ethanol, activity decrease, or hypothermic response among a group of 20 inbred strains of mice. There were significant correlations between (1) home cage activity at baseline versus baseline temperature and versus hypothermic response to ethanol; and (2) home cage ataxia versus hypothermia and versus home cage activity decrease.

As seen in Table 6-1, sleep time correlates with preference in rats but not in mice, with cerebellar Purkinje cell sensitivity in both mice and rats, and with convulsive sensitivity in mice. While ataxia to ethanol correlates with hypothermia in inbred strains of mice, it does not correlate with sleep time. Locomotor activation correlates negatively with sleep time in LSXSS RI strains, but at a low level, not being significant in one study and just significant in another from the same laboratory. One of the more robust correlations is between acute tolerance and preference, which is found in both mice and rats. Waller et al. (1983) found that the alcohol-prefering (P) rats develop acute tolerance more rapidly or to a different degree than do nonpreferring (NP) rats. While it is not possible to calculate genetic correlations in such an experiment, it is consistent with those experiments where correlations between preference and acute tolerance were calculated.

One of the highest correlations found in mice is between sleep time and convulsive sensitivity precipitated by bicuculline, a GABAa antagonist. Given the relationship of GABAa and ethanol actions found in both mice and rats, this is perhaps not surprising. The general conclusions that one can draw from such results is that there are relatively few correlations between various measures of acute sensitivity to ethanol that hold across two species. We are left with Purkinje cell sensitivity correlating with sleep time and acute tolerance correlating with preference for across species studies. The lack of more significant correlations cannot be taken as proof that none exist, just that relatively few have been tested in both mice and rats, and essentially none have been tested in other species.

Genetic Influence on Metabolism of Alcohol

Genetic Correlations between Metabolism and Sensitivity

The metabolism of ethanol is generally considered to be dependent on alcohol and aldehyde dehydrogenase activity (Havre et al., 1977; Crabb et al., 1983; Crabb et al., 1987). Two other pathways, one dependent on the peroxidative activity of catalase and the second dependent on the activity of the microsomal cytochrome P-450, have been proposed as responsible for alcohol dehydrogenase independent ethanol oxidation (Hasumura et al., 1975; Shigeta et al., 1984; Krikun et al., 1984; Glassman et al., 1985; Handler and Thurman, 1985; Handler et al., 1986; Lieber et al., 1987; Knecht et al., 1990). Direct studies between genotype and ethanol elimination rates have centered on alcohol dehydrogenase, although catalase or cytochrome P-450 might make an overall contribution. Genetic variance of ethanol elimination has been demonstrated in both rats and mice. The reported heritability estimates of ethanol elimination rates cover a wide range, from .16 (mice) and .17 (rats) (Gibson and Oakeshott, 1981) to over .90 (rats) (Thurman, 1980). A heritability estimate for alcohol elimination rates across the eight inbred strains used to construct the outbred HS/Ibg line of mice was found to be .49 (Petersen, personal communication). The mice used in this study were all maintained under identical conditions and given the same dose (3 g/kg) of ethanol. There is a significant ($p < .05$) phenotypic correlation ($r = -.75$) between the rate of ethanol metabolism (Petersen, personal communication) and sleep time (Spuhler et al., 1982) in these eight inbred strains.

The correlation between sleep time and ethanol metabolism is not significant in the eight inbred strains of rats used to make up the N/Nih line of rats; however, ($r = -.43$) (Spuhler and Deitrich, 1984). The dose of alcohol has been shown to affect ethanol elimination rate; in addition, inbred rodent strains respond differently to higher doses of ethanol (Petersen and Atkinson, 1980; Thurman et al., 1983; Glassman et al., 1985; Smolen et al., 1986; Smolen and Smolen, 1989). Considering the differential effect of blood ethanol concentration on elimination rates, it is most likely that if the heritability of ethanol elimination in these inbred rodent strains was determined at a second ethanol dose, a different estimate of heritability would be obtained.

Genetic Influences in Alcohol Dehydrogenase Activities

The alcohol dehydrogenases belong to a family of enzymes that are differentially expressed in separate tissues and in individual inbred mouse strains. At least three genes (Adh-1, Adh-2, and Adh-3) encode mouse alcohol dehydrogenase. The three isozymes are designated ADH-A$_2$, ADH-B$_2$, ADH-C$_2$, and exist as dimeric tissue-specific enzymes (Burnett and Felder, 1978; Balak et al., 1982; Holmes, 1985; Rex et al., 1987b; Tussey and Felder, 1989). For mouse alcohol dehydrogenase, ADH-A$_2$ is the primary isozyme implicated in the metabolism of ethanol. Two different forms of ADH-A$_2$ have been identified, ADH-A$_2^1$ and ADH-A$_2^2$. All common inbred mouse strains have the ADH-A$_2^1$ isozyme, since the ADH-A$_2^2$ has only been identified in the Danish (Skive) strain of mice (Rex et al., 1987a). Since the modification is not in the active site and is reported not to influence the oxidation of ethanol, the genotypic-dependent differences in alcohol dehydrogenase activity must be due to the quantity of the enzyme rather that the type (Rex et al., 1987a).

Genetic determination of mouse liver alcohol dehydrogenase synthesis was demonstrated by Balak et al. (1982). These investigators reported a twofold difference in liver alcohol dehydrogenase activity among 10 inbred strains of mice. A locus was identified (Adh-1-t) that contributed to the variation in liver alcohol dehydrogenase activity (Balak et al., 1982; Tussey and Felder, 1989). In another study, genotype-dependent expression of alcohol dehydrogenase as well as differences in the development of alcohol dehydrogenase activity was also reported in six inbred mouse strains (Wang and Singh, 1985).

Although genotype-specific expression of alcohol dehydrogenase is well established in the mouse, a direct relationship between alcohol dehydrogenase activity and ethanol elimination rates is not supported by all studies. Rachamin reported a correlation coefficient of .77 between the rate of ethanol elimination and the activity of alcohol dehydrogenase in C57BL/6 mice, DBA/2 mice, Sprague Dawley, and SH rats (Rachamin and Israel, 1985). A very complex genotype-dependent rate of ethanol elimination was demonstrated for ARK/J, DBA/2J, C$_3$H/HeJ, and C57BL/6J mice (Thurman et al., 1982). The rate of ethanol elimination in these mice was influenced by blood ethanol levels differentially in each strain such that if the strains were ranked in order of increasing ethanol elimination rates, each of the five blood ethanol concentrations would produce a different order (Thurman et al., 1982). Differences in ethanol metabolism between female and male C57BL6/ibg or BALB mice could not be explained on the basis of liver alcohol dehydrogenase activity (Collins et al., 1975). In addition, in several species and strains, the rate of ethanol metabolism may be limited by the rate of mitochondrial reoxidation of NADH (Videla et al., 1975; Rachamin and Israel, 1985).

Environmental factors have been shown to significantly influence total liver alcohol dehydrogenase activity, which in turn may obscure genetic components of ethanol elimination. In fact, studies in which the level of liver alcohol dehydrogenase has been manipulated by environmental conditions, have furnished the most convincing evidence linking ethanol elimination rates to total alcohol dehydrogenase activity. Crabb et al. (1983) determined that the kinetic parameters of alcohol dehydrogenase from fed and fasted rats was identical and that the difference in ethanol elimination rates could be totally accounted for by differences in liver alcohol dehydrogenase activity. The difference in elimination rates observed between high and low ethanol doses can be accounted for by substrate or product inhibition of alcohol dehydrogenase (Crow, 1985). In contrast, no correlation between the rate of ethanol metabolism and alcohol dehydrogenase activity could be demonstrated in the suckling rat (Zorzano and Herrera, 1989) or between several animal species (Zorzano and Herrera, 1989; Zorzano and Herrera, 1990).

Aldehyde dehydrogenase activity has been reported to be the rate-limiting factor in the metabolism of acetaldehyde oxidation (Svanas and Weiner, 1985). In addition, a threefold difference in the rate of aldehyde dehydrogenase activity between inbred strains of mice has been reported (Sheppard et al., 1970). However, there is no evidence that aldehyde dehydrogenase activity determines ethanol elimination rates. Interestingly, a strong correlation between ethanol elimination rates and the low Km (cytosolic) aldehyde dehydrogenase was found in eight inbred mouse strains (Petersen, personal communication). Significant ($p < .05$) correlations of .86 and .76 were found between ethanol elimination rates and low Km cytosolic and high Km cytosolic aldehyde dehydrogenase, respectively, using eight inbred mouse strains plus an outbred mouse line (HS/Ibg) derived from the eight inbred strains. The study suggests a close link between the high Km enzyme and genetic determinants of alcohol elimination, but it is unlikely that the cytosolic aldehyde dehydrogenase is kinetically involved, since this enzyme contributes little to the metabolism of acetaldehyde.

The rate of ethanol metabolism is influenced by dose and prior ethanol exposure, and the extent of both is influenced by the genotype of the experimental animal (Lieber et al., 1975; Thurman et al., 1982; Thurman et al., 1983; Glassman et al., 1985; Wilson et al., 1986). Thurman reported a range in ethanol elimination in outbred female Sprague-Dawley rats from 11.7 to 4.1 mmoles of ethanol/kg/hr, and in male rats from 8.0 g/kg/hr to 2.2 g/kg/hr. The elimination rate was repeated three weeks later. The ethanol elimination rate determined in the second test was found not to vary more than 10% from the original value determined for each individual animal (Thurman, 1980). The same rats were given one 5 g/kg dose of ethanol via gastric intubation and the ethanol elimination rate measured 14 hours later with a 2.5 g/kg dose. The ethanol elimination rate in the treated rats ranged from the same as initially determined to over a 400% increase.

Pairs of animals showing no adaptive increase were bred, as was a pair with a high adaptive increase in ethanol metabolism. The ethanol elimination rate was determined in the offspring. Heritability of .88 to .93 was determined for no adaptive increase; heritabilities of .36 to .64 were found in the high adaptive increase offspring. An increase in ethanol metabolism following 4 hours of ethanol treatment via vapor in four inbred mouse strains was also reported (Thurman et al., 1982). The authors suggested that genotype was a major determinate of the increase in ethanol metabolism in these four inbred mouse strains. An increase in alcohol dehydrogenase-dependent ethanol oxidation was suggested as the mechanism of the immediate increase in ethanol metabolism (Glassman et al., 1985).

Genetic Influences in Other Alcohol Metabolizing Systems

Genotype-specific induction of the microsomal ethanol oxidation has also been demonstrated in mouse lines selected for differential acute sensitivity to ethanol. Microsomal alcohol oxidation is increased in the alcohol-resistant, SS line upon treatment with 3-methylcholanthrene, whereas the alcohol-sensitive, LS line does not respond to 3-methylcholanthrene treatment (French et al., 1979). The LS and SS mice did not differ in the rate of ethanol elimination, however (Petersen and Atkinson, 1980; Hjelle et al., 1981).

Deer mice (*Peromyscus maniculatus*) offer a unique genetic model to investigate the role of alcohol dehydrogenase independent ethanol metabolism. Deer mouse strains have been identified (Burnett and Felder, 1978; Burnett and Felder, 1980), one of which lacks liver alcohol dehydrogenase (Adh^n/Adh^n) (ADH^-), while another corresponding strain (Adh^f/Adh^f) (ADH^+) expresses liver cytosolic alcohol dehydrogenase activity. The animals have been used extensively to evaluate the pathway and extent of nonalcohol dehydrogenase-dependent ethanol elimination. Although it is well established that the elimination of ethanol in ADH^- mice is accomplished primarily through oxidation of ethanol and not by excretion of intact ethanol, the contribution made by either cytochrome P450, catalase, or dehydrogenase activity has not been resolved (Burnett and Felder, 1978; Burnett and Felder, 1980; Shigeta et al., 1984; Handler et al., 1986; Alderman et al., 1987; Handler et al., 1988; Norsten et al., 1989).

The difference in ethanol metabolism demonstrated across inbred strains of laboratory animals and between individual animals of outbred lines all suggest a genetic component to regulation of ethanol oxidation and elimination. However, the differential response of each genotype to environmental factors such as dose, gender, or dietary history makes it very difficult to quantitate the genetic differences that regulate ethanol elimination.

Given the genetic variability among inbred mouse and rate strains that have been used to make up heterogenous lines for selective breeding, it is surprising that, during the process of selective breeding for differential ethanol sensitivity, a large difference in ethanol elimination rates has not been found. Whether or not one could select for differential ethanol metabolic rates is an open question, but the presumption is that this should be possible.

Conclusions

There is little doubt that initial sensitivity to ethanol in rodents, by any measure so far used, is genetically heterogenous. The surprising aspect is that there is so little genetic overlap thus far demonstrated between the various behavioral effects of ethanol sensitivity. It is somewhat interesting and difficult to imagine that there are so many different mechanisms involved in various responses. If that proves to be the case, however, animal genetics will afford one of the best methods to unravel the puzzles.

In the short term, the identification of genes that influence the initial actions of ethanol on the central nervous system provide a starting point to discover the basic mechanisms by which ethanol acts. Only a few years ago it was the dogma that ethanol acted as did the general anesthetics, by bulk effects on the cell membrane, but recent studies show a much smaller target for the actions of ethanol—membrane bound protein receptors or enzymes responsible for posttranslational modification of these receptors. These proteins are direct gene products, and with the explosion in molecular gentics, we are able to study them in ways unthought of a few years ago. Undoubtly, continued study of these receptors and their interactions with ethanol will reveal others that are affected by ethanol. The techniques of animal behavioral genetics, coupled with those of molecular genetics, make a powerful team to investigate the actions of ethanol at the molecular level.

It should be reiterated that the study of genetic variability in the behavioral response of rodents to ethanol is undertaken primarily as a tool to understand how ethanol acts at the cellular and molecular levels. It is an article of faith that such fundamental actions will be common to ethanol's action on all cells, including those in the human central nervous system. It is not necessary, nor even likely, however, that all the genetic polymorphisms with regard to ethanol actions found in rodents will also be present in humans. Quite naturally, any such rodent polymorphic genes will certainly be among the first to be tested in a human population as candidate genes, especially given the paucity of other candidates.

In the longer view, beyond additions to knowledge, the significance of the studies reviewed can be seen either as critical to the understanding of human alcoholism or as being entirely irrelevant. Certainly the toll in human lives, suffering, and economic cost is to some extent due to the initial central nervous system depressant actions of ethanol. The larger issue of chronic abuse of ethanol makes up the balance of those enormous costs. Quite obviously individuals find the initial effects of ethanol on their brain rewarding; it is entirely unlikely that anyone drinks to produce a loss of brain function or to produce a cirrhotic liver. Of what advantage would it be to understand the actions of ethanol on the brain well enough to be able to design the equivalent of a naloxone for ethanol? Such a compound would block the initial effects of ethanol on the brain as well as reverse the effects once they were established. Such a compound presumably would at least decrease the incidence of accidents that intoxicated individuals cause. Would the availability of such an amethystic agent increase or decrease the incidence of alcohol abuse? This is an empirical question that awaits the development of such an agent.

Acknowledgments: The writing of this chapter was partially supported by grants from the National Institutes of Health, AA03527, AA00093, and AA07157.

References

Alderman, J., Takagi, T., and Lieber, C. S. (1987). Ethanol-metabolizing pathways in deer mice. Estimation of flux calculated from isotope effects. *J. Biol. Chem.* **262**:7497–7503.

Allan, A. M., and Harris, R. A. (1986). Gamma-aminobutyric acid and alcohol actions: Neurochemical studies of long sleep and short sleep mice. *Life Sci.* **39**:2005–2015.

Allan, A. M., and Harris, R. A. (1989). Sensitivity to ethanol hypnosis and modulation of chloride channels. Does not cosegregate with pentobarbital sensitivity in HS mice. *Alcohol.: Clin. Exp. Res.* **13**:428–434.

Allan, A. M., Gallaher, E. J., Gionet, S. E., and Harris, R. A. (1988a). Genetic selection for benzodiazepine ataxia produces functional changes in the gamma-aminobutyric acid receptor chloride channel complex. *Brain Res.* **452**:118–126.

Allan, A. M., Spuhler, K. P., and Harris, R. A. (1988b). Gamma-aminobutyric acid-activated chloride channels: Relationship to genetic differences in ethanol sensitivity. *J. Pharmacol. Exp. Ther.* **244**:866–870.

Allan, A. M., Mayes, G. G., and Draski, L. J. (1991). Gamma-aminobutyric acid-activated chloride channels in rats selectively bred for differential acute sensitivity to alcohol. *Alcohol.: Clin. Exp. Res.* **15**:212–218.

Alpern, H. P., and McIntyre, T. D. (1985). Evidence that the selectively bred long- and short-sleep mouse lines display common narcotic reactions to many depressants. *Psychopharmacology* **85**:456–459.

Baker, R., Melchior, C., and Deitrich, R. (1980). The effect of halothane on mice selective bred for differential sensitivity to alcohol. *Pharmacol. Biochem. Behav.* **12**:691–695.

Balak, K. J., Keith, R. H., and Felder, M. R. (1982). Genetic and developmental regulation of mouse liver alcohol dehydrogenase. *J. Biol. Chem.* **257**:15000–15007.

Belknap, J. K. (1975). The grid test: A measure of alcohol and barbiturate-induced impairment in mice. *Behav. Res. Meth. Instrum.* **7**:66–67.

Bowers, B. J., Boxy, T. Z., and Wehner, J. M. (1990). Adrenalectomy increases bicuculline-induced seizure sensitivity in long-sleep and short-sleep mice. *Pharmacol. Biochem. Behav.* **38**:593–600.

Brick, J., Pohorecky, L. A., Faulkner, W., and Adams, M. N. (1984). Circadian variations in behavioral and biological sensitivity to ethanol. *Alcohol.: Clin. Exp. Res.* **8**:204–211.

Burnett, K. G., and Felder, M. R. (1978). Genetic regulation of liver alcohol dehydrogenase in Peromyscus. *Biochem. Genet.* **16**:443–454.

Burnett, K. G., and Felder, M. R. (1980). Ethanol metabolism in Peromyscus genetically deficient in alcohol dehydrogenase. *Biochem. Pharmacol.* **29**:125–130.

Campanelli, C., Le, A. D., Khanna, L. M., and Kalant, H. (1988). Effect of raphe lesions on the development of acute tolerance to ethanol and pentobarbital. *Psychopharmacology* **96**:454–457.

Collins, A. C., Yeager, T. N., Lebsack, M. E., and Panter, S. S. (1975). Variations in alcohol metabolism: Influence of sex and age. *Pharmacol. Biochem. Behav.* **3**:973–978.

Crabb, D. W., Bosron, W. F., and Li, T. K. (1983). Steady-state kinetic properties of purified rat liver alcohol dehydrogenase: Application to predicting alcohol elimination rates in vivo. *Arch. Biochem. Biophys.* **224**:299–309.

Crabb, D. W., Bosron, W. F., and Li, T. K. (1987). Ethanol metabolism. *Pharmacol. Ther.* **34:**59–73.

Crabbe, J. C. (1983). Sensitivity to ethanol in inbred mice: Genotypic correlations among several behavioral responses. *Behav. Neurosci.* **97:**280–289.

Crabbe, J. C. (1986). Genetic differences in locomotor activation in mice. *Pharmacol. Biochem. Behav.* **25:**289–292.

Crabbe, J. C., Feller, D. J., and Phillips, T. J. (1990). Selective breeding for two measures of sensitivity to ethanol. In *Initial Sensitivity to Alcohol,* R. A. Dietrich and A. A. Pawlowski, eds. National Institute of Alcohol Abuse and Alcoholism, Research Monograph No. 20 (DHHS publ. no. (ADM) 90-1611), Washington DC, pp. 123–151.

Crow, K. E. (1985). Ethanol metabolism by the liver. *Rev. Drug Metabol. Drug Interact.* **5:**113–158.

deFiebre, C. M., Romm, E., Collins, J. T., Draski, L., Deitrich, R. A., and Collins A. C. (1991). Responses to cholinergic agonists of rats selectively bred for differential sensitivity to ethanol. *Alcohol.: Clin. Exp. Res.* **15:**270–276.

DeFries, J. C. (1981). Current perspectives on selective breeding: Example and theory. In *Development of Animal Models as Pharmacogenetic Tools,* G. E. McClearn, R. A. Deitrich and V. G. Erwin, eds. National Institute of Alcohol Abuse and Alcoholism, Research Monograph No. 6, (DHHS publ. no. 81-1133), Washington, DC, pp. 11–35.

Deitrich, R. A. (1990). Selective breeding of mice and rats for initial sensitivity to ethanol: Contribution to understanding of ethanol's actions. In *Initial Sensitivity to Alcohol,* R. A. Deitrich and A. A. Pawlowski, eds. National Institute of Alcohol Abuse and Alcoholism, Research Monograph No. 20, (DHHS publ. no. (ADM) 90-1611), Washington, DC pp. 7–59.

Deitrich, R. A., Draski, L. J., and Baker, R. C. (1994). Effect of pentobarbital and gaseous anesthetics on rats selectively bred for ethanol sensitivity. *Pharm. Biochem. Behav.* **41:**721–725.

Draski, L. J., Spuhler, K. P., Erwin, V. G., Baker, R. C., and Deitrich, R. A. (1991). Selective breeding of rats differing in sensitivity to the effects of acute ethanol administration. Submitted.

Durkin, T. P., Hashem-Zadek, H., Mandel, P., and Ebel, A. (1982). A comparative study of the acute effects of ethanol on the cholinergic system in hippocampus and striatum of inbred mouse strains. *J. Pharmacol. Exp. Ther.* **220:**203–208.

Eriksson, K., and Rusi, M. (1981). Finnish selection studies on alcohol related behaviors: General outline. In *Development of Animal Models as Pharmacogenetic Tools,* G. E. McClearn, R. A. Deitrich, and V. G. Erwin, eds. National Institute of Alcohol Abuse and Alcoholism, Research Monograph No. 6, (DHHS publication no. 81-1133), Washington, DC, pp. 87–117.

Erwin, V. G., Heston, W. D. W., McClearn, G. E., and Deitrich, R. A. (1976). Effects of hypnotics on mice genetically selected for sensitivity to ethanol. *Pharmacol. Biochem. Behav.* **4:**679–683.

Erwin, V. G., McClearn, G. E., and Kuse, A. R. (1980). Interrelationships of alcohol consumption, actions of alcohol and biochemical traits. *Pharm. Biochem. Behav.* **13:**297–302.

Erwin, V. G., Jones, B. C., and Radcliffe, R. (1990). Further characterization of LSXSS recombinant inbred strains of mice: Activating and hypothermic effects of ethanol. *Alcohol.: Clin. Exp. Res.* **14:**200–204.

Feller, D. J., and Crabbe, J. C. (1991). Effect of alcohols and other hypnotics in mice selected for differential sensitivity to hypothermic actions of ethanol. *J. Pharmacol. Exp. Ther.* **256:**947–958.

French, T. A., Atkinson, N., Petersen, D. R., and Chung, L. W. (1979). Differential induction of hepatic microsomal ethanol and drug metabolism by 3-methylcholanthrene in "LS" and "SS" mice. *J. Pharmacol. Exp. Ther.* **209:**404–410.

Gallaher, E. J., Parsons, L. M., and Goldstein, D. B. (1982). The rapid onset of tolerance to ataxic effects of ethanol in mice. *Psychopharmacology* **78:**67–70.

Gibson, J. B., and Oakeshott, J. G. (1981). Genetics of biochemical and behavioural aspects of alcohol metabolism. *Aust. N. Z. J. Med.* **11:**128–131.

Glassman, E. B., McLaughlin, G. A., Forman, D. T., Felder, M. R., and Thurman, R. G. (1985). Role of alcohol dehydrogenase in the swift increase in alcohol metabolism (SIAM). Studies with deer mice deficient in alcohol dehydrogenase. *Biochem. Pharmacol.* **34:**3523–3526.

Goldstein, D. B. (1983). *Pharmacology of Alcohol.* New York: Oxford University Press, p. 7.

Grant, K. A., Werner, R., Hoffman, P. L., and Tabakoff, B. (1989). Chronic tolerance to ethanol in the N:NIH rat. *Alcohol.: Clin. Exp. Res.* **13:**402–406.

Greer, C. A., and Alpern, H. P. (1978). Differential neurohumoral modulation of myoclonic and clonic seizures. *Arch. Int. Pharmacol.* **236:**74–85.

Hakkinen, J. D., and Kulonin, E. (1976). Ethanol intoxication and gamma-aminobutyric acid. *J. Neurochem.* **27:**631–633.

Handler, J. A., and Thurman, R. G. (1985). Fatty acid-dependent ethanol metabolism. *Biochem. Biophys. Res. Commun.* **133:**44–51.

Handler, J. A., Bradford, B. U., Glassman, E., Ladine, J. K., and Thurman, R. G. (1986). Catalase-dependent ethanol metabolism in vivo in deer mice lacking alcohol dehydrogenase. *Biochem. Pharmacol.* **35:**4487–4492.

Handler, J. A., Koop, D. R., Coon, M. J., Takei, Y., and Thurman, R. G. (1988). Identification of P-450ALC in microsomes from alcohol dehydrogenase-deficient deer mice: Contribution to ethanol elimination in vivo. *Arch. Biochem. Biophys.* **264:**114–124.

Harris, R. A., and Allan, A. M. (1989). Genetic differences in coupling of benzodiazepine receptors to chloride channels. *Brain Res.* **490:**26–32.

Hasumura, Y., Teschke, R., and Lieber, C. S. (1975). Hepatic microsomal ethanol-oxidizing system (MEOS): Dissociation from reduced nicotinamide adenine dinucleotide phosphate oxidase and possible role of form I of cytochrome P-450. *J. Pharmacol. Exp. Ther.* **194:**469–474.

Havre, P., Abrams, M. A., Corral, R. J., Yu, L. C., Szczepanik, P. A., Feldman, H. B., Klein, P., Kong, M. S., Margolis, J. M., and Landau, B. R. (1977). Quantitation of pathways of ethanol metabolism. *Arch. Biochem. Biophys.* **182:**14–23.

Hellevuo, K., and Kiianmaa, K. (1989). GABA turnover in the brain of rat lines developed for differential ethanol-induced motor impairment. *Pharmacol. Biochem. Behav.* **34:**905–909.

Hellevuo, K., Kiianmaa, K., and Korpi, E. R. (1989). Effect of GABAergic drugs on motor impairment from ethanol, barbital and lorazepam in rat lines selected for differential sensitivity to ethanol. *Pharmacol. Biochem. Behav.* **34:**399–404.

Heston, W. D., Erwin, V. G., Anderson, S. M., and Robbins, H. (1974). A comparison of the effects of alcohol on mice selectively bred for differences in ethanol sleep-time. *Life Sci.* **14:**365–370.

Hjelle, J. J., Atkinson, N., and Petersen, D. R. (1981). The effects of chronic ethanol ingestion on ethanol binding to hepatic cytochrome P-450 and on certain hepatic and renal parameters in the "long sleep" and "short sleep" mouse. *Alcohol.: Clin. Exp. Res.* **5:**198–203.

Holmes, R. S. (1985). Genetic variants of enzymes of alcohol and aldehyde metabolism. *Alcohol.: Clin. Exp. Res.* **9**:535–538.

Howerton, T. C., and Collins, A. C. (1984). Ethanol-induced inhibition of GABA release from LS and SS mouse brain slices. *Alcohol* **1**:471–477.

Howerton, T. C., Marks, M. J., and Collins A. C. (1982). Norepinephrine, gamma-aminobutyric acid and choline reuptake kinetics and the effects of ethanol in long-sleep and short-sleep mice. *Subst. Alcohol Actions/Misuse* **3**:89–99.

Howerten, T. C., Burch, J. B., O'Connor, M. F., Miner, L. L., and Collins, A. C. (1984). A genetic analysis of ethanol, pentobarbital and methyprylon sleep-time response. *Alcohol.: Clin. Exp. Res.* **8**:546–550.

Kakihana, R., Brown, D. R., McClearn, G. E., and Tabershaw, I. R. (1966). Brain sensitivity to alcohol in inbred mouse strains. *Science* **154**:1574–1575.

Keir, W., and Deitrich, R. A. (1990). Development of central nervous system sensitivity to ethanol and pentobarbital in short- and long-sleep mice. *J. Pharmacol. Exp. Ther.* **254**:831–835.

Keir, W., Kozak, C. A., Chakraborti, A., Deitrich, R. A., and Sikela, J. M. (1991). The cDNA sequence and chromosomal location of the murine GABA$_A$α1 receptor gene. *Genomics* **9**:390–395.

Kiianmaa, K., Hellevuo, K., and Korpi, E. R. (1988). The AT (alcohol tolerant) ANT (alcohol non-tolerant) rat lines selected for differences in sensitivity to ethanol: An overview. In *Biomedical and Social Aspects of Alcohol and Alcoholism,* K. Kuriyama, A. Takada, and H. Ishii, eds. Amsterdam: Elsevier Sci. Pub., pp. 415–418.

Knecht, K. T., Bradford, B. U., Mason, R. P., and Thurman, R. G. (1990). In vivo formation of a free radical metabolite of ethanol. *Mol. Pharmacol.* **38**:26–30.

Koblin, D. D., and Deady, J. E. (1981). Anesthetic requirement in mice selectively bred for differences in ethanol sensitivity. *Br. J. Anaesth.* **53**:5–10.

Krikun, G., Lieber, C. S., and Cederbaum, A. I. (1984). Increased microsomal oxidation of ethanol by cytochrome P-450 and hydroxyl radical-dependent pathways after chronic ethanol consumption. *Biochem. Pharmacol.* **33**:3306–3309.

Lewis, M. J., and June, H. L. (1990). Neurobehavioral studies of ethanol reward and activation. *Alcohol* **7**:213–219.

Lieber, C. S., Teschke, R., Hasumura, Y., and Decarli, L. M. (1975). Differences in hepatic and metabolic changes after acute and chronic alcohol consumption. *Fed. Proc.* **34**:2060–2074.

Lieber, C. S., Lasker, J. M., Alderman, J., and Leo, M. A. (1987). The microsomal ethanol oxidizing system and its interaction with other drugs, carcinogens, and vitamins. *Ann. N. Y. Acad. Sci.* **492**:11–24.

Lin, A. M. -Y., Bickford, P. C., and Palmer, M. R. (1993a). The effects of ethanol on gamma-aminobutyric acid-induced depressions of cerebellar Purkinje neurons: Influence of *beta* adrenergic receptor action in young and aged Fischer 344 rats. *J. Pharmacol. Exp. Ther.* **264**:951–957.

Lin, A. M. -Y., Freund, R. K., and Palmer, M. R. (1991). Ethanol potentiation of GABA-induced electrophysiological responses in cerebellum: Requirement for catecholamine modulation. *Neurosci. Lett.* **122**:154–158.

Lin, A. M. -Y., Freund, R. K., and Palmer, M. R. (1993b). Sensitization of gamma-aminobutyric acid-induced depressions of cerebellar Purkinje neurons to the potentiative effects of ethanol by *beta* adrenergic mechanisms in rat brain. *J. Pharmacol. Exp. Ther.* **265**:426–432.

Liu, Y. F., Civelli, O., Grandy, D. K., and Albert, P. R. (1992). Differential sensitivity of the short and long human dopamine D_2 receptor subtypes to protein kinase C. *J. Neurochem.* **59:**2311–2317.

McClearn, G. E., and Kakihana, R. (1981). Selective breeding for ethanol sensitivity: Short-sleep and long-sleep mice. In *Development of Animal Models as Pharmacogenetic Tools,* G. E. McClearn, R. A. Deitrich, and V. G. Erwin, eds. National Institute of Alcohol Abuse and Alcoholism, Research Monograph No. 6 (DHHS publ. no. 81-1133), Washington, DC, pp. 147–159.

McIntyre, T. D., Trullas, R., and Skolnick, P. (1988). Differences in the biophysical properties of the benzodiazepine/γ-aminobutyric acid receptor chloride channel complex in the Long-Sleep and Short-Sleep mouse lines. *J. Neurochem.* **51:**642–647.

Marley, R. J., Miner, L. L., Wehner, J. M., and Collins, A. C. (1986). Differential effects of central nervous depressants in long-sleep and short-sleep mice. *J. Pharmacol. Exp. Ther.* **238:**1028–1033.

Marley, R. J., Stinchcomb, A., and Wehner, J. M. (1988). Further characterization of benzodiazepine receptor differences in long-sleep and short-sleep mice. *Life Sci.* **43:**1223–1231.

Marley, R. J., and Wehner, J. M. (1986). GABA enhancement of flunitrazepam binding in mice selectively bred for differential sensitivity to ethanol. *Alc. and Drug Res.* **7:**25–32.

Martz, A., Deitrich R. A., and Harris, R. A. (1983). Behavioral evidence for the involvement of gamma-aminobutyric acid in the actions of ethanol. *Eur. J. Pharmacol.* **89:**53–62.

Mellanby, E. (1919). Special report. Series no. 31. London: Medical Research Committee.

Norsten, C., Cronholm, T., Ekstrom, G., Handler, J. A., Thurman, R. G., and Ingelman-Sundberg, M. (1989). Dehydrogenase-dependent ethanol metabolism in deer mice (Peromyscus maniculatus) lacking cytosolic alcohol dehydrogenase. Reversibility and isotope effects in vivo and in subcellular fractions. *J. Biol. Chem.* **264:**5593–5597.

O'Connor, M. F., Howerton, T. C., and Collins, A. C. (1982). Effects of pentobarbital in mice selected for differential sensitivity to ethanol. *Pharmacol. Biochem. Behav.* **17:**245–248.

Palmer, M. R., Wong, Y., Fossom, L. H., and Spuhler, K. (1987). Genetic correlation of ethanol induced ataxia and cerebellar Purkinje neuron depression among inbred strains and selected lines of rats. *Alcohol.: Clin. Exp. Res.* **11:**494–501.

Palmer, M. R., Harlan, J. T., and Spuhler, K. (1992). Genetic-covariation in LAS and HAS selected lines of rats: Behavioral and electrophysiological sensitivities to the depressant effects of ethanol and the development of acute tolerance to ethanol *in situ* at generation eight. *J. Pharmacol. Exptl. Therap.* **260:**879–886.

Pato, C. N., Macciardi, F., Pato, M. T., Verga, M., and Kennedy, J. L. (1993). Review of the putative association of dopamine D2 receptor and alcoholism: A meta-analysis. *Am. J. Med. Genet.* **48,** 78–82.

Peris, D. J., Wehner, J. M., and Zahniser, N. R. (1989). [35S]TBPS binding sites are decreased in the colliculi of mice with a genetic predisposition to bicuculline-induced seizures. *Brain Res.* **503:**288–295.

Petersen, D. R., and Atkinson, N. (1980). Genetically mediated responses of microsomal ethanol oxidation in mice. *Adv. Exp. Med. Biol.* **132:**117–128.

Phillips, T. J., Kim, D., and Dudek, B. C. (1989). Convulsant properties of GABA antagonists and anticonvulsant properties of ethanol in selectively bred long- and short-sleep mice. *Psychopharmacology* **98:**544–548.

Rachamin, G., and Israel, Y. (1985). Sex differences in hepatic alcohol dehydrogenase activity in animal species. *Biochem. Pharmacol.* **34:**2385–2386.

Rex, D. K., Bosron, W. F., Dwulet, F., and Li, T. K. (1987a). Purification and characterization of the Danish (Skive) variant of mouse liver alcohol dehydrogenase. *Biochem. Genet.* **25**:111–121.

Rex, D. K., Patterson, L. S., Edenberg, H. J., and Bosron, W. F. (1987b). Structure and expression of mouse liver alcohol dehydrogenase isoenzymes. *Prog. Clin. Biol. Res.* **232**:237–243.

Romm, E., and Collins, A. C. (1987). Body temperature influences on ethanol elimination rates. *Alcohol* **4**:189–198.

Sanders, B., and Sharpless, S. K. (1978). Dissociation between the anticonvulsant action of alcohol and its depressant action in mice of different genotypes. *Life Sci.* **23**:2593–2600.

Sheppard, J. R., Albersheim, P., and McClearn, G. (1970). Aldehyde dehydrogenase and ethanol preference in mice. *J. Biol. Chem.* **245**:2876–2882.

Shigeta, Y., Nomura, F., Iida, S., Leo, M. A., Felder, M. R., and Lieber, C. S. (1984). Ethanol metabolism in vivo by the microsomal ethanol-oxidizing system in deer mice lacking alcohol dehydrogenase (ADH). *Biochem. Pharmacol.* **33**:807–814.

Smolen, A., and Smolen, T. N. (1989). Reproducibility of ethanol elimination rates in long-sleep and short-sleep mice. *J. Stud. Alcohol* **50**:519–524.

Smolen, A., Marks, M. J., Smolen, T. N., and Collins, A. C. (1986). Dose and route of administration alter the relative elimination of ethanol by long-sleep and short-sleep mice. *Alcohol.: Clin. Exp. Res.* **10**:198–204.

Sorensen, S., Palmer, M. R., Dunwiddie, T., and Hoffer, B. (1980). Electrophysiological correlates of ethanol-induced sedation in differentially sensitive lines of mice. *Science* **210**:1143–1145.

Spuhler, K., and Deitrich, R. A. (1984). Correlative analysis of ethanol-related phenotypes in rat inbred strains. *Alcohol.: Clin. Exp. Res.* **8**:480–484.

Spuhler, K., Hoffer, B., Weiner, N., and Palmer, M. (1982). Evidence for genetic correlation of hypnotic effects and cerebellar Purkinje neuron depression in response to ethanol in mice. *Pharm. Biochem. Behav.* **17**:569–578.

Suzdak, P. D., Schwartz, R. D., Sklonick, P., and Paul, S. M. (1986). Ethanol stimulates gamma-aminobutyric acid receptor-mediated chloride transport in rat brain synaptoneurosomes. *Proc. Natl. Acad. Sci. (USA)* **83**:4071–4075.

Svanas, G. W., and Weiner, H. (1985). Aldehyde dehydrogenase activity as the rate-limiting factor for acetaldehyde metabolism in rat liver. *Arch. Biochem. Biophys.* **236**:36–46.

Thurman, R. G. (1980). Ethanol elimination is inherited in the rat. In *Advances in Experimental Medicine and Biology,* vol. 132, R. G. Thurman, ed. New York and London: Plenum Press, pp. 655–661.

Thurman, R. G., Bradford, B. U., and Glassman, E. (1983). The swift increase in alcohol metabolism (SIAM) in four inbred strains of mice. *Pharmacol. Biochem. Behav.* **18**(suppl. 1):171–175.

Thurman, R. G., Paschal, D., Abu-Murad, C., Pekkanen, L., Bradford, B. U., Bullock, K., and Glassman, E. (1982). Swift increase in alcohol metabolism (SIAM) in the mouse: Comparison of the effect of short-term ethanol treatment on ethanol elimination in four inbred strains. *J. Pharmacol. Exp. Ther.* **223**:45–49.

Tuominen, K., Hellevuo, K., and Korpi, E. R. (1990). Plus-maze behavior and susceptibility to 3-mercaptopropionate-induced seizures in rat lines selected for high and low alcohol sensitivity. *Pharmacol. Biochem. Behav.* **35**:721–725.

Tussey, L., and Felder, M. R. (1989). Tissue-specific genetic variation in the level of mouse alcohol dehydrogenase is controlled transcriptionally in kidney and posttranscriptionally in liver. *Proc. Natl. Acad. Sci. (USA)* **86:**5903–5907.

Uusi-Oukari, M., and Korpi, E. R. (1991). Specific alterations in the cerebellar GABAa receptors of an alcohol-sensitive ANT rat line. *Alcohol.: Clin. Exp. Res.* **15:**241–248.

Videla, L., Flattery, K. V., Sellers, E. A., and Israel Y. (1975). Ethanol metabolism and liver oxidative capacity in cold acclimation. *J. Pharmacol. Exp. Ther.* **192:**575–582.

Wafford, K. A., Burnett, D. M., Dunwiddie, T. V., and Harris, R. A. (1990). Genetic differences in the ethanol sensitivity of GABAa receptors expressed in Xenopus oocytes. *Science* **249:**291–293.

Wafford, K. A., Burnett, D. M., Leidenheimer, N. J., Burt, D. R., Wang, J. B., Kofuji, D. P., Dunwiddie, T. V., Harris, R. A., and Sikela, J. M. (1991). Ethanol sensitivity of the GABAa receptor expressed in Xenopus oocytes requires eight amino acids contained in the γ2L subunit. *Neuron* **7:**27–33.

Wafford, K. A., and Whiting, P. J. (1992). Ethanol potentiation of $GABA_A$ receptors requires phosphorylation of the alternatively spliced variant of the gamma2 subunit. *FEBS Lett.* **313:**113–117.

Waller, M. B., McBride, W. J., Lumeng, L., and Li, T. -K. (1983). Initial sensitivity and acute tolerance to ethanol in the P and NP lines of rats. *Pharmacol. Biochem. Behav.* **19:**683–686.

Wang, C. H., and Singh, S. M. (1985). Genetic considerations in the effects of ethanol in mice. I. Genotype-dependent alterations in alcohol dehydrogenase activity. *Can. J. Genet. Cytol.* **27:**158–164.

Wilson, J. S., Korsten, M. A., and Lieber, C. S. (1986). The combined effects of protein deficiency and chronic ethanol administration on rat ethanol metabolism. *Hepatology* **6:**823–829.

Zorzano, A., and Herrera, E. (1989). Decreased in vivo rate of ethanol metabolism in the suckling rat. *Alcohol.: Clin. Exp. Res.* **13:**527–532.

Zorzano, A., and Herrera, E. (1990). In vivo ethanol elimination in man, monkey and rat: A lack of relationship between the ethanol metabolism and the hepatic activities of alcohol and aldehyde dehydrogenases. *Life Sci.* **46:**223–230.

7

Genetic Influences on Alcohol Preference in Animals

LAWRENCE LUMENG, JAMES M. MURPHY, WILLIAM J. MCBRIDE, AND TING-KAI LI

A key objective of alcoholism research is to explain why people drink, why some continue to drink even when alcohol use creates problems for them (i.e., alcohol abuse), and why some are unable to stop drinking even when faced with highly detrimental consequences (i.e., alcohol dependence). The underlying agent of alcoholism, of course, is ethanol; however, it is also clear that the final common behavioral path is the acquisition of ethanol through drinking (or self-administration), and that the central issue of alcoholism research should be the understanding of the psychosocial and biological (genetic and environmental) factors that contribute to aberrant alcohol drinking behavior. Although alcoholism is a disorder unique to humans, considerable efforts have been made to develop animal models of ethanol self-administration and to use them to elucidate the neurobiological substrates of alcohol-seeking behavior. Several species of experimental animals, including subhuman primates, miniature pigs, rats, and mice, have been studied, with the rat being used the most widely. A variety of manipulations, including scheduled availability (Holloway et al., 1984), schedule-induced polydipsia in weight-reduced animals (Meisch, 1976), secondary conditioning with operant procedures (Samson, 1986), and forcible prior induction of physical dependence and tolerance (Deutsch and Eisner, 1977) have been shown to increase alcohol drinking. However, the most successful procedure has been genetic, in particular the use of selective breeding to develop divergent rodent lines that differ in alcohol preference and voluntary alcohol consumption.

Historically, Williams and associates (1949) and Mardones and coworkers (1949) were the first to suggest that genetic factors can influence voluntary alcohol consumption in rodents. In the early 1950s, Mardones and his group (1950, 1953) reported the selective inbreeding of the UChA (low) and the UChB (high) strains of rats that differed in alcohol preference, and calculated a high coefficient of heritability for this phenotype. In 1951, Reed also reported that the spontaneous choice of alcohol by six inbred strains of rats differed markedly among them. These early studies set the stage for a series of papers by McClearn and his associates (McClearn and Rodgers, 1959, 1961; Rodgers and McClearn, 1962; Rodgers, 1972) that emphasized the large and reproducible differences in alcohol preference that could be demonstrated among inbred strains of mice. They reported that in general the C57 sublines exhibited the highest alcohol preference, with mean ratios of volume of 10% (v/v) ethanol to total fluid consumed that ranged from 0.55 to 0.90, while the DBA sublines demonstrated the lowest alcohol preference, i.e., mean ratios that were less than 0.05. They found that most other inbred strains exhibited intermediate mean ratios of alcohol preference: RIII, 0.3–0.6; C3H, about 0.3; BALB/c, about 0.2, and A, 0.06–0.2. These inbred strain differences provided prima facie evidence that voluntary alcohol ingestion in mice is under genetic influence.

Stronger evidence for a genetic influence on alcohol preference was subsequently provided by McClearn and Rodgers (1961) when they examined alcohol preference among several genetic crosses that involved the C57BL, A/2, BALB/C, C3H/2, and DBA inbred strains. They reported that F_1 offspring of these crosses exhibited intermediate preferences between the parent strains without heterosis or complete dominance. This was also true of F_1 and F_2 offspring and all backcrosses, and the mean preference of the C57BL backcross was higher than that of the A backcross. The general pattern clearly demonstrated a genetic effect on alcohol preference.

It was realized in the mid- and late-1960s that inbred mouse and rat strains are not particularly suitable for elucidating the biochemical, physiological, and behavioral factors that may underlie the large variance of alcohol drinking behaviors in rodents and in humans (Eriksson, 1968). This is because inbred strains are raised by brother–sister mating for at least 20 generations. Such extended inbreeding eliminates heterozygosity and results in animals that have their genes fixed by chance. While behavioral differences, such as alcohol preference, between inbred strains raised within the same laboratory environment can be ascribed to genetic differences, these inbred strains are not ideal models to study "correlated traits and responses" because of the high probability of fortuitous associations (Eriksson and Rusi, 1981; Crabbe, 1989).

Whereas many of the correlated traits and responses observed in inbred strains of rodents were brought about by random, nondirectional, chance fixation of genes, it became quite clear to several research groups in the last three decades that selective bidirectional breeding for alcohol preference and nonpreference would be a much more powerful tool for conducting research on the factors that affect alcohol drinking. The thesis is that by avoiding inbreeding and by systematic mating of animals that exhibit the most extreme levels of high and low alcohol preference from a heterogeneous stock, selection over many generations should yield divergent lines that possess a high and a low frequency of genes that impact on alcohol preference, while the frequency of trait-irrelevant genes remains randomly distributed and uninfluenced by selective breeding. To date, five separate sets of alcohol-preferring and -nonpreferring lines of rats have been raised through selective breeding (Table 7-1): the ALKO alco-

Table 7-1 Selectively Bred Rat Lines that Differ in Alcohol Preference

Line	Foundation Stock	Location	Control Line	Replicate Lines	Generation Reached and Year	Extent of Inbreeding
UChB/UChA	Wistar (Chilean Bacteriol. Institute)	University of Chile, Santiago	No	No	S61 UCHA, S53 UChB (1990)	High
AA/ANA	Wistar (ALKO outbred); S37 rats were revitalized with F1 hybrids of Brown Norwegian × Lewis	ALKO, Helsinki, Finland	No	No	S55 (1989)	Low
P/NP	Wistar (W-rm: WRC(WI) BR, Walter Reed)	Indiana University, Indianapolis	No	No	S-33 (1991)	Low
HAD/LAD	N/Nih[a] heterogeneous stock (NCI)	Indiana University, Indianapolis	No	Yes	S13–S15 (1991)	Least
sP/sNP	Wistar (University of Cagliari)	University of Cagliari, Italy	No	No	S16–S17 (1990)	Uncertain

[a]Derived from crossing eight inbred strains, i.e., ACI, BN, BUF, F344, M520, MR, WKY, and WN (Hansen and Spuhler, 1984).

hol/nonalcohol (AA/ANA) lines developed in Helsinki, Finland (Eriksson, 1968); the alcohol-preferring/-nonpreferring (P/NP) lines developed at Indiana University (Lumeng et al., 1977); the University of Chile B and A (UChB/UChA) line raised in Santiago, Chile (Mardones et al., 1953); the high-/low-alcohol-drinking (HAD/LAD) replicate lines also developed in Indiana (Lumeng et al., 1986a; Gongwer et al., 1989; Li et al., 1993); and the Sardinian alcohol preferring/nonpreferring (sP/sNP) lines raised in Cagliari, Italy (Fadda et al., 1989). As summarized by Table 7-1, only the HAD/LAD lines have been selectively bred in replicate from a heterogeneous foundation stock (i.e., the N/Nih rat) that is more heterogeneous than the Wistar rat. Additionally, the extent of inbreeding is probably most intense in the selection for the UChB/A lines, but is probably the least in the selection for the HAD/LAD lines. With the latter selection experiment, a within-family selection and a rotational breeding design was used from the beginning of the selection experiment to slow down inbreeding. To maintain adequate sample size in the HAD/LAD replicate selection, eight breeding families were set up for each of the lines. Owing to financial constraints, none of the selection experiments for alcohol preference in rats (including the HAD/LAD selection) had included a nonselected control line. Selection for the HAD_1 and LAD_1 lines has now reached generation S-15, while selection for the HAD_2 and LAD_2 lines lags behind by two generations. As depicted in Fig. 7-1, divergence of drinking scores in the replicate HAD and LAD lines has been progressing steadily but more slowly than

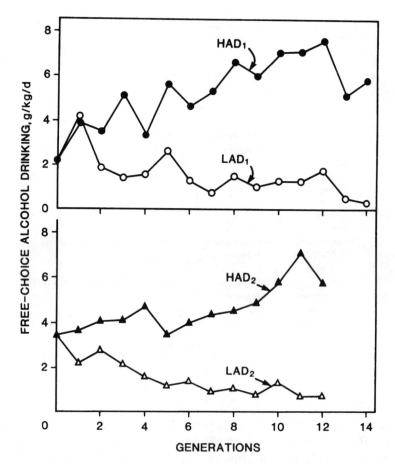

Fig. 7-1 Bidirectional selection for the replicate HAD₁/LAD₁ and HAD₂/LAD₂ lines starting from the N/Nih heterogeneous stock.

the P and NP rats because within-family selection rather than mass selection (used for the P/NP lines) was used for the HAD/LAD replicate selection.

Among the selectively bred rat lines that differ in alcohol preference, the P and NP lines have been most extensively characterized with regard to associated behavioral and neurobiological traits, and the P rats have been shown to satisfy all the major criteria of an animal model of alcoholism. While the sociocultural and psychosocial variables unique to humans cannot be incorporated into an animal model, the mouse and the rat are the most practical and useful animals in which invasive neurobiological experiments can be performed.

In this chapter, we review the behavioral, biochemical, and neuropharmacologic differences found in the P and NP rats. Where appropriate, pertinent findings in the P and NP rats will be compared to those reported in other rodent models and in the other pairs of selectively bred alcohol-preferring and nonpreferring rat lines. It is beyond the scope of this chapter, however, to cover all the experimental results obtained with all the selectively bred rat lines and inbred mouse strains that differ in alcohol preference. For more specific information, the reader should consult the reviews by Rodgers (1972), Li et al. (1981, 1986, 1987), Eriksson and Rusi (1981), Eriksson (1981), Mardones et al. (1983), Lumeng et al. (1988, 1989), McBride et al. (1989a, 1991a, 1991b), and Sinclair et al. (1989).

Alcohol Preference as a Heritable Phenotypic Trait

Alcohol preference is generally defined as ethanol consumption in the presence of food, an ethanol solution, and another equally palatable fluid or water. Experimentally, alcohol preference is tested over several weeks by either a two-bottle or a three-bottle test design and with food available ad libitum. In the two-bottle test, only water and a 10% (v/v) ethanol solution are available as drinking fluids, while in the three-bottle test, water, an empty bottle, and increasing concentrations (3% to 30% v/v) of ethanol are provided on each successive day. The positions of the drinking bottles are changed daily at random. In the selection of AA/ANA, P/NP, and HAD/LAD rats, the two-bottle preference test was used and, in addition, preference testing was preceded by a variable period (4 to 10 days of adaptation) wherein 10% ethanol was given as the sole source of fluid. In the past, these experimental procedures were impugned; however, it is now clear that both the initial adaptation period and the two-bottle test are valid. P/NP and AA/ANA rats displayed their characteristic alcohol-drinking behavior regardless of whether they were tested with or without the initial adaptation period and whether the two-bottle or the three-bottle preference test was used (Lankford et al., 1991).

Alcohol preference has been scored by different phenotypic measures, i.e., amount of ethanol solution consumed as a percentage of total fluid consumption (preference ratio, ml %), ethanol consumption as absolute amount of ethanol in relation to body weight (g ethanol/kg/day), and ethanol caloric intake in relation to total caloric intake (preference ratio, cal %) (Sinclair et al., 1989). In the selection of P/NP and HAD/LAD rats, ethanol intake (g ethanol/kg/day) has been used as the primary selection criterion, with preference ratio (ml %) the secondary criterion. The use of both these criteria tended to eliminate bias such as animals with high alcohol consumption due to small body weights or animals with polydipsia with high volume intake of both the 10% alcohol solution and water. In the ALKO selection of AA/ANA rats, different single phenotypic measures were used for different generations and, at this point in their selective breeding, a combination of all three measures are used with equal weighting (Sinclair et al., 1989).

McClearn (1968) earlier had explored other methods of testing for alcohol preference in mice. In this endeavor, he developed another phenotypic measurement called *alcohol acceptance*. Alcohol acceptance was measured by recording daily water intake for the first two days. This was then followed by subjecting the mouse to total fluid deprivation for 24 hours, and finally recording the ingestion of a 10% ethanol solution on the fourth day of the test period. Solid food was made available ad libitum. An alcohol acceptance score was calculated by dividing the amount of ethanol consumed on day 4 to the mean daily water intake on days 1 and 2. McClearn (1968) compared the strain rank order of alcohol acceptance with that of alcohol preference in six different inbred strains of mice and found that their rank order was the same, i.e., C57BL > RIII > C3H/2 > Balb/c > A > DBA/2. Following this study, Anderson and McClearn (1981) employed mass selection and raised duplicate lines of high ethanol acceptance (HEA) and low ethanol acceptance (LEA) mice starting from the heterogeneous (HS) stock maintained at the Institute for Behavioral Genetics in Boulder, Colorado. Selective breeding for alcohol acceptance reached S14 generations, and quite divergent ethanol acceptance scores were found with little overlap, e.g., 0.38 for the LEA line and 1.19 for the HEA line (Anderson and McClearn, 1981). The divergence was symmetrical and the estimate of realized heritability for each line was 0.21. Selective breeding for the HEA and LEA lines was discontinued subsequently because alcohol acceptance as a phenotype was not equivalent to alcohol preference (Anderson and McClearn, 1981). Although the two phenotypes were significantly correlated (McClearn, 1968), the extent of correlation was low (Anderson and McClearn, 1981). At best, based on present knowledge, ethanol acceptance may be an initial step to alcohol preference; at worst, it is a reflection of thirst. Nonetheless, there has been considerable interest recently on alcohol acceptance as a phenotype, because high alcohol acceptance correlates well with the basic allele of a brain protein called LTW-4 in 11 of 15 C57BL × DBA (or B × D) recombinant inbred strains and 8 of 19 distantly related inbred mouse strains (Goldman et al., 1987; McClearn et al., 1991). Further studies including segregation analysis will be needed to better document this interesting and potentially important correlation.

Realized heritability for alcohol preference has been calculated in several of the selection experiments as the regression of cumulative response to selection on cumulative selections differential. Data from the selection of the HAD and LAD replicate rat lines indicate that $h^2 = 0.15$ for the upward selection and $h^2 = 0.23$ for the downward selection in the HAD_1/LAD_1 lines, and $h^2 = 0.12$ for upward selection and $h^2 = 0.25$ for downward selection in the HAD_2/LAD_2 lines (unpublished results). These values are similar to the realized heritability estimates obtained earlier for the AA and ANA rat lines when they were initially raised (Eriksson, 1969) and those obtained recently when they were revitalized by crossing them with F_1 hybrids from Brown Norwegian and Lewis rats (Hyytia et al., 1987). It should be noted that for selection studies in behavioral genetics, almost all the heritability estimates have been <50%. For instance, in DeFries' selection of mice with high and low open-field activity, the line difference between mice selected for high and low activity was 30-fold after 30 generations, even though the realized heritability was only moderate, i.e., about 0.25 for each line (DeFries and Hegmann, 1970). Similarly, the realized heritability for the selection of the short-sleep (SS) and long-sleep (LS) mice was calculated to be only 0.18 for each of the lines (McClearn and Kakihana, 1973).

Alcohol Preference in Rodents as a Relevant Model for Studying Alcoholism

In an excellent review entitled, "A Critique of Animal Analogues of Alcoholism," Cicero (1979) discussed the criteria that an animal model of alcoholism should ideally satisfy. With the exception of sociocultural variables that influence alcohol drinking in humans, which cannot be incorporated into an animal model, he proposed the following criteria:

1. The animal should self-administer alcohol orally.
2. The amount of alcohol ingested should be pharmacologically significant, i.e., approach or exceed the limit of metabolic capacity and elevate blood alcohol concentrations to meaningful levels.
3. Alcohol should be consumed for its pharmacologic effects, not its caloric value, taste, or smell.
4. Ethanol should be positively reinforcing, i.e., the animals should be willing to overcome obstacles or work to obtain the ethanol.
5. Tolerance to ethanol, both metabolic and neuronal, should be demonstrated after a period of continuous consumption.
6. Dependence on ethanol should also develop after a period of continuous consumption.

The P line of rats has been characterized with respect to these criteria for animal models of alcoholism. The accumulated evidence demonstrates that the P rats meet all the requirements of a relevant animal model. Some of the major findings that have been uncovered with the P rats are as follows.

1. *Most of the P rats consume >5 g of ethanol/kg/day.* As shown in Table 7-2, many of the replicate HAD rats now in the thirteenth to fifteenth generations of selection also drink >5 g of ethanol/kg/day. P rats usually consume between 20% and 30% of their total daily calories as ethanol. They substitute the ethanol calories for a part of the food calories and gain weight at the same rate as control animals not given access to an ethanol solution (Lumeng et al., 1977).

2. *Blood alcohol concentrations (BACs) up to 200 mg% (mean of about 65 mg%).* These concentrations have been measured in P rats during free-choice alcohol drinking when blood was sampled at regular intervals, e.g., at the third and eleventh hours of the

Table 7-2 Free-Choice Ethanol Consumption (g/kg/day, mean ±SD) in P/NP and HAD/LAD Lines

	P Line		NP Line	
Generation	Male	Female	Male	Female
S-8	5.3 ± 1.9	5.0 ± 2.5	1.6 ± 0.9	1.7 ± 0.9
S-16	5.3 ± 1.8	6.5 ± 2.3	0.9 ± 1.0	0.8 ± 1.3
S-20	5.5 ± 1.2	7.3 ± 1.9	1.1 ± 0.6	1.0 ± 0.9
S-31	5.7 ± 0.16	6.6 ± 0.19	0.5 ± 0.08	0.4 ± 0.08
	HAD_1 Line		LAD_1 Line	
	Male	Female	Male	Female
S-15	6.9 ± 2.1	6.6 ± 3.1	0.6 ± 1.0	0.4 ± 0.4
	HAD_2 Line		LAD_2 Line	
	Male	Female	Male	Female
S-13	7.6 ± 2.2	7.8 ± 3.3	0.3 ± 0.4	0.8 ± 1.3

12-hr dark cycle (Murphy et al., 1986a). The P rats drink about 70% of the ethanol in the dark when they also eat most of the food. In the dark, alcohol drinking occurs in bursts at irregularly spaced intervals (Murphy et al., 1986a). We have also monitored alcohol drinking by P rats by drinkometer and have measured BACs 5 minutes after the completion of an alcohol-drinking episode; BACs of 43 to 122 mg% (mean of 62 mg%) were obtained (Li et al., 1979; Lumeng and Li, 1986b). At one hour after each drinking episode, BACs reached 42–218% (mean of about 87 mg%) (Murphy et al., 1986a). These data clearly indicate that P rats attain BACs that are pharmacologically active, at least for humans, during free-choice drinking.

The relationship of BAC to the regulation of voluntary ethanol drinking in the P rats has been studied. In one study, BACs were experimentally elevated either by intravenous infusion of ethanol or by the administration of 4-methylpyrazole, a specific alcohol dehydrogenase inhibitor (Waller et al., 1982a). With intravenous infusions of ethanol given hourly for 24 hours and in amounts equal to or 50% higher than that of their preinfusion daily oral alcohol intake, an inverse correlation between the amounts of ethanol infused and ingested was obtained. Similarly, after a single intraperitoneal injection of 4-methylpyrazole (90 mg/kg), BACs measured every 6 hours following drug injection increased from a mean value of about 10 mg% to about 50–65 mg% for 2–3 days, and P rats decreased their drinking of 10% ethanol and proportionately increased their water intake. Both kinds of experiments indicated that, on the average, BACs of 50–70 mg% would bring about cessation of voluntary alcohol drinking in P rats. They also suggested that the reinforcing action of ethanol for P rats may be at concentrations below 100 mg%.

In another kind of experiment, the relationship of BAC to spontaneous motor activity in P and NP rats was examined after intraperitoneal injection of ethanol (Waller *et al.,* 1986). The P rats, but not NPs, exhibited increased spontaneous motor activity following the administration of ethanol, 0.07 to 0.5 g/kg body weight. BACs reached 15–75 mg%. These data indicate that BACs in this range are pharmacologically active and probably reflect the positive reinforcing effect of ethanol. It is interesting that with repeated daily injections of ethanol at 0.25 g/kg doses for up to 7 days, the increase of spontaneous motor activity in the P rats was as much as 50% after each daily injection and there was no tolerance or reverse tolerance.

3. *The alcohol preference exhibited by P rats is inelastic to dietary manipulations.* In one experiment (Li et al., 1987), P rats were offered the choice of three powdered diets of different carbohydrate content along with water and 10% ethanol. All the diets contained 4.34 kcal/g and 10% fat, while the carbohydrate content was varied from 78% to 59% to 22%. Regardless of whether all three diets were presented together or individually with water and 10% ethanol available ad libitum, alcohol consumption by the P rats was inelastic to the dietary manipulation, i.e., P rats maintained a high alcohol preference under all test conditions and they substituted ethanol calories for the solid food calories.

An extreme example of inelasticity of alcohol consumption to dietary manipulation in the P rats was reported by Lankford et al. (1991). These investigators presented the P rats with free-choice laboratory chow, water, the most preferred concentration (21 ±

2%) of ethanol, and one of two strongly flavored solutions as a third drinking fluid, i.e., a 2:1 diluted chocolate-flavored Slender drink that was calorically fortified and a 5 g/1 Nutrasweet solution, an artificially sweetened solution devoid of calories. With the diluted Slender as the third fluid, P rats became polydipsic and consumed large volumes of the Slender solution but ethanol intake was unaffected at all and it remained high at about 7.7 g/kg/day. With Nutrasweet as the third fluid available ad libitum, P rats were not polydipsic; nevertheless, ethanol consumption during free-choice drinking was also unaltered (ethanol intake averaged 7.8 g/kg/day). These data clearly demonstrated that alcohol drinking in P rats is inelastic to dietary influences.

4. *Ethanol is positively reinforcing to the P line of rats by operant responding experiments.* Experiments have been performed with either a one- or two-lever operant design to test whether P rats will bar press to obtain alcohol when food and water are freely available. With the one-lever design (Penn et al., 1978), response rates in excess of 1000 bar presses per 24 hours to obtain ethanol as a reinforcer were recorded in each of the free-fed P rats tested. With the two-lever design, laboratory chow was offered ad libitum along with operant responding to obtain water and different concentrations of ethanol (Murphy et al., 1989). P rats self-administered more of the ethanol solution than water, even when ethanol concentration in the drinking solution was increased to 30%. With 15% and 20% ethanol, P rats self-administered up to 9.5 g ethanol/kg/day. By comparison, NP rats showed a preference for water as soon as the alcohol concentration exceeded 5%.

Additionally, studies have been performed to determine whether for P rats the reinforcing properties of ethanol arise from its central nervous system (CNS) pharmacologic actions or its taste or smell. These studies have included experiments conducted to discern whether P rats would self-administer ethanol by the intragastric route (Waller et al., 1984) or by direct infusion of nanoliter amounts of ethanol solutions into the ventral tegmental area of the brain (Gatto et al., 1990a; Gatto et al., 1992). In intragastric self-administration studies, the experimental design originally reported by Deutsch and coworkers (Deutsch and Hardy, 1976; Deutsch and Eisner, 1977) was used. The results of this experiment indicate that the P rats consistently self-infused greater volumes of an ethanol solution and lesser volumes of water than did the NP rats (Waller et al, 1984). This difference was observed regardless of whether the concentration of ethanol infused intragastrically was 10, 20, 30, or 40%. The amount of ethanol infused by the NP rats was always less than 1 g/kg/day at all concentrations of ethanol tested. By contrast, the amount of ethanol self-infused by the P rats increased from 3.0 ± 0.3 g/kg/day with 10% ethanol to 9.4 ± 1.7 g/kg/day with 40% ethanol. The BACs measured 30 minutes after observed episodes of self-infusion of 20% ethanol reached 116 to 303 mg% (mean of 199 mg%), while with 40% ethanol, BACs attained 92 to 415 mg% (mean of 231 mg%). These data indicate that P rats will work to obtain ethanol for CNS positive reinforcing effects and not for its calories, taste, or smell.

In another series of experiments, the role of the ventral tegmental area (VTA) in the CNS mechanism that mediates the rewarding properties of ethanol was examined (Gatto et al., 1990a). Alcohol-naive P rats were implanted with a guide cannula in the

VTA that was connected to an electrolytic microinfusion transducer system. Experiments were conducted to determine whether the P rats would self-administer ethanol directly into the VTA. The rats were placed in a 2-lever operant chamber and were allowed to self-administer 25–200 mg% ethanol in artificial cerebrospinal fluid (100 nl over 5 sec) in a FR1 schedule by pressing an active lever that resulted in response-contingent intracranial self-administration (ICSA) of ethanol. Pressing the active lever also activated a red cue light. Response on a second lever was inactive and was not reinforcing. In each 6-hourly session, the P rats responded significantly more (as high as 13-fold) on the active lever than on the inactive lever. Responses on the active lever increased with increasing ethanol concentration, and maximum response rates were recorded at 100–150 mg%. These data clearly indicate that P rats will work to obtain ethanol for CNS effect and not for its calories, taste, or smell.

Since these initial experiments with ICSA of ethanol, additional experiments have been done to show that P rats will press the active lever for ICSA of ethanol even without the red cue light as a neutral stimulus (Gatto et al., 1992). These data provide additional support that ethanol has CNS positive reinforcing actions in the P rat and, furthermore, indicate that the VTA may be a major CNS site where alcohol initiates these positive effects.

5. *The P rats develop metabolic and neuronal tolerance.* This has been shown (Lumeng et al., 1986b) with chronic free-choice drinking of 10% (v/v) ethanol. After six weeks, ethanol elimination rate of the alcohol-consuming P rats was 15% higher than that of control P rats. The mechanism for the development of metabolic tolerance has not been studied in the P line of rats, but presumably the induction of cytochrome P450IIE1 (CYP450IIE1) is at least partially involved. Recently, Winters and Cederbaum (1992) measured the constitutive levels of CYP450IIE1 in the liver of P and NP rats and its inducibility by agents such as pyrazole and 4-methylpyrazole. These investigators measured both enzyme activities and immunoreactive protein content of CYP450IIE1 and found no difference between the two lines. A difference in CYP450IIE1 has been found in selectively bred LS and SS mice, lines that differ in ethanol-induced sleep time or righting reflex (French et al., 1979).

With chronic free-choice drinking of 10% alcohol, and food and water available at all times, it has also been demonstrated that P rats develop behavioral or neuronal tolerance as assessed by a jump test that required the animals to jump onto a descending platform to escape foot shock (Gatto et al., 1987a). Neuronal tolerance was demonstrated by a significantly shorter time for the tolerant P rats to recover to criterion performance on the jump test after an intraperitoneal injection of ethanol and by a significantly higher BAC at the time of recovery.

6. *Chronic free-choice drinking for 20 weeks by the P rats produces physical dependence.* This physical dependence, shown in a study by Waller (1982b), was evidenced by the development of signs of withdrawal in 18 of 19 ethanol-exposed P rats within the first 24 hours following removal of ethanol. These signs included Straub tail, broad-based gait, tremulousness, hyperactivity, wet-dog shakes, teeth-chattering, sound-induced running, and bizarre behavior. These manifestations abated within 72 hours.

Table 7-3 Selectively Bred Alcohol-Preferring Lines of Rats as Animal Models of Alcoholism

	P	HAD	AA	sP	UChB
1. Alcohol drinking exceeding 5g/kg/day	Most	Most	Most[a]	Most[b]	Most[c]
2. BACs reach >100 mg% during free-choice alcohol drinking	Yes[d]		Yes[e]		
3. Ethanol is reinforcing as shown by operant responding or other means	Yes[f]		Yes[g]	Yes[h]	
4. Metabolic tolerance with chronic free-choice drinking	Yes[i]				
5. Behavioral or neuronal tolerance with chronic free-choice drinking	Yes[j]		Yes[k]		No[l]
6. Alcohol dependence with chronic free-choice drinking	Yes[m]				

[a]Sinclair et al., 1989.

[b]Fadda et al., 1989

[c]Mardones and Segovia-Riquelme, 1983.

[d]Murphy et al., 1986a

[e]Aalto, 1986.

[f]Penn et al., 1978

[j]Murphy et al., 1989.

[g]Hyytia and Sinclair, 1989.

[h]Colombo et al., 1990.

[i]Lumeng et al., 1986.

[j]Gatto et al., 1987a, Gatto et al 1987b.

[k]Kalant, 1987.

[l]Tampier et al., 1980.

[m]Waller et al., 1982b.

Table 7-3 compares the extent to which the P line of rats has been shown to meet the criteria of an animal model of alcoholism with that in the other selected rat lines that exhibit high alcohol preference. It is clear that there is to date a high degree of concordance among the rat lines selectively bred by different laboratories, i.e., most of the alcohol-preferring rats drink >5 g of ethanol/kg/day, they raise their BACs to >100 mg% during free-choice drinking, and they demonstrate that alcohol is positively reinforcing. Both the P and the AA lines have been shown to develop behavioral or neuronal tolerance with chronic free-choice alcohol consumption, although the UChB rats have been shown not to develop tolerance.

It should be noted that the P/NP rats do not differ in ethanol elimination rates (Li and Lumeng, 1977) and in acetaldehyde concentrations attainable after alcohol administration (unpublished data). However, an interesting polymorphism of the rat liver mitochondrial aldehyde dehydrogenase (ALDH2) was observed that involves a G for A exchange in the cDNA of NP rats that changes amino acid 67 from Gln (CAG codon; $ALDH2^Q$ allele) to Arg (CGG codon; $ALDH2^R$ allele) (Carr et al., 1990, 1991). In a study of 37 P and 49 NP rats, it was found that the frequency of the $ALDH2^R$ allele was 63% in the NP line and only 18% in the P line; the frequency of the $ALDH2^Q$ allele was 82% in the P and 37% in the NP line. Whether these polymorphisms will produce ALDH2 enzymes with different kinetic properties is the subject of ongoing investigation. In contrast to the P/NP lines, differences in the rates of ethanol and acetaldehyde metabolism have been demonstrated in the AA/ANA lines (Sinclair et al., 1989). The rates of ethanol metabolism and BACs at 30 minutes after ethanol administration have been reported to be higher in ethanol-naive F_{17}, F_{40}, F_{43}, and F_{48} AAs than in ANAs. The accumulation of acetaldehyde in blood has been demonstrated to be higher in F_{17}, F_{29}, F_{40}, and F_{43} ANAs when compared with AAs. While total liver ALDH activities do not differ between ethanol-naive AA/ANA lines (Inoue et al., 1981), a recent report indicated that AAs exhibited lower ALDH activity in the olfactory tubercle than the ANAs, and that AAs had higher ALDH activity in their spinal cord motor neurons, Purkinje cells, and capillary endothelial cells of the cerebellum (Sinclair et al., 1989). The significance of these findings is still unclear. Recently, two different alleles of the mitochondrial ALDH gene (ALDH2), ALDH2^R and ALDH2^Q, have been found in rats, but studies with AA and ANA indicate that there are no line differences in their frequencies of ALDH2^R and ALDH2^Q alleles. Thus, a known polymorphism in the ALDH2 gene in rats does not explain the acetaldehyde accumulations in the ANA rats (Koivisto et al., 1993). One should recall that in humans a variant of mitochondrial ALDH2 is found in about 50% of Asians in which a Lys is substituted for Glu at position 487, and that the resultant enzyme subunit is inactive, causing a deficiency of liver ALDH activity and the alcohol-induced flush reaction with drinking (Yoshida et al., 1984). The latter is a major deterrent factor against alcohol abuse among Asians (Thomasson et al., 1991). Whether high blood acetaldehyde levels in ANA rats or a high frequency of ALDH2^R allele in NP rats actually produces alcohol aversion has not been experimentally tested.

Contrary to the findings with selectively bred rat lines such as the P and AA lines, Dole et al. (1984, 1985, 1988) have pointed out that the inbred C57BL mouse strain may not be a suitable animal model of alcoholism. They questioned whether the motivation of alcohol drinking in the C57BL mice is the same as that of humans who drink excessive amounts of alcohol. Although most C57BL mice consume large amounts of alcohol on free-choice and frequently raise their BACs to levels >100 mg%, Dole et al. (1985) found that the alcohol consumption of these mice was "elastic" to dietary influences, i.e., free-choice alcohol drinking decreased when their lab chow was supplemented with either sucrose or fat. This elasticity in alcohol ingestion infers that C57BL mice have a strong nutritional need to drink alcohol and do not drink because of drug-seeking behavior. Gentry et al. (1983) have also observed that alcohol intake of C57BL mice was insensitive to BACs. In one experiment, these investigators found that C57BL mice treated with 4-methylpyrazole developed mean BACs up to the range of 116 mg%, while control mice treated with saline exhibited mean BACs in the range of 11 mg%. Despite these large differences in BACs, alcohol consumption measured as daily alcohol intake and preference ratio was the same between the two groups. Thus, C57BL mice apparently did not appear to seek bouts of intoxication or to avoid it. An extreme situation was the observation that some 4-methylpyrazole-treated mice, being accustomed to drinking large volumes of 10% ethanol and seemingly insensitive to the accumulation of ethanol in their blood, actually drank alcohol during free-choice to the point of coma (Gentry, 1985). Of note, a relative insensitivity of C57BL mice to the taste of alcohol has also been reported (Nachman et al., 1971). These observations led Dole et al. (1988) to conclude that the genetic component that influences alcohol ingestion in the C57BL mice is only permissive in nature and that it can be explained by their relative insensitivity to the aversive orosensory and pharmacological effects of 10% ethanol rather than as a specific drug-seeking predisposition.

Behavioral and Neurophysiological Differences in Alcohol-Preferring and -Nonpreferring Rats

The factors that determine the amount of drug an animal consumes can be divided into those that encourage drug intake (reinforcing effects) and those that limit drug intake (aversive effects). Whether alcohol is positively reinforcing or aversive depends on its dose, i.e., low doses are reinforcing but high doses are aversive (the so-called biphasic effects of ethanol).

It is clear from the preceding section that ethanol is much more positively reinforcing to the P rats than to the NPs. This statement is supported by the fact that P rats will self-administer ethanol in a free-choice situation by oral and intragastric routes, and they will work by bar-pressing in an operant chamber to obtain ethanol by either the oral route or by intracranial self-administration into the VTA. Additionally, low doses of ethanol (0.07 to 0.50 g/kg intraperitoneal doses or BACs less than 75 mg%) will cause arousal for the P rats but not the NPs. Low-dose ethanol-induced arousal in P rats was first demonstrated by increased spontaneous motor activities detected within 30 minutes of intraperitoneal injection of ethanol. Recently, electrophysiological measures have further documented an arousing effect of ethanol in the P rats. Morzorati et al. (1988) reported that, during non-REM sleep, 0.5 g of ethanol/kg given intragastrically produced a persistent increase in EEG spectral power in NP rats, but that the power decreased initially in P rats and then returned to baseline. Since it is known that the amplitude and power of the EEG increase as rats cycle in a continuum from wakefulness to drowsiness and finally to deep non-REM sleep, the initial decrease in EEG power in the P rats immediately after ethanol administration indicates that they were aroused by ethanol but that the NP rats were sedated.

Additionally, Ehlers et al. (1991) recently implanted electrodes in the frontal cortex and dorsal hippocampus of P and NP rats and used a passive auditory "oddball" paradigm to record event-related potentials (ERP) following intraperitoneal injection of either saline, 0.5 g, or 1.0 g ethanol/kg. With saline injections, P rats exhibited smaller N1-like ERP components and larger P2 waves in both the cortex and hippocampus when compared with NP rats. With ethanol injections, P rats also exhibited different ERP responses when compared with NP rats, i.e., NP rats displayed a dose-dependent decrease in ERP component amplitudes, such as the N1 recorded from the cortex, whereas P rats showed increased N1 amplitudes, particularly in the hippocampus. These data suggested that ethanol produces more arousal in the P rats than in the NP rats.

There is a popularly held belief that alcohol has a tension-reducing or anxiolytic property when consumed by humans. Baldwin and his colleagues (1991) used the conflict test of Geller-Seifter to test whether P, NP, and outbred Wistar rats differ in punished responding when given different doses of ethanol. In this test, anxiolytics such as the benzodiazepines and chlordiazepoxide are known to increase the rate of lever responses in the punished component of the test. P rats did not show a significant increase in punished responding until the dosage of ethanol reached 0.75 g/kg. By comparison, NP rats displayed significant increases in punished responding with much lower doses of ethanol, 0.25 g/kg, and Wistar rats exhibited significant increases in punished responding with doses of 0.5, 0.75, and 1 g/kg ethanol. Thus, similar to family history-positive human subjects, P rats are less sensitive to the anticonflict effects of ethanol and they need to drink more ethanol to obtain an adequate tension-reducing effect. This conclusion is in general agreement with the report by Stewart et al. (1989) that P rats may be more "anxious" and more sensitive to stress-producing stimuli.

While ethanol may be consumed by the P and AA rats mainly for its hedonic and anxiety-reducing properties, there is also a considerable body of data that indicates that ethanol is less aversive to the alcohol-preferring lines than to the nonpreferring lines. In the case of the P and NP rats, several important innate differences in responses to ethanol have been reported (Table 7-4).

Bice and Kiefer (1990) used orofacial reactivity to tastants to examine ethanol responses of P and NP rats. In the initial exposure, P and NP rats were tested for reactivity to five concentrations of ethanol (5, 10, 20, 30, and 40% v/v), water, a sucrose solution, and a quinine solution. A two-bottle preference test with 10% ethanol and water was then given to both the P and NP rats for three weeks. A second taste reactivity test was done using the same solutions as in the initial test. These investigators did not find any significant differences in taste reactivity between P and NP rats on initial exposure. During alcohol preference testing, P rats consistently drank more ethanol

Table 7-4 Innate Differences in Responses to Aversive Effects of Ethanol and Tolerance Development (or Persistence) in P/NP and HAD/LAD Rats Given Different Doses of Ethanol

Correlated Response	Innate Difference	Tolerance Development/Persistence
1. Aversive taste	No differences between P and NP	Less aversion (tolerance development) in P but not in NP with free-choice alcohol drinking for 3 weeks
2. Conditioned place avoidance	Less avoidance of place paired with ethanol in P relative to NP	Tolerance to aversion in P rats after chronic free-choice alcohol drinking
3. Conditioned taste aversion	1 g/kg ethanol, less conditioned taste aversion in P; 0.25 g/kg ethanol, facilitation in P but not in NP	Tolerance to aversion in P after chronic free-choice alcohol drinking
4. Jump test to avoid footshock	Faster recovery in P and HAD rats due to within session acute tolerance	Persistence of tolerance in P and HAD, but less so in NP and LAD
5. Sleep time (loss of righting reflex)	Faster recovery in P rats due to within session acute tolerance	Persistence of tolerance in P, but sensitization in NP when 2 doses of ethanol (3 g/kg) were given separated by 1 day
6. Hypothermia	—	Persistence of larger tolerance in P than NP (2 doses, 3.5 g/kg, separated by 1 day); sensitization in NP rats (2 doses 3.5 g/kg, separated by 3 days)
7. Loss of aerial righting reflex	No difference in initial sensitivity	—

than NP rats. On the second taste reactivity test, P rats showed considerably fewer aversive responses (passive drips, gapes, head shakes, forelimb flails, and fluid expulsion) to alcohol than NP rats. Between the initial and the second reactivity tests, taste reactivity of NP rats to alcohol did not change, and responses of P and NP rats to sucrose and quinine also did not differ. These data indicated that alcohol-naive NP and P rats do not innately differ in taste reactivity to ethanol but that the taste of alcohol becomes more palatable to P rats (though not to the NPs) after ethanol exposure, and that this factor may play a role in maintaining high alcohol consumption in the P rats.

Stewart et al. (1992a) employed a place-conditioning procedure to study innate differences to the positive and negative reinforcing properties of alcohol as well as tolerance development to the aversive effects of ethanol in P and NP rats. A two-compartment apparatus was used. Four ethanol conditioning trials were administered on alternate days in which groups of P and NP rats received intraperitoneal injections of 0.5, 1.0, or 1.5 g ethanol/kg or saline and were confined for 15 minutes in one compartment of a two-compartment apparatus. On the intervening days, the same animals received saline injections preceding a 15-min confinement in the other compartment. It was found that, while a dose-dependent avoidance of the compartment previously paired with ethanol injection was seen in both P and NP rats, the magnitude of the avoidance with 1.0 and 1.5 g/kg doses of ethanol was considerably less in the P relative to the NP rats. Thus, ethanol was less aversive to P than to NP rats with doses that produced peaked BACs of about 200 to 250 mg%.

Stewart et al. (1992b) also tested the possibility that P rats might develop tolerance to the aversive effects of ethanol after chronic free-choice alcohol drinking. For this experiment, one group of P rats was offered free-choice ethanol for 33 days, while another group was treated identically but had no ethanol to drink. Conditioned place-avoidance was tested on day 34, and it was again found that a dose-dependent avoidance of the ethanol-paired compartment was evident, but the place-avoidance was attenuated at the 1.0-g/kg ethanol dose in the group of P rats that had been chronically exposed to alcohol. Thus, as in the taste reactivity studies conducted by Bice and Kiefer (1990), tolerance to the aversive effects of ethanol develops in P rats during chronic alcohol drinking.

Froehlich et al. (1988) used a conditioned taste aversion paradigm to compare P and NP rats in their response to ethanol. Injections of different doses of ethanol was paired with the drinking of a saccharin solution. The P and NP rats were then tested for drinking preference in a choice between the saccharin solution and water. With a low dose of ethanol (0.25 g/kg), P rats exhibited conditioned facilitation, whereas NP rats showed no effect. At the 1.0-g/kg dose, NP rats began to show conditioned aversion to drinking the saccharin solution, but the P rats were unaffected. At higher doses, ethanol produced conditioned taste aversion equally in both the P and NP rats. These data suggest low-dose ethanol is rewarding to the P rats, but not the NP rats, and indicate that P rats are less affected than NP rats by the high-dose aversive actions of ethanol.

Stewart et al. (1990) have tested whether chronic free-choice alcohol consumption in P rats can attenuate subsequent conditioned taste aversion produced by ethanol injections. Following 33 days of continuous availability of food, water, and 10% ethanol, five daily conditioned taste aversion trials were given to a group of alcohol-drinking P rats and to a group of alcohol-naive control P rats. During this period, the P rats increased ethanol consumption by 50%. The conditioned taste aversion trials consisted of access to a polycose solution for 20 minutes, followed by intraperitoneal injections of either saline, 0.5, 1.0, or 1.5g ethanol/kg body weight. The alcohol-exposed P rats developed an increased preference for the polycose solution when paired with 0.5-g ethanol/kg injections, but the control P rats did not. At the 1.0-g/kg dose, the alcohol-exposed group exhibited an attenuated conditioned taste aversion response relative to the control group. At 1.5-g ethanol/kg, both the alcohol-exposed and alcohol-naive groups displayed similar conditioned taste aversion responses. Thus, as with the taste reactivity responses and conditioned place avoidance studies, P rats develop tolerance to the aversive effects of ethanol during chronic free-choice alcohol drinking, and this tolerance could contribute at least partly to their high alcohol intake.

In addition to chronic tolerance, a series of studies has shown that P rats can develop acute tolerance to a single sedative-hypnotic dose of ethanol more quickly and/or to a greater extent than NP rats. It was found that the acquisition of acute tolerance can explain why P rats recovered much more quickly than NP rats in a number of behavioral tests that measured the depressant action of ethanol. These tests include a performance test that required trained rats to jump onto a descending platform to avoid foot-shock (Lumeng et al., 1982; Waller et al., 1983); hypothermia induced by high-dose ethanol (Froehlich et al., 1989); and regain of righting-reflex (sleep time) produced by a single injection of a sedative-hypnotic dose of ethanol (Kurtz et al., 1990, 1991). Following an injection of a single intraperitoneal dose (2.0 g ethanol/kg body weight) of ethanol given to both P and NP rats, P rats recovered to a criterion of 75% of preethanol training performance in the jumping apparatus within 33 ± 0.5 minutes and with BACs of 250 ± 5 mg%, but NP rats recovered much more slowly, i.e., in 74 ± 6 minutes and with BACs of 234 ± 5 mg%. Similar results have also been obtained in studies using sleep time as a test of acute tolerance. Interestingly, using the jump test, Gatto et al. (1987b) have further reported that the acute tolerance that developed in the P rats to a single dose of ethanol could persist for as long as 10 days, whereas such tolerance, which was much smaller in the NP rats, dissipated within 3 days. Hitherto, acute tolerance development is the most robust association in rodents with high voluntary alcohol consumption (Murphy et al., 1990). In addition to the P and NP rats, disparate acquisition of acute tolerance has been described in the alcohol-preferring C57BL and the alcohol-nonpreferring DBA mouse strains (Tabakoff and Ritzman, 1979; Tabakoff et al., 1980), in the HS/Ibg heterogenous stock mice with high and low alcohol preference (Erwin et al., 1980), and in the selectively bred AA and ANA rats (Nikander and Pekkanen, 1977).

The most plausible explanation for why P and NP (or AA and ANA) rats differ in alcohol-seeking behavior is summarized in the following list and in Fig. 7-2.

1. Ethanol is more positively reinforcing to P than NP and to AA than ANA rats.
2. In alcohol-naive animals, aversive effects of ethanol are only evident at BACs that are significantly higher in P than NP rats.

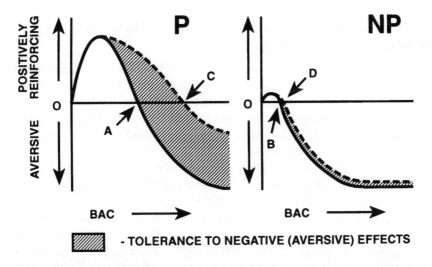

Fig. 7-2 Innately, the crossover point in BAC between the reinforcing and aversive properties of ethanol is shifted to the right in the P rats (point A vs. point B). Additionally, P rats find alcohol much more positively reinforcing at low BACs than do NP rats. P rats develop both acute and chronic tolerance to the aversive effects of high-dose alcohol to a much greater extent than do NP rats (point C vs. point D). Moreover, the acute tolerance acquired by P rats is more persistent than that acquired by NP rats.

3. Acute tolerance development to a single high (aversive) dose of ethanol is more robust and more persistent in the P than NP rats.
4. Chronic tolerance to the high-dose, aversive effects of ethanol develops in P rats (but not NPs) during chronic free-choice alcohol drinking. This effect can lead to a progressive increase in alcohol intake with time in the P rats. Based on accumulated data, the alcohol-preferring and -nonpreferring rats differ considerably in sensitivity to BACs when alcohol is reinforcing and aversive, i.e., the crossover point in BAC between the reinforcing and aversive properties of alcohol is shifted to the right in the P (and AA) rats (Fig. 7-2). In addition to innate differences in the rewarding features of alcohol, the development of both acute and chronic tolerance makes an important contribution to the aversive actions of alcohol in alcohol-preferring rats. Tolerance development moves the crossover points toward a higher BAC in the P (and AA) rats than in the NP (and ANA) rats (Fig. 7-2). As described before, the alcohol-preferring lines also develop and maintain tolerance to a greater extent than the contrasting lines. Because the alcohol-preferring lines drink much more ethanol and can raise their BACs to much higher levels than the nonpreferring lines, the preferring rats can develop chronic tolerance to the aversive effects of ethanol, while the nonpreferring lines cannot. Thus, a combination of an increased sensitivity to the low-dose reinforcing effects of ethanol and the development of acute and chronic tolerance to the aversive effects of ethanol at a high threshold provides the most attractive hypothesis to explain the development of excessive alcohol-drinking behavior (Fig. 7-2). As tolerance to the high-dose effects of ethanol develops, the reinforcing/rewarding actions of ethanol become progressively extended into a higher BAC range, leading to increased consumption. Future efforts should be devoted to testing this hypothesis in humans and to determining the neurochemical substrates that explain this process in alcohol-preferring lines.

Neurochemical and Neuroanatomical Differences in Alcohol-Preferring and -Nonpreferring Animals

Neurochemical and neuroanatomical studies to date have elucidated major innate differences in the alcohol-preferring relative to the nonpreferring lines, and to a lesser extent some differences in response to ethanol as well. The neurotransmitter systems that have been most extensively investigated are the serotonin (5HT), dopamine (DA), and gamma-aminobutyric acid (GABA) systems. Neuropeptide studies have also been conducted by various investigators.

The relationship between alcohol preference and a deficiency in the 5HT system has been extensively studied in the selectively bred P and NP lines of rats. One of the most positive findings was that the contents of 5-HT and 5-hydroxyindoleacetic acid (5-HIAA) were 12–26% lower for the P than for the NP rats in several CNS regions, including the cerebral cortex, hippocampus, corpus striatum, thalamus, and hypothalamus (Murphy et al., 1982). Similar differences were not found in the midbrain or pons–medulla. In a follow-up study, Murphy et al. (1987) also found 20–30% lower levels of 5-HT in the frontal cortex, nucleus accumbens, and anterior striatum. Since several of these CNS regions (e.g., the frontal cortex, nucleus accumbens, hypothalamus) might be involved in mediating the rewarding properties of abusive drugs, including ethanol, these data indicate a strong relationship of the serotonin systems to alcohol preference. These data, however, do not indicate whether the lower contents of 5-HT and/or 5-HIAA are due to decreased synthesis, lower functional activity, and/or lower 5-HT innervations in the CNS of the P line of rats.

If a deficiency in the CNS 5-HT system is associated with alcohol preference, then similar differences in the contents of 5-HT and 5-HIAA may be expected to be found in the CNS between other lines of animals with high- and low-alcohol preference. Early studies on the C57BL (alcohol preferrers) and DBA (alcohol nonpreferrers) strains of mice indicated that there were no differences between the two groups in whole-brain content of 5-HT (Ho et al., 1975; Pickett and Collins, 1975). In contrast to the findings with the P and NP rats, early studies with the AA and ANA lines of rats indicated that higher levels of 5-HT were found in many brain regions of the AA rats (Ahtee and Eriksson, 1972, 1973). These findings of were recently confirmed after revitalization of the two lines (Korpi et al., 1988).

Other recent studies, on the other hand, have provided additional evidence supporting a relationship between lower CNS 5-HT levels and alcohol preference. Yoshimoto and Komura (1987) examined the relationship between voluntary alcohol consumption and brain monoamine levels in several inbred strains of mice and found an inverse relationship between alcohol intake and brain 5-HT levels. In agreement with this latter finding, a lower brain content of 5-HT and 5-HIAA in the alcohol-preferring C57BL compared with the nonpreferring CBA mice has been reported (Badaway et al., 1989). Three separate studies with other rat lines also support the idea that a CNS 5-HT deficiency is associated with high alcohol intake. Murphy et al. (1986b) found lower contents of 5-HT and 5-HIAA in the thalamus and hypothalamus of N/Nih heterogeneous stock rats that had been tested and found to consume high amounts of alcohol (>5.0 g ethanol/kg/day) in comparison to N/Nih heterogeneous stock rats that were tested and found to consume low quantities of alcohol (<0.5 g/kg/day). This study was extended by selectively breeding the high and low alcohol drinkers from the N/Nih heterogeneous stock rats to produce the replicate HAD and LAD lines, respectively (Li et al., 1988). The contents of 5-HT and 5-HIAA were examined in several CNS regions of the HAD and LAD lines after the eighth generation. In excellent agreement with the data for the P and NP rats, Gongwer et al. (1989) found that the contents of 5-HT and/or 5-HIAA were approximately 10–20% lower (P < 0.05) in several CNS regions (cerebral cortex, striatum, nucleus accumbens, septal nuclei, hippocampus, and hypothalamus) of the HAD line compared with the LAD rats. Finally, Fawn Hooded rats have recently been reported to have high alcohol drinking behavior and to exhibit a deficiency in the brain 5-HT system (Rezvani et al., 1990a).

Additional studies have been undertaken with the P and NP lines to better understand the reasons for the differences in 5-HT CNS regional contents and to examine some of the possible neurobiological consequences of this apparent 5-HT deficiency. Immunocytochemical experiments demonstrated that there were fewer 5-HT immunostained fibers in several CNS regions (e.g., anterior frontal cortex, nucleus accumbens, and portions of the ventral hippocampus) of the P than in the NP (Zhou et al., 1991a, 1991b). These findings suggest that the lower contents of 5-HT observed in the CNS of the P rat are due to decreased 5-HT innervations in these areas. Furthermore, the lower 5-HT fiber densities appear to be due to fewer 5-HT immunostained neurons in the dorsal and median raphe of the P rat (Zhou et al., 1991c).

As a result of the decreased 5-HT innervations in the P line, there appears to be an upregulation of 5-HT$_{1A}$ receptors. Wong et al. (1990, 1993) reported a higher density of 5-HT$_{1A}$ receptors in membrane preparations from the hippocampus and frontal cortex of the P compared to the NP rats. Autoradiography experiments confirmed these findings, i.e., that in frontal cortical areas and certain hippocampal regions the densities of 5-HT$_{1A}$ receptors were higher in the alcohol-preferring rats (McBride et al., 1990, 1991a, 1991b, 1992).

Recent biochemical studies reported by Badaway et al (1989) on the C57BL mice have offered a different mechanism for the low 5-HT and 5HIAA levels in the brain of these mice. These investigators found that C57BL mice (when compared with CBA/Ca mice) possessed lower serum levels of total and free tryptophan as well as lower brain contents of tryptophan. They further observed that C57BL mice exhibited much higher serum corticosterone levels than the CBA/Ca mice plus higher hepatic tryptophan pyrrolase activities (an enzyme induced by corticosterone). They concluded that the lower brain content of 5HT in C57BL mice can be explained by a decrease in circulating tryptophan availability to the brain, and that the latter can in turn be explained by a higher liver tryptophan pyrrolase activity associated with a higher circulating corticosterone concentration. These findings in the C57BL mice are different from those in the P rats since the mechanism responsible for decreased 5HT content in the brain of P rats seems to be caused by a decrease in the number of 5HT fibers in certain brain areas important in drug reward (Zhou et al, 1991a, 1991b, 1991c).

Although the majority of data favors the hypothesis of an innate serotonergic deficiency being an underlying factor in high alcohol drinking, data from the AA and ANA rats suggest that elevated levels of brain 5-HT are associated with high ethanol preference. Alcohol drinking is likely to be a very complex behavior involving the interactions of multiple transmitter systems, of which the serotonin system plays only one part. An imbalance in one or more of these interactions could produce abnormal alcohol drinking behavior. Thus, in some cases, a deficient 5-HT system may create an imbalance in the circuitries that regulate alcohol drinking. In other cases, the abnormality may be in a different system (e.g., peptidergic), which produces alterations in the other circuitries involved in regulating alcohol intake. This hypothesis is consistent with the notion that there are subtypes of alcoholic patients (Cloninger et al, 1981; Bohman et al., 1981).

In most CNS regions thus far studied, there appears to be no significant innate differences in the contents of DA between rodents with high alcohol preference and those with low alcohol preference with two important exceptions. Among the several CNS regions examined in the P versus the NP rats (Murphy et al., 1982; 1987) and in the HAD versus the LAD rats (Gongwer et al., 1989), there was a 10–30% lower content (P < 0.05) of DA, DOPAC (3,4-dihydroxyphenylacetic acid) and HVA (homovanillic acid) in the nucleus accumbens and a 15–20% lower content of DA, DOPAC, and/or HVA in the anterior striatum of the groups with high alcohol preference. These data suggest that there is a deficiency in the DA pathway that projects from the VTA to these two regions. Moreover, since other regions that receive DA projections from the VTA (e.g., septal nuclei) or from the substantia nigra (e.g., posterior striatum) do not exhibit an innate difference in the content of DA, it would appear that a specific population of DA neurons within the VTA may be abnormal. The nature of this deficiency is unknown but could be due to a number of factors, i.e., decreased synthesis, reduced innervation, and/or lower functional activity.

In addition to differences in DA contents in several CNS regions of the P and NP rats, two independent reports from separate laboratories have shown decreased densities of DA D_2 receptors in the limbic systems of the alcohol-preferring rats (Stefanini et al., 1992; McBride et al., 1993). In the P rats, quantitative autoradiography revealed that the binding of [^{3}H] sulpiride was 20–25% lower in the caudate-putamen, medial and lateral nucleus accumbens, and the ventral tegmental area of the P compared with the NP rats. With standard membrane preparations and Scatchard analysis, it was found that the decreased [^{3}H] sulpiride binding in the caudate-putamen was due to lower Bmax values for the P line (McBride et al., 1993). Similar data have also been reported for the Sardinian sP and sNP rats, i.e., approximately 20% lower Bmax values were reported in the caudate nucleus, nucleus accumbens, and olfactory tubercle of sP rats compared with the sNP rats (Stefanini et al., 1992). Of note, several studies have indicated that the VTA DA system projecting to the nucleus accumbens is involved in mediating the actions of alcohol and alcohol-seeking behavior (Levy et al., 1991b; Weiss et al., 1992; Samson et al., 1993).

Other studies with inbred strains of mice or selected lines of rats, with either high or low alcohol preference, do not provide evidence supporting an innate abnormal functioning of the DA systems being associated with high alcohol drinking behavior. However, none of these studies examined the nucleus accumbens specifically. With their revitalized AA and ANA lines, Korpi et al. (1988) found no difference in the DA contents in the hypothalamus, midbrain–brainstem, frontal cortex, hippocampus, or striatum. Similarly, there was no difference in the contents of DA in the caudate nucleus, medial prefrontal cortex, and olfactory tubercles between the selectively bred Sardinian alcohol-preferring (sP) and -nonpreferring (sNP) lines of rats (Fadda et al., 1989). In addition, Yoshimoto and Komura (1987) found no clear correlation between the brain content of DA and alcohol intake among several inbred strains of mice.

There is some evidence that an innate abnormality in the noradrenergic (NE) system is associated with high alcohol consumption. Yoshimoto and Komura (1987) reported a significant positive correlation between brain NE levels and alcohol intake among several inbred strains of mice. Murphy et al. (1982) also reported that the NE content was 20% higher ($P < 0.05$) in the cerebral cortex of the P compared to the NP rats. However, no differences were observed in the NE content between the P and NP lines in several other forebrain regions examined (e.g., striatum, thalamus, hypothalamus, and hippocampus). In contrast to the preceding NE differences, with the revitalized AA and ANA lines, Korpi et al. (1988) found that NE levels were 15% lower ($P < 0.05$) in the frontal cortex of the alcohol preferrers. However, NE levels in the hypothalamus were approximately 25% higher in the AA than ANA line; no differences were observed between those two lines in the hippocampus and striatum (Korpi et al., 1988). A higher NE level could indicate increased NE innervation and/or a metabolic or storage anomaly. However, additional information will need to be obtained to establish the possibility that an innate abnormality in the NE system is involved with high alcohol intake. Other evidence gathered thus far does not support this idea. Wong et al., (1988) examined the binding of [^{3}H]-ligands to membrane preparations of the posterior cerebral cortex and found no differences between P and NP rats in K_D or B_{max} values for α-1- α-2-, and β-adrenergic receptors.

There is now considerable evidence that ethanol can exert some of its effects by potentiating the actions of GABA at the GABA$_A$ receptor complex (Suzdak et al., 1986a, 1986b, 1986c) and that this receptor might be involved in mediating alcohol drinking behavior of the P line of rats (McBride et al., 1988). However, very little has been published to indicate that an innate abnormality may exist in the GABA system that could be associated with alcohol preference. A recent immunocytochemical and morphometric study examined the densities of GABAergic terminals in the nucleus accumbens, corpus striatum, nucleus tractus solitarius, and lateral septum of the selectively bred P and NP rats and of the HAD and LAD lines (Hwang et al., 1990). The results of this study indicated a higher density of GABAergic terminals in the nucleus accumbens of the P compared with the NP line and of the HAD relative to the LAD rats. There were no differences between the respective lines in the other regions. These results suggest that an innate, abnormal GABAergic inhibitory system within the nucleus accumbens may be a factor involved in the alcohol preference of P and HAD rats.

There have been several studies indicating that alcohol can stimulate the activity of certain DA and 5-HT pathways. Following acute intraperitoneal administration of ethanol, the tissue levels of DOPAC increase in the striatum (Bustos et al., 1976; Fadda et al., 1980) and nucleus accumbens (Khatib et al., 1988) of nonselected rats. In addition, using a brain transdialysis technique, increased extracellular levels of DA in the caudate nucleus and nucleus accumbens were demonstrated following systemic ethanol administration to nonselected rats (Imperato and DiChiara, 1986). In a similar manner, intraperitoneal ethanol administration has been reported to elevate the level of 5-HIAA in the tissue of the striatum and nucleus accumbens (Khatib et al., 1988) and to increase the extracellular concentration of 5-HT in the nucleus accumbens (Yoshimoto et al., 1991) of Wistar rats. These studies indicate that in certain regions where innate abnormalities of certain neurotransmitter systems exist, these same systems appear to be activated by alcohol. However, only recently have there been attempts to determine if the dopamine and serotonin systems are uniquely affected by ethanol in alcohol-preferring animals.

There is some evidence that the VTA and substantia nigra DA systems respond to systemic ethanol administration to a greater degree in the alcohol-preferring sP than in the alcohol-nonpreferring sNP line (Fadda et al., 1990). These investigators reported that the levels of DOPAC and HVA in the tissue of caudate nucleus, medial prefrontal cortex, and olfactory tubercles one hour after the administration of alcohol by gavage were higher in the sP rats than in the sNP line. Although these data do not indicate a difference in sensitivity to ethanol, since dose-response effects were not compared, the results are encouraging in suggesting a difference in response of the DA systems to alcohol between the lines. In addition, another study by this group (Fadda et al., 1989) established that voluntary ingestion of ethanol by the selectively bred sP line can also increase the level of DOPAC in the tissue of the caudate nucleus, medial prefrontal cortex, and olfactory tubercles.

Comparison of the effects of ethanol on the metabolism of DA or 5-HT in the CNS of P versus NP rats has not been reported. There is evidence, however, that both acute intraparitoneal administration of ethanol and chronic alcohol drinking can affect certain DA and 5-HT pathways in the P rat (Murphy et al., 1988a). Acute intraperitoneal injection of 2.5 g ethanol/kg body weight can significantly increase the levels of DOPAC, HVA, and 5-HIAA by 20–50% in the tissue of the nucleus accumbens, frontal cortex, and anterior striatum of alcohol-nontolerant P rats (Murphy et al., 1988a). An identical dose of ethanol given to alcohol-tolerant P rat, however, produces a significantly smaller response for (a) DOPAC and/or HVA in all 3 CNS regions and (b) 5-HIAA in the nucleus accumbens. These data suggest that alcohol can activate certain DA and 5-HT pathways in the P rats and that this action can be desensitized with chronic ethanol exposure. In addition, dose-response studies with the HAD and LAD lines indicated that intraperitoneal administration of ethanol could increase the release of both DA and 5-HT in the nucleus accumbens of both lines, but there was no evidence for a differential sensitivity to ethanol between the lines (Yoshimoto et al., 1992).

In conclusion, the accumulated data support the hypothesis that a genetic deficiency in certain CNS 5-HT systems may be involved in the high alcohol preference of certain selectively bred lines of rodents. Additionally, the evidence indicates that the VTA DA system may be involved in regulating alcohol drinking behavior and that a genetic deficiency in this DA system could be a major factor contributing to high alcohol preference in certain selectively bred lines of rats. An innate abnormality of the nucleus accumbens GABA system could also be a factor contributing to high alcohol-drinking behavior. Although there is a suggestion of an innate abnormality in the NE system that may be associated with high alcohol preference, additional experimentation will need to be done to obtain more convincing data. Overall, the results support the notion that an innate abnormality in one or more neurotransmitter systems is a major neurobiological factor involved in excessive alcohol-drinking behavior.

Although less extensively studied than the serotonin or monoamine systems, there are now several reports that point to the involvement of peptidergic pathways in governing alcohol-drinking behavior. Ehlers et al. (1992) injected corticotropin releasing factor (CRF) intracerebroventricularly (0.15 nmoles vs. saline) into P and NP rats. They found that there was a significantly increased EEG response to CRF in the theta frequency range in the frontal cortex in the P rats as compared with the NP rats. The P rats also exhibited decreased CRF levels in the hypothalamus, amygdala, prefrontal cortex, and cingulate cortex. Taken together, the findings suggest increased regulation of CRF receptors in the P animals. This conclusion agreed in general with the report by Stewart et al. (1989) that P rats may be more anxious and more sensitive to stress-producing stimuli. If ethanol is anxiolytic, one should expect that higher doses of ethanol will be needed in the P rats in order to produce an adequate tension-reducing effect (cf. Baldwin et al., 1991). This mechanism may explain why P rats drink more alcohol than NP rats.

Another peptidergic system that might be involved in regulating alcohol preference is the renin–angiotensin system. In a series of experiments, Grupp et al. (Grupp, 1988; N Grupp et al., 1991) have shown with randomly bred Wistar rats that manipulations that alter activity of the renin–angiotensin system can produce significant changes in voluntary alcohol drinking. Grupp and Kalant (1989) measured plasma renin activity (PRA) in alcohol-naive P and NP rats. They found that the mean PRA in P rats was about 50% of that in NP rats and that the PRA levels were inversely related to voluntary alcohol consumption. Grupp (1992) also examined the effects of intraperitoneal injections of Ceranapril (an angiotensin-converting enzyme inhibitor) and intravenous (iv) infusion of angiotensin II on alcohol drinking in the P and NP rats, and found that both chemicals reduced alcohol drinking in these rat lines.

Pharmacological Manipulations of Ethanol Intake in Selectively Bred Rats with High Alcohol-Drinking Preference

An expanding area of research in recent years has been the testing of pharmacological agents for their capacity to alter alcohol drinking. The eventual goal is to identify potential therapeutic agents that can be used to treat alcohol abuse and alcoholism. From a basic experimental standpoint, however, the testing of these agents is also of theoretical interest as one approach to studying neurochemical systems involved in the genetic predisposition to alcohol preference and the rewarding properties of ethanol.

To date, the selectively bred alcohol-preferring P and HAD rats have been most extensively used for testing the effects of pharmacologic agents on alcohol intake. Since these rats consistently have a high voluntary intake of alcohol (10% v/v) without food and water restrictions, the effects of agents on concurrent food, water, and alcohol consumption can be easily determined. One approach has been the testing of effects of pharmacological agents on continuous free-choice access to ethanol (10% v/v), food, and water. Another method has been limited-access paradigm, in which food and water are available ad libitum, but access to the ethanol solution is restricted, usually to 2–4 hours/day. Limited access offers the advantages that the alcohol intake can be regularized, and the effects and time course of pharmacological manipulations can be more precisely delineated (Murphy et al., 1986a).

Pharmacological compounds that have selective effects on CNS serotonergic systems have been studied most extensively for their capacity to alter alcohol intake. This is partly because the possible involvement of 5-HT systems has an extensive history (Myers and Melchior, 1977) and because of the documented lower contents of 5-HT in several CNS regions of the selectively bred P and HAD rats compared with the respective NP and LAD nonpreferring lines (McBride et al., 1990). Thus, if the lower contents of 5-HT are associated with high alcohol-seeking behavior, increasing the physiological pool of 5-HT in the CNS or mimicking the actions of 5-HT pharmacologically would be expected to decrease alcohol drinking. Intraperitoneal injections of the 5-HT uptake inhibitor fluoxetine (5 and 10 mg/kg) significantly decreased the 24-hour intake of ethanol in P rats to 71 and 56% of saline control values, respectively, but had only mild anorectic effects on food intake (Murphy et al., 1985). When injected before the 4-hour scheduled access to ethanol, fluoxetine at 10 mg/kg almost completely abolished alcohol drinking, indicating a rapid onset of action that lasts for at least 4 hours but lessens within 24 hours. Similar results with fluoxetine have been observed for the HAD rats (McBride et al., 1990, 1992). In another study, P rats were trained to self-administer ethanol (20% v/v) intragastrically, and the effects of intragastric fluoxetine at 10 mg/kg/day for seven days were assessed (Murphy et al., 1988b). The fluoxetine treatment attenuated ethanol self-administration, while water self-administration showed a compensatory increase. Food intake was slightly but not significantly decreased. The findings with P rats are generally consistent with studies by other investigators that 5-HT uptake inhibitors decrease alcohol intake in rats not selectively bred for alcohol preference (see reviews by McBride et al., 1990, 1992). In the P rat, agents that enhance functioning of 5-HT systems by other mechanisms have also been tested. The 5-HT releasor fenfluramine and precursor D,L-5-hydroxytryptophan both reduce the oral consumption of ethanol (see reviews by McBride et al., 1989a, 1990, 1992).

Agonists at different 5-HT receptor subtypes have been tested in the P and HAD rats, and all have been found to significantly reduce alcohol intake during a four-hour scheduled access. 1-(3-trifluoromethylphenyl)piperazine (TFMPP), an agent that has some agonist activity at 5-HT$_{1B}$ receptors (Schecter, 1988), and the 5-HT$_{1A}$ agonists, 8-hydroxy-2-(di-n-propylamino)tetralin (8-OH-DPAT) and buspirone (Hoyer, 1988; Glennon, 1990) significantly decreased alcohol drinking, but the effects were usually short acting in that the reduction of alcohol intake would abate by the end of 4 hours (Rezvani et al., 1991; McBride et al., 1992; Murphy, et al., 1992). When microinjected directly into the nucleus accumbens, however, 8-OH-DPAT had little effect on alcohol intake, whereas low, but not high doses of TFMPP enhanced alcohol drinking

(McBride et al., 1991a, 1991b, 1992). These observations suggest that local regulation of the reinforcing effects of ethanol within the nucleus accumbens may be mediated partly by 5-HT_{1B} receptors in P rats.

The 5-HT_2 agonist, 1-(2,5-dimethoxy-4-iodophenyl)-2-aminopropane (DOI), also has been shown to reduce alcohol intake in P rats, but it produced a biphasic dose response in HAD rats. Low doses increased and high doses decreased alcohol drinking (McBride et al., 1992). Since agonists and other agents that potentiate functioning within 5-HT systems seem to consistently decrease alcohol intake, antagonists at 5-HT receptors might be expected to have the opposite effect. This expectation has not been the case, however, when antagonists are given intraperitoneal before a scheduled access to ethanol. Pindolol blocks 5-HT_{1A} receptors in addition to adrenergic receptors (Glennon, 1990), but it failed to alter alcohol consumption (Rezvani et al., 1991; McBride et al., 1992). Spiroxatrine has some antagonist actions at 5-HT_{1A} receptors, but also failed to decrease alcohol intake by itself (McBride et al., 1989b). However, spiroxatrine proved to act like a partial agonist, since it potentiated the effects of fluoxetine on alcohol intake in P and HAD rats (McBride et al., 1989b).

The 5-HT_2 antagonist, LY53857, was found to significantly reduce alcohol consumption in HAD rats (McBride et al., 1992). This observation together with the finding that the 5-HT_2 agonist DOI caused a biphasic action on alcohol intake in the HAD rats could indicate that 5-HT_2 receptors are involved in the circuitry mediating the rewarding properties of ethanol in HAD rats. Reduced alcohol consumption may occur because the 5-HT_2 antagonist blocks any reinforcing effects, while high doses of the agonist maximally activate the 5-HT_2 receptor and prevent further positive actions of ethanol. Low doses of the agonist may potentiate the positive effects of ethanol and tend to increase consumption. However, neither LY53857 nor methysergide, a less specific 5-HT antagonist, blocked the reduction of ethanol intake caused by fluoxetine treatment of P rats (Murphy et al., 1985). Taken together, the findings suggest that 5-HT systems and receptor subtypes are involved in alcohol preference, but the exact nature of the role is still uncertain.

Another reliable neurochemical difference observed for the alcohol-preferring P and HAD lines is lower content of dopamine (DA) and its metabolites in the nucleus accumbens compared with the respective alcohol-nonpreferring NP and LAD lines (Murphy et al., 1987; Gongwer et al., 1989). The mesolimbic DA system has been implicated in the reinforcing effects of several abusive drugs, including ethanol (DiChiara and Imperato, 1988; Koob and Bloom, 1988), and DA systems appear to be involved in the rewarding effects of ethanol in the selectively bred sP rats (Fadda et al., 1991). The hypothesis that the mesolimbic DA system is involved in the rewarding effects of alcohol is supported by the observation that P but not NP rats will self-administer ethanol directly into the ventral tegmental area (Gatto et al., 1990a). In addition, agents that increase the extracellular levels of DA (such as the reuptake inhibitor GBR12909 and the releasor amphetamine) or mimic the action of DA (such as the $D_1\text{–}D_2$ agonist bromocriptine) also decrease alcohol intake of the P line of rats (McBride et al., 1990). Moreover, Weiss et al. (1990) reported that bromocriptine produced a significant dose-dependent shift in preference of P rats from alcohol toward water by inhibiting operant responding for ethanol while increasing responding for water.

The role of the DA mesolimbic system in alcohol drinking of the P rats has also been investigated by microinjecting D_1 and D_2 antagonists directly into the nucleus accumbens (Levy et al., 1991). The D_2 antagonist sulpiride caused a statistically significant dose-dependent increase in alcohol drinking. While the D_1 antagonist SCH23390 tended to increase alcohol intake, this effect was not statistically significant.

Although agents that alter DA and 5-HT functioning have received the most attention, pharmacological manipulations of other neurotransmitter systems have also been studied for the capacity to alter alcohol drinking in selectively bred lines. The noradrenergic (NE) uptake inhibitor desipramine has been observed to decrease alcohol intake in P rats given ad libitum access to 10% (v/v) ethanol as well as in NP rats that were drinking a very palatable solution containing ethanol (Murphy et al., 1985; McBride et al., 1988; Gatto et al., 1990b). However, this effect was not selective for ethanol, since the ingestion of food or another palatable solution without ethanol was also decreased. Additionally, the alpha- and beta-NE antagonists phentolamine and propranolol, respectively, did not alter alcohol intake in P rats during a 4-hour scheduled access (Murphy et al., 1985).

The inverse benzodiazepine agonist RO15-4513 has been reported to block the in vivo and in vitro effects of ethanol at the $GABA_A$-benzodiazepine-Cl^- receptor complex (Suzdak et al., 1986a, 1986b). To test whether this receptor complex might be involved in the reinforcing effects of ethanol, P rats were injected with RO15-4513 before scheduled access to alcohol (McBride et al., 1988). The results indicated a selective reduction of alcohol intake without any effect on food or water consumption. Similar findings have been reported with RO19-4603 given to sP rats (Balakleevsky et al., 1990). A reduction of alcohol intake by RO15-4513 has also been reported in unselected rats (June et al., 1991). These findings provide evidence that the $GABA_A$ receptor complex may be involved in the reinforcing properties of alcohol.

Ethanol is known to modulate endorphinergic activity in the brain and pituitary (Tabakoff and Hoffman, 1987; Patel and Poherecky, 1989), and there is evidence that the reinforcing effects of ethanol can be mediated by the endogenous opioid system (Volpicelli *et al.,* 1986). Based on these observations, Froehlich et al. (1988, 1990a, 1990b) postulated that alcohol drinking may result in the release of endogenous opioid peptides that can serve to reinforce and maintain subsequent alcohol drinking. If this postulate is correct, opioid receptor antagonists such as naloxone should decrease voluntary alcohol drinking. Indeed, this was found to be the case. HAD rats were treated with naloxone (0.05 to 18 mg/kg) or saline before access to either water alone or to a free-choice between 10% ethanol and water in a scheduled access paradigm. Naloxone suppressed water intake when water was presented by itself; however, it selectively produced a dose-dependent decrease in ethanol ingestion without changing water intake when both ethanol and water were presented concurrently. Thus, ethanol ingestion as a subset of consummatory behaviors is unusually sensitive to opioid receptor blockade. A similar finding has also been reported in the AA rats by Sinclair (1990).

At least two other agents have been tested for their effects on alcohol consumption in P rats and in the Fawn-hooded rats, which may have a 5-HT deficiency (Rezvani et al., 1991). Scopolamine, a cholinergic antimuscarinic drug, and verapamil, a calcium channel antagonist, were both found to decrease alcohol drinking during 24-hour free-choice access in the P and Fawn-hooded rats. Verapramil has numerous effects on neurotransmitters and may be acting through any number of CNS systems. Whether the scopolamine effect implicates a CNS cholinergic systems in the reinforcing effects of ethanol has yet to be unequivocally determined, but a peripheral cholinergic mechanisms appears to contribute to the scopolamine effect (Rezvani et al., 1990b).

In conclusion selectively bred alcohol-preferring rats, such as the P and HAD lines (as well as AA lines, although few pharmacologic studies have been done by the Finnish research group), can serve as useful models for testing the effects of pharmacological agents on genetically predisposed abnormal alcohol-seeking behavior. From the studies performed thus far, it appears that pharmacological manipulations of several neurotransmitter systems can reliably decrease alcohol intake. These findings have already produced important practical implications in delineating potential agents for testing in the clinical treatment of alcohol abuse and alcoholism. For instance, four clinical, double-blind placebo-controlled trials have demonstrated that citalopram, fluoxetine, and zimelidine can all significantly curtail ethanol intake by about 10% to 26% and that this action of 5-HT neuronal uptake blockers is independent of their known antidepressive, sedative, or anxiolytic effects (see review by Ferreira and Soares-da-Silva, 1991).

Summary

Selective breeding for high and low alcohol drinking preference has produced several rat lines that have been shown to be instrumental for studying the biological nature of excessive alcohol-seeking behavior. These selective breeding experiments provide strong evidence, as do family, twins, and adoption human studies, that alcohol-seeking behavior and alcoholism are highly heritable. Compared with alcohol nonpreferring lines, the preferring rats exhibit increased responsivity to the low-dose activating effects of alcohol and enhanced capacity to develop tolerance to the behaviorally aversive effects of high-dose alcohol. Furthermore, the preferring rats exhibit lower brain serotonin and dopamine neurotransmitter activities as well as alterations in other neurotransmitter modulator systems as compared with the alcohol nonpreferring lines.

References

Aalto, J. (1986). Circadian drinking rhythms and blood alcohol levels in two rat lines developed for their alcohol consumption. *Alcohol* 3:73–75.

Ahtee, L., and Eriksson, K. (1972). 5-hydroxytryptamine and 5-hydroxyindoleacetic acid content in brain of rat strains selected for their alcohol intake. *Physiol. Behav.* 8:123–126.

Ahtee, L., and Eriksson, K. (1973). Regional distribution of brain 5-hydroxytryptamine in rat strains selected for their alcohol intake. *Ann. N. Y. Acad. Sci.* 215:126–134.

Anderson, S. M., and McClearn, G. E. (1981). Ethanol consumption: Selective breeding in mice. *Behav. Genet.* 11:291–301.

Badawy, A. A. -B., Morgan, C. J., Lane, J., Dhaliwal, K., and Bradley, D. M. (1989). Liver tryp-
    tophan pyrrolase: A major determinant of the lower brain 5-hydroxytryptamine concen-
    tration in alcohol-preferring C57BL mice. *Biochem. J.* **264:**597–599.
Balakleevsky, A., Colombo, G., Fadda, F., and Gessa, G. L. (1990). RO19-4603, a benzodi-
    azepine receptor inverse agonist, attenuates voluntary ethanol consumption in rats selec-
    tively bred for high ethanol preference. *Alcohol Alcohol.* **25:**449–452.
Baldwin, H. A., Wall, T. L., Shuckit, M. A., and Koob, G. F. (1991). Differential effects of
    ethanol on punished responding in the P and NP rats. *Alcohol.: Clin. Exp. Res.*
    15:700–704.
Bice, P. J., and Kiefer, S. W. (1990). Taste reactivity in alcohol preferring and non-preferring
    rats. *Alcohol.: Clin. Exp. Res.* **14:**721–727.
Bohman, M., Sigvardson, S., and Cloninger, C. R. (1981). Maternal inheritance of alcohol
    abuse. Cross-fostering analysis of adopted women. *Arch. Gen. Psychiatr.* **38:**965–969.
Bustos, G., and Roth, R. H. (1976). Effect of acute ethanol treatment on transmitter synthesis
    and metabolism in central dopaminergic neurons. *J. Pharm. Pharmacol.* **28:**580–581.
Carr, L., Mellencamp, B., Crabb, D., Lumeng, L., and Li, T. -K. (1990). A polymorphism in the
    rat liver mitochondrial ALDH2 gene is associated with alcohol drinking behavior. In
    Enzymology and Molecular Biology of Carbonyl Metabolism, 3. H. Weiner, ed. N. Y:
    Plenum Press, pp. 61–65.
Carr, L., Mellencamp, B., Crabb, D., Weiner, H., Lumeng, L., and Li, T. -K. (1991). Polymor-
    phism of the rat liver mitochondrial aldehyde dehydrogenase cDNA. *Alcohol.: Clin. Exp.
    Res.* **15:**753–756.
Cicero, T. J. (1979). A critique of animal analogue of alcoholism. In *Biochemistry and Pharma-
    cology of Ethanol,* E. Majchrowicz and E. P. Noble, eds. New York: Plenum Press,
    2:533–560.
Cloninger, C. R., Bohman, M., and Sigvardson, S. (1981). Inheritance of alcohol abuse of cross-
    fostering analysis of adopted men. *Arch. Gen. Psychiatr.* **38:**965–969.
Colombo, G., Kuzmin, A., Fadda, F., Pani, L., and Gessa, G. L. (1990). Conditioned place pref-
    erence induced by ethanol in a rat line selected for ethanol preference. *Pharmacol. Res.*
    22:48.
Crabbe, J. C. (1989). Genetic animal models in the study of alcoholism. *Alcohol.: Clin. Exp.
    Res.* **13:**120–127.
DeFries, J. C., and Hegmann, J. P. (1970). Genetic analysis of open-field behavior. In *Contribu-
    tions to Behavior-Genetic Analysis: The Mouse as a Prototype,* G. Lindzey and D. D.
    Thiessen, eds. New York: Appleton-Century-Crofts, pp. 23–56.
Deutsch, J. A., and Eisner, A. (1977). Ethanol self-administration in the rat induced by forced
    drinking of ethanol. *Behav. Biol.* **20:**81–90.
Deutsch, J. A., and Hardy, W. T. (1976). Ethanol tolerance in the rat measured by the untasted
    intake of alcohol. *Behav. Biol.* **17:**379–389.
DiChiara, G., and Imperato, A. (1988). Drugs abused by humans preferentially increase synaptic
    dopamine concentrations in the mesolimbic system of freely moving rats. *Proc. Natl.
    Acad. Sci.* (USA) **85:**5274–5278.
Dole, V. P., and Gentry, R. T. (1984). Toward an analogue of alcoholism in mice: Scale factors
    in the model. *Proc. Natl. Acad. Sci.* (USA) **81:**3543–3546.
Dole, V. P., Ho, A., and Gentry, R. T. (1985). Toward an analogue of alcoholism in mice: Crite-
    ria for recognition of pharmacologically motivated drinking. *Proc. Natl. Acad. Sci.*
    (USA) **82:**3469–3471.
Dole, V. P., Ho, A., Gentry, R. T., and Chin, A. (1988). Toward an analogue of alcoholism in

mice: Analysis of nongenetic variance in consumption of alcohol. *Proc. Natl. Acad. Sci.* (USA) **85**:827–830.

Ehlers, C. L., Chaplin, R. I., Lumeng, L., and Li, T. -K. (1991). Electrophysiological response to ethanol in P and NP rats. *Alcohol.: Clin. Exp. Res.* **15**:739–744.

Ehlers, C. L., Chaplin, R. I., Wall, T. L., Lumeng, L., Li, T. -K., Owens, M. J., and Nemeroff, C. B. (1992). Corticotropin releasing factor (CRF): Studies in alcohol, preferring and non-preferring rats. *Psychopharmacology* **106**:359–364.

Eriksson, K. (1968). Genetic selection for voluntary alcohol consumption in the albino rat. *Science* **159**:739–741.

Eriksson, K. (1969). The estimation of heritability for the self-selection of alcohol in the albino rat. *Ann. Med. Exp. Biol. Fenn.* **47**:172–174.

Eriksson, C. J. P. (1981). Finnish selection studies on alcohol-related behaviors: Factors regulating voluntary alcohol consumption. In *Development of Animal Models as Pharmacogenetic Tools,* G. E. McClearn, R. A. Deitrich, and V. G. Erwin, eds. Washington, DC: U.S. Government Printing Office, pp. 119–145.

Eriksson, K., and Rusi, M. (1981). Finnish selection studies on alcohol-related behaviors: General outline. In *Development of Animal Models as Pharmacogenetic Tools,* G. E. McClearn, R. A. Deitrich, and V. G. Erwin, eds. Washington, DC: U.S. Government Printing Office, pp. 87–117.

Erwin, V. G., McClearn, G. E. and Kuse, A. R. (1980). Interrelationships of alcohol consumption actions of alcohol and biochemical traits. *Pharmacol. Biochem. Behav.* **13**(suppl.1):297–302.

Fadda, F., Argiolas, A., Melis, M. R., Serra, G., and Gessa, G. L. (1980). Differential effect of acute and chronic ethanol on dopamine metabolism in frontal cortex, caudate nucleus and substantia nigra. *Life Sci.* **27**:979–986.

Fadda, F., Mosca, E., Colombo, G., and Gessa, G. L. (1989). Effect of spontaneous ingestion of ethanol on brain dopamine metabolism. *Life Sci.* **44**:281–287.

Fadda, F., Mosca, E., Colombo, G., and Gessa, G. L. (1990). Alcohol-preferring rats: Genetic sensitivity to alcohol-induced stimulation of dopamine metabolism. *Physiol. Behav.* **47**:727–729.

Fadda, F., Colombo, G., and Gessa, G. L. (1991). Genetic sensitivity to effect of ethanol on dopaminergic system in alcohol preferring rats. *Alcohol Alcohol.* **1**(suppl.):439–442.

Ferreira, L., and Soares-da-Silva, P. (1991). 5-hydroxytryptamine and alcoholism. *Human Psychopharmacol.* **6**:521–524.

French, T. A., Atkinson, N., Petersen, D. R., and Chung, L. W. K. (1979). Differential induction of hepatic microsomal ethanol and drug metabolism by 3-methylcholanthrene in LS and SS mice. *J. Pharmacol. Exp. Ther.* **209**:404–410.

Froehlich, J. C., Harts, J., Lumeng, L., and Li, T. -K. (1988). Differences in response to the aversive properties of ethanol in rats selectively bred for oral ethanol preference. *Pharmacol. Biochem. Behav.* **31**:215–222.

Froehlich, J. C., Stewart, R., Kurtz, D., Zweifel, M., Lumeng, L., and Li, T. -K. (1989). Genetic differences in hypothermic effects of ethanol. *Alcohol.: Clin. Exp. Res.* **13**:306 (abstract).

Froehlich, J. C., Harts, J., Lumeng, L., and Li, T. -K. (1990a). Naloxone attenuates voluntary ethanol intake in rats selectively bred for high ethanol preference. *Pharmacol. Biochem. Behav.* **35**:385–390.

Froehlich, J. C., and Li, T. -K. (1990b). Enkephalinergic involvement in voluntary drinking of alcohol. In *Opioids, Bulimia, Alcohol Abuse and Alcoholism* L. Reid, ed. New York: Springer-Verlag, pp. 217–228.

Froehlich, J. C., Zweifel, M., Harts, J., Lumeng, L., and Li, T. -K. (1991). Importance of delta opioid receptors in maintaining alcohol drinking. *Psychopharmacology* **103:** 467–472.

Gatto, G. J., Murphy, J. M., Waller, M. B., McBride, W. J., Lumeng, L., and Li, T. -K. (1987a). Chronic ethanol tolerance through free-choice drinking in the P line of alcohol-preferring rats. *Pharmacol. Biochem. Behav.* **28:**111–115.

Gatto, G. J., Murphy, J. M., Waller, M. B., McBride, W. J., Lumeng, L., and Li, T. -K. (1987b). Persistence of tolerance to a single dose of ethanol in the selectively-bred alcohol preferring P rat. *Pharmacol. Biochem. Behav.* **28:**105–110.

Gatto, G. J., Murphy, J. M., McBride, W. J., Lumeng, L., and Li, T. -K. (1990a). Intracranial self-administration of ethanol into the ventral tegmental area of alcohol-preferring (P) rats. *Alcohol.: Clin. Exp. Res.* **14:**291 (abstract).

Gatto, G. J., Murphy, J. M., McBride, W. J., Lumeng, L., and Li, T. -K. (1990b). Effects of fluoxetine and desipramine on palatability-induced ethanol consumption in the alcohol-nonpreferring (NP) line of rats. *Alcohol* **7:**531–536.

Gatto, G. J., Murphy, J. M., McBride, W. J., Lumeng, L., and Li, T. -K. (1991). Ethanol-associated conditioned reinforcement in alcohol-preferring (P) rats. *Alcohol.: Clin. Exp. Res.* **15:**313 (abstract).

Gatto, G. J., Murphy, J. M., Lumeng, L., Li, T. -K., and McBride, W. J. (1993). Extinction of intracranial self-administration (ICSA) of ethanol into the ventral tegmental area (VTA) in alcohol-preferring (P) rats. Submitted.

Gentry, R. T. (1985). An experimental model of self-intoxication in C57 mice. *Alcohol* **2:**671–675.

Gentry, R. T., Rappaport, M. S., and Dole, V. P. (1983). Elevated concentrations of ethanol in plasma do not suppress voluntary ethanol consumption in C57BL mice. *Alcohol.: Clin. Exp. Res.* **7:**420–423.

Glennon, R. A. (1990). Serotonin receptors: Clinical implications. *Neurosci. Biobehav. Rev.* **14:**35–47.

Goldman, D., Lister, R. G., and Crabbe, J. C. (1987). Mapping of a putative genetic locus determining ethanol intake in the mouse. *Brain Res.* **420:**220–226.

Gongwer, M. A., Murphy, J. M., McBride, W. J., Lumeng, L., and Li, T. -K. (1989). Regional brain contents of serotonin, dopamine and their metabolites in the selectively bred high- and low-alcohol drinking lines of rats. *Alcohol* **6:**317–320.

Grupp, L. A. (1988). Alcohol satiety, hypertension and the renin-angiotensin system. *Med. Hypoth.* **24:**11–19.

Grupp, L. A. (1992). Reduction of alcohol intake in alcohol-preferring (P) and alcohol-nonpreferring (NP) rats: Effects of angiotensin II and an angiotensin converting enzyme inhibitor. *Pharmacol. Biochem. Behav.* **41:**105–108.

Grupp, L. A., and Kalant, H. (1989). Alcohol intake is inversely related to plasma renin activity in the genetically selected alcohol-preferring and -nonpreferring lines of rats. *Pharmacol. Biochem. Behav.* **32:**1061–1063.

Grupp, L. A., Perlanski, E., and Stewart, R. B. (1991). Regulation of alcohol consumption by the renin-angiotensin system: A review of recent findings and a possible mechanism of action. *Neurosci. Biobehav. Rev.* **15:**265–275.

Hansen, C., and Spuhler, K. (1984). Development of the National Institute of Health genetically heterogeneous rat stock. *Alcohol.: Clin. Exp. Res.* **8:**477–479.

Ho, A. K. S., Tsai, C. S., and Kissin, B. (1975). Neurochemical correlates of alcohol preference in inbred strains of mice. *Pharmacol. Biochem. Behav.* **3:**1073–1076.

Holloway, F. A., Bird, D. C., and Devenport, J. A. (1984). Periodic availability: Factors affecting alcohol selection in rats. *Alcohol* **1**:19–25.

Hoyer, D. (1988). Functional correlates of serotonin 5-HT1 recognition sites. *J. Receptor Res.* **8**:59–81.

Hwang, B. H., Lumeng, L., Wu, J. -Y., and Li, T. -K. (1990). Increased number of GABAergic terminals in the nucleus accumbens is associated with alcohol preference in rats. *Alcohol.: Clin. Exp. Res.* **14**:503–507.

Hyytia, P., and Sinclair, J. D. (1989). Demonstration of lever pressing for oral ethanol by rats with no prior training or ethanol experience. *Alcohol* **6**:161–164.

Hyytia, P., Halkka, O., Sarviharju, M., and Eriksson, K. (1987). Alcohol-preferring (AA) and alcohol-avoiding (ANA) lines of rats after introgession of alien genes. *Alcohol Alcohol.,* **1**(supp.):351–355.

Imperato, A., and DiChiara, G. (1986). Preferential stimulation of dopamine release in the nucleus accumbens of freely moving rats by ethanol. *J. Pharmacol. Exp. Ther.* **239**:219–228.

Inoue, K., Rusi, M., and Lindros, K. O. (1981). Brain aldehyde dehydrogenase activity in rat strains with high and low ethanol preferences. *Pharmacol. Biochem. Behav.* **14**:107–111.

June, H. L., Lummis, G. H., Colker, R. E., Moore, T. O., and Lewis, M. J. (1991), RO15-4513 attenuates the consumption of ethanol in deprived rats. *Alcohol.: Clin. Exp. Res.* **15**:406–411.

Kalant, H. (1987). Free choice consumption of ethanol by AA and ANA rats in an operant model. In *Problems of Drug Dependence,* L. S. Harris, ed. Washington, DC: U.S. Government Printing Office, 307.

Khatib, S. A., Murphy, J. M., and McBride, W. J. (1988). Biochemical evidence for activation of specific monoamine pathways by ethanol. *Alcohol* **5**:295–299.

Koivisto T., Carr L. G., Li, T. -K., and Eriksson, C. J. (1993). Mitochondrial aldehyde dehydrogenase (ALDH$_2$) polymorphism in AA and ANA rats: Lack of genotype and phenotype line differences. *Pharmacol. Biochem. Behav.* **45**:215–220.

Koob, G. F., and Bloom, F. E. (1988). Cellular and molecular mechanisms of drug dependence. *Science* **242**:715–723.

Korpi, E. R., Sinclair, J. D., Kaheinen, P., Viitamaa, T., Hellevuo, K., and Kiianmaa, K. (1988). Brain regional and adrenal monoamine concentrations and behavioral responses to stress in alcohol-preferring AA and alcohol-avoiding ANA rats. *Alcohol* **5**:417–425.

Kurtz, D., Stewart, R. B., Zweifel, M., Li, T. -K., and Froehlich, J. C. (1990). Genetic differences in tolerance and sensitization to the sedative/hypnotic effects of ethanol. *Alcohol.: Clin. Exp. Res.* **14**:307 (abstract).

Kurtz, D. L., Stewart, R. B., Zweifel, M. J., Li, T. -K., and Froehlich, J. C. (1995). Genetic differences in response to the sedative/hypnotic effects of ethanol. *Psychopharmacology,* in press.

Lankford, M. F., Roscoe, A. K., Pennington, S. N., and Myers, R. D. (1991). Drinking of high concentrations of ethanol versus palatable fluids in alcohol-preferring (P) rats: Valid animal model of alcoholism. *Alcohol* **8**:293–299.

Levy, A. D., Murphy, J. M., McBride, W. J., Lumeng, L., and Li, T. -K. (1991). Microinjection of sulpiride into the nucleus accumbens increase ethanol intake of alcohol-preferring (P) rats. *Alcohol Alcohol.* **1**(suppl.):417–420.

Li, T. -K., and Lumeng, L. (1977). Alcohol metabolism of inbred strains of rats with alcohol preference and non-preference. In *Alcohol and Aldehyde Metabolizing Systems,* Vol. III,

R. G. Thurman, J. R. Williamson, H. Drott, and B. Chance, eds. New York: Academic Press, 625–633.

Li, T. -K., Lumeng, L., McBride, W. J., Waller, M. B., and Hawkins, D. T. (1979). Progress toward a voluntary oral-consumption model of alcoholism. *Drug Alcohol Depend.* **4**:45–60.

Li, T. -K., Lumeng, L., McBride, W. J., and Waller, M. B. (1981). Indiana selection studies on alcohol-related behaviors. In *Development of Animal Models as Pharmacogenetic Tools. Rockville, MD: U.S. Depart. of Health and Health Sciences, NIAAA Research Monograph No. 6*, pp. 171–191.

Li, T. -K., Lumeng, L., McBride, W. J., Waller, M. B., and Murphy, J. M. (1986). Studies on an animal model of alcoholism. In *Genetic and Biological Markers for Drug Abuse and Alcoholism.* DHHS Publications: U. S. Government Printing Office, NIDA/NIAAA Research Monograph Series, pp. 41–49.

Li, T. -K., Lumeng, L., McBride, W. J., and Murphy, J. M. (1987). Alcoholism: Is it a model for the study of disorders of mood and consummatory behavior? *Ann. N.Y. Acad. Sci.* **499**:239–249.

Li, T. -K., Lumeng, L., Doolittle, D. P., McBride, W. J., Murphy, J. M., Froehlich, J. C., and Morzorati, S. (1988). Behavioral and neurochemical associations of alcohol-seeking behavior. *Excerpta Med. Int. Congr. Ser.* **805**:435–438.

Li, T. -K., Lumeng, L., and Doolittle, D. P. (1993). Selective breeding for alcohol preference and associated responses. *Behav. Genet.* **23**:163–170.

Lumeng, L. and Li, T. -K. (1986). The development of metabolic tolerance in the alcohol-preferring P rats: Comparison of forced and free-choice drinking of ethanol. *Pharmacol. Biochem. Behav.* **25**:1013–1020.

Lumeng, L., Hawkins, T. D., and Li, T. -K. (1977). New strains of rats with alcohol preference and non-preference. In *Alcohol and Aldehyde Metabolizing Systems,* Vol. III, R. G. Thurman, J. R. Williamson, H. Drott, and B. Chance, eds. New York Academic Press,: pp. 537–544.

Lumeng, L., Waller, M. B., McBride, W. J., and Li, T. -K. (1982). Different sensitivities to ethanol in alcohol-preferring and nonpreferring rats. *Pharmacol. Biochem. Behav.* **16**:125–130.

Lumeng, L., Doolittle, D. P., and Li, T. -K. (1986). New duplicate lines of rats that differ in voluntary alcohol consumption. *Alcohol Alcohol.* **21**:A37 (abstract).

Lumeng, L., Murphy, J. M., McBride, W. J., and Li, T. -K. (1988). Basic neurochemical mechanisms of modulation of alcohol consumption in the P and NP rats. *Pharmacol.: Excerpta Med. Int. Congr. Ser.* **750**:727–730.

Lumeng, L., Li, T. -K., McBride, W. J., Murphy, J. M., Morzorati, S. L., and Froehlich, J. C. (1989). Mechanisms(s) of modulation of alcohol consumption: Studies on the P and NP rats. In *Molecular Mechanisms of Alcohol,* G. Y. Sun, ed. New Jersey: Humana Press, pp. 359–370.

Mardones, J., and Segovia-Riquelme, N. (1983), Thirty-two years of selection of rats by ethanol preference: UChA and UChB strains. *Neurobehav. Toxicol. Teratol.* **5**: 171–178.

McBride, W. J., Murphy, J. M., Lumeng, L., and Li, T. -K. (1988). Effects of Ro 15-4513, fluoxetine and desipramine on the intake of ethanol, water and food by the alcohol-preferring (P) and -nonpreferring (NP) lines of rats. *Pharmacol. Biochem. Behav.* **30**:1045–1050.

McBride, W. J., Murphy, J. M., Lumeng, L., and Li, T. -K. (1989a). Serotonin and ethanol preference. In *Recent Developments in Alcoholism,* M. Galanter, ed. Plenum New York: pp. 187–209.

McBride, W. J., Murphy, J. M., Lumeng, L., and Li, T. -K. (1989b). Spiroxatrine augments flu-oxetine-induced reduction of ethanol intake by the P line of rats. *Pharmacol. Biochem. Behav.* **34:**381–386.

McBride, W. J., Murphy, J. M., Lumeng, L., and Li, T. -K. (1990). Serotonin, dopamine and GABA involvement in alcohol drinking of selectively bred rats. *Alcohol* **7:** 199–205.

McBride, W. J., Murphy, J. M., Gatto, G. J., Levy, A. D., Lumeng, L., and Li, T. -K. (1991a). Serotonin and dopamine systems regulating alcohol intake. In *Proceedings, 5th Congress of the International Society for Biomedical Research on Alcoholism,* H. Kalant, ed. N.Y.: Pergamon Press, pp. 411–416.

McBride, W. J., Murphy, J. M., Gatto, G. J., Levy, A. D., Lumeng, L., and Li, T. -K. (1991b). Serotonin and dopamine systems regulating alcohol intake. *Alcohol Alcoholism.* **1**(suppl.):411–416.

McBride, W. J., Murphy, J. M., Lumeng, L., and Li, T. -K. (1992). Serotonin and alcohol con-sumption. In *Novel Pharmacological Interventions for Alcoholism,* C. A. Naranjo and E. M. Sellers, eds. New York: Springer-Verlag, pp. 59–67.

McBride, W. J., Chernet, E., Dyr, W., Lumeng, L., and Li, T. -K., (1993). Densities of dopamine D2 receptors are reduced in CNS regions of alcohol-preferring P rats. *Alcohol* **10:**387–390.

McClearn, G. E. (1968). The use of strain rank orders in assessing equivalence of techniques. *Behav. Res. Meth. Instrum.* **1**:49–51.

McClearn, G. E., and Rodgers, D. A. (1959). Differences in alcohol preference among inbred strains of mice. *Q. J. Stud. Alcohol* **20:**691–695.

McClearn, G. E., and Rodgers, D. A. (1961). Genetic factors in alcohol preference of laboratory mice. *J. Comp. Physiol. Psychol.* **54:**116–119.

McClearn, G. E., and Kakihana, R. (1973). Selective breeding for ethanol sensitivity in mice. *Behav. Genet.* **3:**409–410.

McClearn, G. E., Plomin, R., Gora-Maslak, G., and Crabbe, J. C. (1991). The gene chase in behavioral science. *Psychol. Sci.* **2:**222–229.

Meisch, R. A. (1976). The function of schedule-induced polydipsia in establishing ethanol as a positive reinforcer. *Pharmacol. Rev.* **27:**465–473.

Morzorati, S., Lamishaw, B., Clemens, J., Lumeng, L., and Li, T. -K. (1988). Effect of low dose ethanol on the EEG of alcohol-preferring and nonpreferring rats. *Brain Res. Bull.* **21:**101–104.

Murphy, J. M., McBride, W. J., Lumeng, L., and Li, T. -K. (1982). Regional brain levels of monoamines in alcohol-preferring and -nonpreferring rats. *Pharmacol. Biochem. Behav.* **16:**145–149.

Murphy, J. M., Waller, M. B., Gatto, G. J., McBride, W. J., Lumeng, L., and Li, T. -K. (1985). Monoamine uptake inhibitors attenuate ethanol intake in alcohol-preferring (P) rats. *Alcohol* **2:**349–352.

Murphy, J. M., Gatto, G. J., Waller, M. B., McBride, W. J., Lumeng, L., and Li, T. -K. (1986a). Effects of scheduled access on ethanol intake by the alcohol-preferring P line of rats. *Alcohol* **3:**331–336.

Murphy, J. M., McBride, W. J., Lumeng, L., and Li, T. -K. (1986b). Alcohol preference and regional brain monoamine contents of N/Nih heterogeneous stock rats. *Alcohol Drug Res.* **7:**33–39.

Murphy, J. M., McBride, W. J., Lumeng, L., and Li, T. -K. (1987). Contents of monoamines in forebrain regions of alcohol-preferring (P) and -nonpreferring (NP) lines of rats. *Pharmacol. Biochem. Behav.* **26:**389–392.

Murphy, J. M., McBride, W. J., Gatto, G. J., Lumeng, L., and Li, T. -K. (1988a). Effects of acute ethanol administration on monoamine and metabolite contents in forebrain regions of ethanol tolerant and nontolerant alcohol-preferring (P) rats. *Pharmacol. Biochem. Behav.* **29:**169–174.

Murphy, J. M., Waller, M. B., Gatto, G. J., McBride, W. J., Lumeng, L., and Li, T. -K. (1988b). Effects of fluoxetine on the intragastric self-administration of ethanol in the alcohol preferring P line of rats. *Alcohol* **5:**283–286.

Murphy, J. M., Gatto, G. J., McBride, W. J., Lumeng, L., and Li, T. -K. (1989). Operant responding for oral ethanol in the alcohol-preferring P and alcohol-nonpreferring NP lines of rats. *Alcohol* **6:**127–131.

Murphy, J. M., Gatto, G. J., McBride, W. J., Lumeng, L., and Li, T. -K. (1990). Persistence of tolerance in the P line of alcohol-preferring rats does not require performance while intoxicated. *Alcohol* **7:**367–369.

Murphy, J. M., McBride, W. J., Lumeng, L., and Li, T. -K. (1992). Monoamine and metabolite levels in CNS regions of the P line of alcohol-preferring rats after acute and chronic ethanol treatment. *Pharmacol. Biochem. Behav.* **19:**849–856.

Myers, R. D., and Melchior, C. L. (1977). Alcohol and alcoholism: Role of serotonin. In *Serotonin in Health and Disease,* Vol.2. *Physiological Regulation and Pharmacological Action,* W. B. Essman, ed. New York: Spectrum, pp. 373–430.

Nachman, M., Larue, C., and LeMagnen, J. (1971). The role of olfactory and orosensory factors in the alcohol preference of inbred strains of mice. *Physiol. Behav.* **6:**53–59.

Nikander, P., and Pekkanen, L. (1977). An inborn alcohol tolerance in alcohol-preferring rats. The lack of relationship between tolerance to ethanol and brain microsomal Na$^+$, K$^+$-ATPase activity. *Psychopharmacology* (Berlin) **51:**219–233.

Patel, V. A., and Pohorecky, L. A. (1989). Acute and chronic ethanol treatment on β-endorphin and catecholamine levels. *Alcohol* **6:**59–63.

Penn, P. E., McBride, W. J., Lumeng, L., Gaff, T. M., and Li, T. -K. (1978). Neurochemical and operant behavior studies of a strain of alcohol-preferring rats. *Pharmacol. Biochem. Behav.* **8:**475–481.

Pickett, R. A., and Collins, A. C. (1975). Use of genetic analysis to test the potential role of serotonin in alcohol preference. *Life Sci.* **17:**1291–1296.

Reed, J. G. (1951). A study of the alcoholic consumption and amino acid excretion patterns of rats of different inbred strains. *Texas Univ. Publ.* **5109:**144–149.

Rezvani, A. H., Overstreet, D. H., and Janowsky, D. S. (1990a). Genetic serotonin deficiency and alcohol preference in the fawn hooded rats. *Alcohol Alcohol.* **25:**573–575.

Rezvani, A. H., Overstreet, D. H., and Janowsky, D. S. (1990b). Reduction in ethanol preference following injection of centrally and peripherally acting muscarinic agents. *Alcohol Alcohol.* **25:**3–7.

Rezvani, A. H., Overstreet, D. H., and Janowsky, D. S. (1991). Drug-induced reductions in ethanol intake in alcohol preferring and fawn-hooded rats. *Alcohol Alcohol.* **1**(suppl):433–437.

Rodgers, D. A. (1972). Factors underlying differences in alcohol preference of inbred strains of mice. In *The Biology of Alcoholism,* Vol. 2, B. Kissin and H. Begleiter, eds. New York: Plenum Press, pp. 107–130.

Rodgers, D. A., and McClearn, G. E. (1962). Alcohol preference of mice. In *Roots of Behavior,* E. L. Bliss, ed. New York: Hoeber, pp. 68–95.

Samson, H. H. (1986). Initiation of ethanol reinforcement using a sucrose-substitution procedure in food and water-sated rats. *Alcohol.: Clin. Exp. Res.* **10**:436–442.

Samson, H. H., Hodge, C. W., Tolliver, G. A., and Haraguchi, M. (1993). Effect of dopamine agonists and antagonists on ethanol-reinforced behavior: The involvement of the nucleus accumbens. *Brain Res. Bull.* **30**:133–141.

Schecter, M. D. (1988). Use of TFMPP stimulus properties as a model of 5-HT1B receptor activation. *Pharmacol. Biochem. Behav.* **31**:53–57.

Sinclair, J. D. (1990). Drugs to decrease alcohol drinking. *Ann. Med.* **22**:357–362.

Sinclair, J. D., Le, A. D., and Kiianmaa, K. (1989). The AA and ANA rat lines, selected for differences in voluntary alcohol consumption. *Experientia* **45**:798–805.

Stewart, R. B., Murphy, J. M., Lumeng, L., and Li, T. -K. (1989). Differences in performance on anxiety tests in rats genetically selected for ethanol preference. *Soc. Neurosci. Abstr.* **15**:61(abstract).

Stewart, R. B., Murphy, J. M., McBride, W. J., Lumeng, L., and Li, T. -K. (1990) Tolerance to the aversive effects of ethanol in selectively-bred alcohol-preferring (P) rats. *Alcohol.: Clin. Exp. Res.* **14**:342 (abstract).

Stewart, R. B., Kurtz, D. L., Zweifel, M., Li, T. -K. and Froehlich, J. C. (1991a). Differences in the hypothermic response to ethanol in rats selectively bred for oral ethanol preference and nonpreference. *Psychopharmacology* **106**:169–174.

Stewart, R. B., McBride, W. J., Lumeng, L., Li, T. -K., and Murphy, J. M. (1991b). Chronic alcohol consumption in alcohol-preferring rats attenuates subsequent conditioned taste aversion produced by ethanol injections. *Psychopharmacology* **105**:530–534.

Stewart, R. B., Li, T. -K., McBride, W. J., Lumeng, L., and Murphy, J. M. (1992a). Place aversion conditioning: Genetic differences in the aversive effects of ethanol in alcohol-preferring P and -nonpreferring NP rats. *Alcohol.: Clin. Exp. Res.* **16**: (abstract).

Stewart, R. B., Li, T. -K., McBride, W. J., Lumeng, L., and Murphy, J. M. (1992b). Chronic ethanol consumption in alcohol-preferring P rats attenuates subsequent conditioned place aversion produced by ethanol injections. *Alcohol.: Clin. Exp. Res.* **16**:395 (abstract).

Suzdak, P. D., Glowa, J. R., Crawley, J. N., Schwartz, R. D., and Skolnick, P. (1986a). A selective imidazobenzodiazepine antagonist of ethanol in the rat. *Science* **234:**1243–1247.

Suzdak, P. D., Schwartz, R. D., Skolnick, P., and Paul, S. M. (1986b). Ethanol stimulates gamma-aminobutyric acid receptor-mediated chloride transport in rat brain synaptoneurosomes. *Proc. Natl. Acad. Sci. (USA),* **83:**4071–4075.

Tabakoff, B., and Ritzman, R. F. (1979). Acute tolerance in inbred and selected lines of mice. *Drug Alcohol Depend.* **4**:87–90.

Tabakoff, B., Ritzman, R. F., Raju T. S., and Deitrich, R. A. (1980). Characterization of acute and chronic tolerance in mice selected for inherent differences in sensitivity to ethanol. *Alcohol.: Clin. Exp. Res.* **4**:70–73.

Tabakoff, B., and Hoffman, P. L. (1987). Interactions of ethanol with opiate receptors: implications for the mechanisms of action of ethanol. In *Brain Reward Systems and Abuse,* J. Engel, L. Oreland, D. H. Ingvar, B. Pernow, S. Rossner, and L. A. Pellborn, eds. New York: Raven Press, pp. 99–107.

Tampier, L., Quintanilla, M. E., and Mardones, J. (1980). Genetic differences in tolerance to ethanol: A study in UChA and UChB rats. *Pharmacol. Biochem. Behav.* **14**:165–168.

Thomasson, H. R., Edenberg, H. J., Crabb, D. W., Mai, X. -L., Jerome, R. E., Li, T. -K., Wang, K., **S. -P.** Lin, Y. -T., Lu, R. -B., and Yin, S. -J. (1991). Alcohol and aldehyde dehydrogenase genotypes and alcoholism in Chinese men. *Am. J. Hum. Genet.* **48:**677–681.

Volpicelli, J. R., Davis, M. A., and Olgin, J. E. (1986). Naltrexone blocks the post-shock increase of ethanol consumption. *Life Sci.* **38**:841–847.

Waller, M. B., McBride, W. J., Lumeng, L., and Li, T. -K. (1982a). Effects of intravenous ethanol and of 4-methylpyrazole on alcohol drinking of alcohol-preferring rats. *Pharmacol. Biochem. Behav.* **17**:763–768.

Waller, M. B., McBride, W. J., Lumeng, L., and Li, T. -K. (1982b). Induction of dependence on ethanol by free-choice drinking in alcohol-preferring rats. *Pharmacol. Biochem. Behav.* **16**:501–507.

Waller, M. B., McBride, W. J., Lumeng, L., and Li, T. -K. (1983). Initial sensitivity and acute tolerance to ethanol in P and NP lines of rats. *Pharmacol. Biochem. Behav.* **19**:683–686.

Waller, M. B., McBride, W. J., Gatto, G. J., Lumeng, L., and Li, T. -K. (1984). Intragastric self-infusion of ethanol by ethanol-preferring and -nonpreferring lines of rats. *Science* **225**:78–80.

Waller, M. B., Murphy, J. M., McBride, W. J., Lumeng, L., and Li, T. -K. (1986). Effect of low dose ethanol on spontaneous motor activity in alcohol-preferring and -nonpreferring lines of rats. *Pharmacol. Biochem. Behav.* **24**:617–623.

Weiss, F., Mitchiner, M., Bloom, F. E., and Koob, G. F. (1990). Free-choice responding for ethanol versus water in alcohol-preferring (P) and unselected Wistar rats is differentially modified by naloxone, bromocriptine, and methysergide. *Psychopharmacology* **101**:178–186.

Weiss, F., Hurd, Y. L., Ungerstedt, U., Markou, A., Plotsky, P. M., and Koob, G. F. (1992). Neurochemical correlates of cocaine and ethanol self-administration. *Ann. N.Y. Acad. Sci.* **654**:220–241.

Williams, R. J., Berry, L. J., and Beerstecher, Jr., E. (1949). Individual metabolic patterns, alcoholism, genetotrophic diseases. *Proc. Nat. Acad. Sci. (USA)* **35**:265–271.

Winters, D. K., and Cederbaum, A. I. (1992). The content and activity of cyt P450IIE1 in liver microsomes from alcohol-preferring and non-preferring rats. *Alcohol Alcohol.* **27**:63–70.

Wise, R. A. (1981). Brain dopamine and reward. In *Theory in Psychopharmacology,* S. J. Cooper, ed. New York: Academic Press, pp. 103–122.

Wong, D. T., Lumeng, L., Threlkeld, P. G., Reid, L. R., and Li, T. -K. (1988). Serotonergic and adrenergic receptors in alcohol-preferring and non-preferring rats. *J. Neural Trans.* **71**:207–218.

Wong, D. T., Threlkeld, P. G., Lumeng, L., and Li, T. -K. (1990). Higher density of serotonin 1-A receptors in the hippocampus and cerebral cortex of alcohol-preferring P rats. *Life Sci.* **46**:231–235.

Wong, D. T., Reid, L. R., Li, T. -K., and Lumeng, L. 1993. Greater abundance of serotomin IA receptor in some brain areas of alcohol-preferring (P) than of -nonpreferring (NP) rats. *Pharmacol. Biochem. Behav.* **46**:173–177.

Yoshida, A., Huang, I. -Y., and Ikawa, M. (1984). Molecular abnormality of an inactive aldehyde dehydrogenase variant commonly found in Orientals. *Proc. Natl. Acad. Sci, (USA)* **81**:258–261.

Yoshimoto, K., and Komura, S. (1987). Re-examination of the relationship between alcohol preference and brain monamines in inbred strains of mice including senescence-accelerated mice. *Pharmacol. Biochem. Behav.* **27**:317–322.

Yoshimoto, K., McBride, W. J., Lumeng, L., and Li, T. -K. (1991). Alcohol stimulates the release of dopamine and serotonin in the nucleus accumbens. *Alcohol* **9**:17–22.

Yoshimoto, K., McBride, W. J., Lumeng, L., and Li, T. -K. (1992). Ethanol enhances the release of dopamine and serotonin in the nucleus accumbens of HAD and LAD lines of rats. *Alcohol. Clin. Exp. Res.* **16**:781–785.

Zhou, F. C., Bledsoe, S., Lumeng, L., and Li, T. -K. (1991a). Immunostained serotonergic fi-
    bers are decreased in selected brain regions of alcohol-preferring rats. *Alcohol* **8**:
    425–431.
Zhou, F. C., Bledsoe, S., Lumeng, L., and Li, T. -K. (1991b). Serotonergic immunostained ter-
    minal fibers are lower in selected forebrain areas of alcohol-preferring rats. *Alcohol*
    8:1–7.
Zhou, F. C., Pu, C. F., Lumeng, L., and Li, T. -K. (1991c). Fewer number of immunostained
    serotonergic neurons in raphe of alcohol-preferring rats. *Alcohol.: Clin. Exp. Res.*
    15:315.

Genetic Factors That Reduce Risk for Developing Alcoholism in Animals and Humans

DAVID W. CRABB, HOWARD J. EDENBERG,
HOLLY R. THOMASSON, AND TING-KAI LI

Alcohol drinking behavior is influenced by a host of biological and environmental factors, some of which contribute to making the experience pleasant or rewarding while others make the experience unpleasant or aversive. The quantity and frequency of drinking are governed by the interaction of these positive and negative reactions to alcohol consumption. During the last 15 years, a great deal of attention has been paid to demonstrating that there is genetic as well as psychosocial risk for "drinking too much." In humans, adoption studies have pointed to the existence of genetic determinants that increase the risk of developing alcoholism in children of alcoholics (Cotton, 1979; Cloninger et al., 1981). Recent studies of twins have shown that patterns of social drinking are also influenced by both environmental and genetic factors (Heath et al., 1991a, 1991b).

In the laboratory, it has been demonstrated that rats can be selectively bred to self-administer large quantities of alcohol orally, intragastrically, and intracerebrally for its pharmacological effects (Li, et al., 1988; McBride et al., 1990). The neurobiological basis for this alcohol-seeking behavior is an area of intense research. On the other hand, relatively little is known about specific biological factors that deter individuals from drinking heavily. For one thing, individuals who are in some way deterred from drinking do not typically come to the attention of clinicians and researchers in the alcohol field. Protective factors could be as important as risk factors in determining an individual's chances of becoming an alcohol abuser. The alcohol-flush reaction is one such deterrent factor; it is the best characterized genetic trait that appears to protect against alcohol-use disorders. We discuss the enzymological and genetic basis of this reaction, and summarize population genetic studies on the contribution of the alcohol-flush reaction to reducing the risk of alcoholism. We also discuss a possible role of alcohol dehydrogenase isozymes in modifying that risk.

The Enzymology of Alcohol Metabolizing Systems

Ethanol is first oxidized to acetaldehyde, which is then oxidized to acetate:

Alcohol dehydrogenase   Aldehyde dehydrogenase

ETHANOL ———————————→ ACETALDEHYDE ———————————→ ACETATE

Cytochrome P450IIE1

Ethanol can be oxidized by alcohol dehydrogenases (Ehrig et al., 1990), cytochrome P450IIE1 and possibly other cytochromes (Lieber, 1987), and perhaps by catalase. Quantitatively, the greatest fraction of alcohol is metabolized by the alcohol dehydrogenase pathway. Minor pathways of ethanol metabolism include the reactions catalyzed by catalase, fatty acid ethyl ester synthases, and phospholipase D, but these contribute little to alcohol elimination and will not be considered further.

Alcohol Dehydrogenase

Alcohol dehydrogenases (ADH, E.C. 1.1.1.1) exist in the cytosol of cells of the liver, kidney, stomach, lung, and other organs; by far the greatest activity is in the liver. These enzymes are dimers of subunits having molecular weights of 40 kDa. There are as many as five different classes of ADH (Table 8-1). Class I isozymes arise from three closely related subunits, α, β, and γ, which can hybridize to form homo- and heterodimers. They have a low K_m for ethanol and are highly sensitive to inhibition by pyrazole (Ehrig et al., 1990). Class II ADH was first found in human liver, has a higher K_m for ethanol, and is less sensitive to pyrazole inhibition (Bosron et al., 1979; Hoog et

Table 8-1 Properties of Ethanol Oxidizing Enzymes in Humans

Gene Locus	Subunit Type	K_m (Ethanol)	Tissue Distribution
Alcohol Dehydrogenases			
Class I			
ADH1	α	4	Liver
ADH2	β	0.05–36	Liver, lung
ADH3	γ	0.5–1	Liver, stomach
Class II			
ADH4	π	34	Liver, cornea
Class III			
ADH5	χ	>500	All tissues
Class IV[a]			
—	σ, μ	20	Liver, stomach
Class V[a]			
ADH6	—	?	Liver, stomach
Cytochrome P450			
CYP2E1	—	10	Liver, kidney

[a]Tentative assignments based upon sequence similarities or differences. See text for details about the class IV and V enzymes. K_m values are given in millimolar. For tissue distribution only major sites are listed.

al., 1987). Class III ADH is found in all tissues thus far studied; it is virtually inactive with ethanol but acts on long-chain alcohols (Wagner et al., 1984). This enzyme also exhibits glutathione-dependent formaldehyde dehydrogenase activity (Koivusalo et al., 1989). The class I, II, and III enzyme subunits are sufficiently different from one another that heterodimers of subunits from the different classes are not found. The most recent additions to this family of enzymes are class IV and (tentatively) class V. The class IV enzymes have been purified from the stomach. Also called μ ADH (Yin et al., 1990) and σ ADH (Moreno and Pares, 1991), its partial amino acid sequence suggests that it probably belongs in a class distinct from I, II, and III (Pares et al., 1990). An additional ADH gene (named *ADH6*) and cDNA have been cloned by screening genomic and cDNA libraries with conserved oligonucleotides. The deduced protein sequence from analysis of the cDNA indicates about 60% homology to class I, II, and III enzymes, and to the σ ADH (Yasunami et al., 1991). The mRNA for this gene has been identified in liver and in stomach (Yasunami et al., 1991), but the enzyme itself has not been purified or expressed. Therefore, its kinetic properties are unknown. Of these different enzymes, classes I, II, and possibly IV participate in the oxidation of ethanol.

There are three class I loci, two of which (*ADH2* and *ADH3*) are polymorphic (Burnell and Bosron, 1989). *ADH1* encodes the α subunit, and is the first gene to be activated in the liver during fetal development (Smith, 1986). *ADH2* encodes the β subunits. Several β polypeptides are known, each differing from the others at a single amino acid residue. Most common in Caucasians, $\beta 1$ has a very low K_m for ethanol and a relatively low V_{max}. Found commonly in Asians, $\beta 2$ was originally designated "atypical" ADH because of a lower pH-optimum for ethanol oxidation (van Wartburg et al., 1964; Yin et al., 1984). It is notable for its considerably higher V_{max} and somewhat higher K_m compared with $\beta 1$. Later, a third form, $\beta 3$, was detected in liver extracts from African-Americans (Bosron et al., 1980). It has a much lower pH-optimum than the other ADH isozymes, has a high K_m for ethanol, and high V_{max}. The *ADH3* gene encodes the γ polypeptides and it, too, is polymorphic. The $\gamma 1$ isozyme has about twice the V_{max} of the $\gamma 2$ isozyme; the K_m for ethanol are similar for the two forms. $\gamma 1$ ADH is found at high frequency in Asians and Blacks; Caucasians have about equal frequency for $\gamma 1$ and $\gamma 2$ ADH (Bosron and Li, 1987). The kinetic properties of these isozymes are summarized in Table 8-2. The other ADH loci have not been shown to be polymorphic to date.

Cytochrome P450

Cytochrome P450IIE1 (encoded by the *CYP2E1* gene) is located in the endoplasmic reticulum, especially in hepatocytes of the centrilobular zone of the liver (Lieber and DeCarli, 1970; Lieber, 1987; Tsutsumi et al., 1989). It has a relatively high K_m for ethanol (Table 8-1). This enzyme is important because it metabolizes many xenobiotics as well as ethanol, and hence is a site for drug–alcohol interactions (Lieber, 1990). Because it is induced several fold in the liver of heavy drinkers, it accounts in part for the increased rate of alcohol metabolism in alcoholics (Lieber, 1987).

Table 8-2 Properties of Polymorphic Forms of Human Alcohol Dehydrogenase

Gene Locus	Subunit Type	K_m (Ethanol)	V_{max}
*ADH2*1*	β1	0.05	9
*ADH2*2*	β2	0.9	400
*ADH2*3*	β3	36	300
*ADH3*1*	γ1	1.0	87
*ADH3*2*	γ2	0.5	35

Note: The kinetic constants given are for the homodimers of the subunits listed (Bosron and Li, 1987). The K_m values are in millimolar, and the V_{max} values are given in terms of turnover number (min⁻¹).

Aldehyde Dehydrogenase

The enzymes that oxidize acetaldehyde are the aldehyde dehydrogenases (ALDH, E.C. 1.2.1.3). Several different ALDHs exist (Table 8-3). There was recently a suggestion for a classification of the nonspecific ALDHs based upon the protein sequences that are becoming available (Anonymous, 1989; Lindahl and Hempel, 1990). The class I and II proteins exist as tetramers with subunit molecular weights of about 54 kDa. They generally utilize NAD^+ in preference to $NADP^+$ as coenzyme, and are thought to form an acyl-enzyme intermediate during catalysis. ALDH1 is the major cytosolic form of the enzyme; it has a relatively low K_m for aldehydes and is very sensitive to inhibition by disulfiram *in vitro* (Ferencz-Biro and Pietruszko, 1984; Goedde and Agarwal, 1987). This isozyme is present in most cells, including erythrocytes (Goedde and Agarwal, 1987). ALDH2 is the mitochondrial form of the enzyme. It has a very low K_m for acetaldehyde (1 μM). This enzyme is expressed differentially in the liver, with lesser amounts in the kidney, lung, and other tissues (Goedde and Agarwal, 1987; Dipple and Crabb, 1993).

ALDH3 and ALDH4 have been described in tissue extracts. These isozymes have considerably lower affinity for aliphatic aldehydes than the class I and II enzymes and

Table 8-3 Properties of Human Aldehyde Dehydrogenases

Gene Locus	Structure	K_m (Acetaldehyde)	Tissue Distribution
Class I			
ALDH1	α4	30 μM	Most tissues
Class II			
ALDH2	α4	< 1 μM	Liver > kidney > lung
Class III			
ALDH3	α2	11 mM	Stomach, liver
Other enzymes			
ALDH4	α2	—	Liver
ALDHₓ	—	—	Liver, testis

Note: The various classes of aldehyde dehydrogenases characterized in humans are shown. $ALDH_x$ has been cloned, but the kinetic properties of the enzyme have not been reported. ALDH4 appears to be identical to glutamic γ-semialdehyde dehydrogenase. The structure of the enzymes is indicated by α2 for dimers and α4 for tetramers.

have higher affinity for aromatic aldehyde substrates. The ALDH3 family includes the cytosolic, TCDD (dioxin)-inducible ALDH, the hepatoma-associated ALDH, and the stomach ALDH3 (Lindahl and Hempel, 1990). The stomach form might participate in the oxidation of acetaldehyde generated during gastric metabolism of ethanol. ALDH4 appears to be the mitochondrial glutamic γ-semialdehyde dehydrogenase (Forte-McRobbie and Peitruszko, 1986). Other mitochondrial aldehyde dehydrogenases include succinic and methylmalonyl semialdehyde dehydrogenases. One additional ALDH, $ALDH_x$, was cloned by screening libraries at reduced stringency. This ALDH is 72% identical to ALDH2 and 65% identical to ALDH1 (Hsu and Chang, 1991). The kinetic properties of this enzyme are unknown; mRNA for this enzyme is found in liver and testis (Hsu and Chang, 1991).

Both ALDH1 and ALDH2 could participate in acetaldehyde oxidation in vivo. The predominant role of ALDH2 in acetaldehyde disposal is demonstrated by a naturally occuring mutation. A variant of the *ALDH2* gene results in deficiency of this enzyme activity. When individuals with this variant drink, they accumulate acetaldehyde in the bloodstream and tissues, attesting to the importance of this form of ALDH in normal alcohol metabolism. This deficiency state is discussed in the following section.

The Asian (or Oriental) Alcohol Flush Reaction

Clinical Description

It had been known since ancient times that alcohol consumption results in facial flushing in certain individuals. This appears to be most marked in individuals of Asian background. Wolff's report in 1972 indicated that about 80% of Japanese, Chinese, and Koreans had visible facial flushing and increased blood flow to the ear lobe after consuming a small amount of alcohol, while only an occasional Caucasian had a similar reaction (Wolff, 1972; Wolff, 1973). Since the reaction was also observed in infants given a dose of alcohol, the reaction was presumed to be genetic in origin. A family study suggested that the flush reaction was inherited as a dominant trait in several Hawaiian families (Schwitters et al., 1982). Although facial and anterior chest wall flushing is the most obvious reaction of these individuals to alcohol, it is only one symptom of this syndrome. Subjects with the reaction also report tachycardia, dizziness, headache, swelling of the face, nausea and occasionally vomiting, and sometimes hypotension.

In the late 1940s, the flushing reaction associated with drinking while taking the drug disulfiram was recognized as being due to elevated blood acetaldehyde levels, and infusion of acetaldehyde was shown to produce tachycardia, hyperventilation, and cutaneous flushing (Asmussen et al., 1948). In recent years, elevated acetaldehyde levels have been found in individuals with the flush reaction when given alcohol to drink (Ijiri, 1974; Zeiner et al., 1979; Mizoi et al., 1979; Mizoi et al., 1983). It has been technically difficult to determine acetaldehyde levels in blood, but the published reports indicated a large difference in blood levels of acetaldehyde between the nonflushers and flushers. For example, in nonflushers, drinking elicited an increase in acetaldehyde levels to perhaps 5–10 µM; in flushers the levels are highly variable, but may exceed 100 µM within an hour of drinking (Enomoto et al., 1991b). Some of the variability in these studies may be due to different classes of flushing subjects, since there are now at least two known genetic mechanisms to account for the flush reaction (see below).

Physiology of the Alcohol Flush Reaction

It is commonly observed that the intensity of the flush reaction in Asians varies among individuals. The physiological factors that control cutaneous skin flow in subjects with normal ALDH2 or with the deficiency are not well understood. First, the flush is not uniform; it appears to be most pronounced in the face and chest. The reason for this is unknown. We do not know if additional vascular beds, such as the splanchnic, coronary, or cerebral circulations are also involved. Second, the changes observed in skin blood flow are probably the result of both central and peripheral reactions. The contribution of central mechanisms was shown elegantly in experiments with individuals with transected spinal cords (Malpas et al., 1990). In most normal subjects, including individuals with active ALDH2, there is an increase in skin blood flow after drinking, although rare instances of subjects who have cutaneous blanching after alcohol have been recorded. In individuals with spinal cord transection, there was no change in skin blood flow (as assessed by changes in the skin temperature) when they drank alcohol (Malpas et al., 1990). Until additional studies are performed, we cannot be sure of the relative contributions of central (neurally mediated vasodilation) and peripheral (local vasodilation due to circulating substances) mechanisms to the flush reaction. However, there is probably some purely local response of the skin to acetaldehyde, since the application of alcohol or acetaldehyde to the skin produces erythema (Muramatsu et al., 1989). This is the basis for patch tests devised to determine the phenotype of individuals without requiring them to drink.

Acetaldehyde may not cause the flush reaction directly. Pharmacologic studies have indicated that the flush can be attenuated with antihistamines (H1 and H2 antagonists) (Miller et al., 1987), nalmefene (an opiate antagonist) (Ho et al., 1988), and nonsteroidal anti-inflammatory agents (Truitt et al., 1985). Acetaldehyde levels were either unchanged or not measured in these studies. Thus, flushing may be mediated by vasoactive substances released when cells (possibly mast or endothelial cells) are exposed to elevated concentrations of acetaldehyde. Presumably, individuals might show different sensitivities of these cells to acetaldehyde, and the vascular responses to these compounds could differ. All of these intermediate steps could, therefore, contribute to the variability in flushing.

Enzymatic Defects in Acetaldehyde Metabolism

At the time the early studies on alcohol flushing were performed, the only known genetic variant in the pathway of alcohol metabolism was the "atypical" alcohol dehydrogenase described originally by von Wartburg et al. (1964), now named β2 ADH

(Ehrig et al., 1990). This isozyme has a high V_{max} due to a mutation of an active site arginine to histidine, which accelerates the release of NADH produced in the reaction (Table 8–2). It was first suggested that the presence of this variant isozyme of ADH in Asians might be responsible for the flush reaction, since it would be expected to metabolize ethanol more rapidly than does the usual Caucasian form of ADH, β1, and would thus generate acetaldehyde more rapidly (Stamatoyannopoulos et al., 1975). We now know that the majority of flushers have a different enzymatic abnormality, although some individuals do appear to flush mildly on the basis of being homozygous for ADH2*2 (see below).

Harada et al. first reported that individuals with the flush reaction lacked aldehyde dehydrogenase activity in extracts of hair roots. The ALDH2 found in hair roots is identical to that found in liver. These and other researchers found that ALDH2 activity was absent only in the flushing individuals (Goedde et al., 1983b; Harada et al., 1982). Subsequent studies have repeatedly confirmed this association, and have documented that ALDH2-deficient individuals have high blood acetaldehyde after drinking (Enomoto et al., 1991b). These data demonstrate the importance of the ALDH2 isozyme in disposing of acetaldehyde generated during alcohol metabolism. Thus, the elevated acetaldehyde levels that occur during a flush reaction result primarily from the impaired ability to remove acetaldehyde rather than from an increased rate of production.

Molecular Basis for ALDH2 Deficiency

The biochemical basis for the deficiency in ALDH2 activity has been demonstrated by protein and cDNA sequencing. The glutamate at position 487, a residue previously not suspected to play a role in the catalytic function of the enzyme and not generally conserved among aldehyde dehydrogenases, was a lysine in the individuals with the enzyme deficiency (Yoshida et al., 1984).

The lysine for glutamate substitution is the result of a single nucleotide change. The normal allele is termed ALDH2*1 and the mutant allele is ALDH2*2. The different alleles can be detected using allele-specific oligonucleotides (ASOs). One method utilizes Southern blotting of restriction enzyme-digested genomic DNA with the ASOs (Hsu et al., 1987). A more robust method utilizes the polymerase chain reaction (PCR) to amplify the exon containing the site of the mutation; the DNA is then hybridized with ASOs to determine the genotype (Crabb et al., 1989).

Determination of the genotypes of liver samples known to be either normal or ALDH2 deficient revealed an unexpected, interesting phenomenon: the deficient phenotype appears as a dominant trait (Crabb et al., 1989). Most of the Japanese (Crabb et al., 1989) and Korean subjects (Goedde et al., 1989) with the deficient phenotype are heterozygous for the ALDH2*2 allele.

In the humans with ALDH2 deficiency, liver extracts showed no activity when assayed at high NAD^+ concentrations or when activity stained on isoelectric focusing or starch gels (Johnson et al., 1987). However, one laboratory has reported the presence of about 15% of expected activity in partially purified fractions of ALDH2 from an ALDH2-deficient liver (Ferencz-Biro and Pietruszko, 1984). The ALDH2 enzyme is a tetrameric protein (Tu and Weiner, 1987). If individuals who are heterozygous for the *ALDH2*2* allele produce equal amounts of the normal and variant forms of the protein subunits and they associate randomly, about 94% of the tetramers would contain at least one mutant subunit. We hypothesized that the presence of even a single defective subunit renders the tetramer inactive (Crabb et al., 1989). It is also possible that transport into and assembly of ALDH2 within the mitochondria cannot proceed normally when the mutant polypeptide is present. Conceivably, interactions between the normal and mutant peptide could prevent the transport of both peptides. The half-life of the mitochondrial enzyme might also be altered if a mutant polypeptide is present in the tetramer. This issue is unresolved.

Population Genetics of ALDH2 Deficiency and Its Association with Alcohol-Drinking Behavior

To date, a high prevalence of ALDH2 deficiency and the variant *ALDH2*2* allele has been detected only in certain Asian populations (Table 8-4). We have looked for the *ALDH2*2* allele in Caucasians in the United States, Great Britain, and Byelorussia, but have not found individuals with it (Day et al., 1991). There are differences in the prevalence of this allele in China, Japan, and Korea, and the prevalence apparently is considerably lower among Filipinos (Goedde et al., 1983b; Goedde and Agarwal, 1987) and native Atayal in Taiwan (below). There is disagreement about ALDH2 deficiency in certain Ecuadoran Indian tribes: hair root analysis showed that approximately 40% of the Indians were ALDH2 deficient (Goedde et al., 1983b; Goedde et al., 1986), whereas the *ALDH2*2* allele was not detected by a PCR-ASO method (O'Dowd et al., 1990). Of course, the genotyping method is designed only to evaluate differences at codon 487; it is therefore possible that a different mutation is present in these Indian populations. Clearly, a direct comparison of phenotype with genotype needs to be performed.

Among several Asian populations, it has been observed in cross-sectional studies that individuals who are alcoholic (Harada et al., 1982; Goedde et al., 1983a; Harada et al., 1983), or who have alcoholic liver disease (Shibuya and Yoshida, 1989) rarely had

Table 8-4 Population Genetics of ALDH2 in Asians

Population	Allele Frequency (*ALDH2*2*)	ALDH2 Deficiency (%)
Japanese (Shibuya and Yoshida, 1988)	0.35	50
Korean (Goedde et al., 1989)	0.15	28
Chinese (Thomasson et al., 1991)	0.30	30–50
Atayal (Thomasson et al., 1990b)	0.05	—
Vietnamese (Goedde and Agarwal, 1987)	—	53
Indonesian (Goedde and Agarwal, 1987)	—	39
Filipino (Goedde and Agarwal, 1987)	—	13

Note: The frequency of the *ALDH2*2* allele determined by genotyping and the frequency of ALDH2 deficiency (phenotypes) determined by hair root analysis are shown.

ALDH2 deficiency or an *ALDH2*2* allele. Among Japanese alcoholics with liver disease, only 7% had an *ALDH2*2* allele (Shibuya and Yoshida, 1989). In a study we performed on Chinese males living in Taiwan, the frequency of the *ALDH2*2* allele was 30% in a nonalcoholic control group, and 6% in a group of alcoholic individuals (Thomasson et al., 1991). The native Atayal tribe of Taiwan exhibited a much lower frequency of the mutation in the nonalcoholic group (5%) and a somewhat, but not statistically significantly, lower frequency in the alcoholic group (2%). The low frequency of this allele in the Atayal population is of interest. They also have a reduced frequency of self-reported flushing and higher rates of alcoholism compared with the Chinese in Taiwan. Although there are many social and economic differences between these groups, it is interesting to speculate that, as a group, the Atayal lack the protective effect of the *ALDH2*2* allele against heavy drinking and alcoholism. It would also be interesting to carry out longitudinal studies to see if there is a protective effect of the *ALDH2*2* allele in the Atayals who possess that allele.

The reduction in the prevalence of alcohol-use disorders is presumed to be the result of the aversive reaction evoked by acetaldehyde. In effect, these individuals have an inborn error of alcohol metabolism or pharmacogenetic disorder that renders them sensitive to the aversive effects of alcohol and they learn to avoid it. This is conceptually similar to the learned avoidance of protein exhibited by individuals with disorders of urea cycle enzymes, avoidance of milk products by individuals with lactase deficiency, and the avoidance of fruit by individuals with hereditary fructose intolerance. These are interesting examples of genetic influences on behavior (ecogenetic disorders). It should be noted, however, that at least one study of socially drinking Asians who have an *ALDH2*2* allele indicated that some experience more positive feelings after they drink alcohol than did a control group of Asians with only *ALDH2*1* alleles (Ehlers, personal communication).

The alcohol flush reaction, of course, is only one countervailing influence in individuals who are ALDH2 deficient. They may experience the usual biological and environmental influences that promote heavy drinking, and they may sometimes become alcoholic. Furthermore, the intensity of the flush reaction is quite variable. It is possible that those ALDH2-deficient individuals who become alcoholic have milder degrees of flushing; alternatively, the rewarding properties of alcohol for them may be greater than the presumed aversive effect of the flush reaction.

If ALDH2 deficiency does not deter heavy drinking, it may actually be a risk factor for complications of alcohol abuse. It has been noted in the Japanese that, among individuals with ALDH2 deficiency and alcoholic liver disease, the estimated daily intake of ethanol was lower (88 ± 9 g/day) than among individuals with normal ALDH2 genotype [136 ± 34 g/day (Enomoto et al., 1991a)]. The ALDH2-deficient individuals also had a higher prevalence of alcoholic hepatitis. These authors suggested that ALDH2 deficiency moderated their intake of alcohol, but that increased levels of acetaldehyde were generated in their livers when they drank. This may render them more susceptible to the liver complications of drinking, since acetaldehyde appears to play a major role in the hepatotoxicity of alcohol.

Pharmacogenetics of the Flush Reaction

Among individuals who flush, the peak acetaldehyde level varies widely (Enomoto et al., 1991b); however, correlation of the acetaldehyde level with the flush intensity has, to our knowledge, not yet been performed. The difference in the intensity of the flush reaction was originally attributed to differences between homozygotes and heterozygotes for the mutant *ALDH2* alleles. The earlier models of the genetics of ALDH2 deficiency suggested that mild flushing resulted from the heterozygous state and more severe flushing from the homozygous *ALDH2*2* state. With our understanding that heterozygotes have very low ALDH2 activity and may flush intensely (above), this has had to be reevaluated (see the section on the role of ADH genotype in the flush reaction. Although only a few have been tested, homozygotes for *ALDH2*2* ascertained by the new genotyping methods have very severe, almost anaphylactic responses to even small amounts of alcohol. The reaction is so severe that they rarely drink.

Other Possible Defects in Aldehyde Metabolism and Causes of Alcohol-Induced Flushing

There have been isolated reports of abnormal ALDH1 isozymes in Asians and Caucasians. Yoshida and coworkers observed one of ten Japanese livers to be deficient in ALDH1 activity despite the presence of immunologically cross-reacting material (Yoshida, 1983). Flushing after drinking is reported rather uncommonly among Caucasians (6–10%, Wilson et al., 1978). Caucasians who flush and have an ALDH1 with altered mobility on gel electrophoresis have been reported (Yoshida et al., 1989). The basis for the altered mobility is unknown but, perhaps more importantly, the presence of flushing was not unequivocally established in the published report.

We recently tested 10 Caucasians who claimed to flush after they drank various alcoholic beverages, but were *ALDH2*1* homozygotes. These individuals were given ethanol and their blood alcohol levels and the change in blood flow in facial skin were measured. None of these individuals had a greater change in skin blood flow than did controls who did not report flushing (about a 2-fold increase in all individuals, Thomasson, unpublished data). These findings emphasize the need to adequately establish the flushing phenotype of such individuals before proceeding with biochemical analyses.

American Indians are reported to flush after drinking (Wolff, 1973). However, the prevalence of ALDH2 deficiency in the Indians studied to date has been quite low (2–5% in one study (Goedde et al., 1986) and 0% in another (Rex et al., 1985)). Other studies have shown that Indians generally have the β1 form of ADH that is usually found in Caucasians (Rex et al., 1985). We do not understand the basis for flushing in American Indian subjects.

Alcoholic Caucasians also exhibit elevated acetaldehyde levels after drinking (to as high as 40–50 μM) (Korsten et al., 1975) and may flush, but apparently do not experience this as an aversive reaction. The elevation in acetaldehyde level probably results from higher rates of acetaldehyde formation by cytochrome P450IIE1, which is induced by heavy drinking, and reduced ability of the mitochondria to oxidize the acetaldehyde due to toxic effects of ethanol or acetaldehyde itself. Alcoholics are not deterred from drinking by this flushing; hence, there appears to be a difference in the response to acetaldehyde depending upon whether the elevated acetaldehyde accompanies every drinking episode from a young age (as in the case of Asians with the flush reaction) or only occurs after the rewarding effects of alcohol have been experienced and the patient is gradually habituated to the elevated acetaldehyde concentration (as may occur in alcoholics). Differences such as these may help explain why aversive therapy with ALDH inhibitors like disulfiram or cyanamide has not been very successful (although the major problem appears to be lack of compliance). These differences may now be experimentally testable in the rat models of alcohol preference now available.

ALDH2 Polymorphism in Rats Selected for Alcohol Preference

There is a difference in the electrophoretic mobility of ALDH2 in extracts of liver from the P (alcohol-preferring) and NP (alcohol-nonpreferring) lines of rats (Carr et al., 1991). The ALDH2 cDNA from the two lines was cloned (by reverse PCR) and sequenced. A single base difference between the two forms was found: the P rats have a glutamine at position 67, while the NP rats have an arginine. By establishing genotyping methods for this variant, it was found that the arginine allele of ALDH2 is present at a frequency of 18% in P rats and at a frequency of 63% in NP rats (Carr et al., 1991). At present it is not known if the two forms differ in catalytic properties. Based on staining of isoelectric focusing gels, the forms do not differ in activity with saturating concentrations of aldehyde and NAD^+. Hence, these variants of ALDH2 in the rat may not modulate different drinking behaviors in these lines.

The Role of ADH Genotype in the Alcohol Flush Reaction

Effect of ADH Genotype on Intensity of the Flush Reaction

The acetaldehyde-producing enzymes, ADH and cytochrome P450IIE1, are obvious candidates as modifiers of intensity of the flush reaction. To date, there have been no reported polymorphisms in the P450IIE1 protein among humans, although the gene contains an RFLP (Williamson et al., 1990) that could be tested for association with flushing intensity. An additional polymorphism in the 5' flanking region of the human CYP2E1 gene was reported to modify the transcriptional activity of the gene (Hayashi et al., 1991). Since different forms of ADH have substantial differences in kinetic properties *in vitro,* we measured alcohol elimination rates and the intensity of flushing after drinking in a group of Chinese subjects whom we had genotyped at the *ALDH2* and *ADH* loci (Thomasson et al., unpublished data). A number of interesting findings emerged. First, the *ADH* genotype did not correlate strongly with the intensity of the flush reaction. Simply stated, individual flush reactions varied widely in a manner that could not be accounted for by the *ADH* genotype. There was, however, an influence of both *ADH* and *ALDH2* genotypes on the rate of alcohol elimination. Individuals with *ALDH2*2* had decreased rates of alcohol elimination, possibly due to product inhibition of ADH by acetaldehyde (Thomasson et al., 1990a). Others have reported that acetaldehyde concentrations in peripheral blood reach 100 μM in flushers, compared with 5–10 μM in nonflushers; intrahepatic concentrations of acetaldehyde are presumed to be considerably higher. This may be sufficient to inhibit human class I ADHs, which have inhibition constants for acetaldehyde in the range of 500 μM (Bosron, W. F., unpublished data).

Of interest, some individuals homozygous for *ADH2*2* (but with normal ALDH2) had a greater degree of flushing as measured by laser Doppler velocimetry than did the heterozygotes or Caucasians homozygous for *ADH2*1*. This suggested that more rapid rates of alcohol metabolism may result in increases in blood acetaldehyde, although acetaldehyde levels were not measured in these pilot studies. By analogy, one would predict that the ADH form found in African-Americans (*ADH2*3*) might also lead to flushing, especially in homozygous individuals. Because of the relatively low overall frequency of the *ADH2*3* allele, homozygotes are rare. This ADH form has a higher K_m for ethanol, and thus will mainly be active (and flushing might only occur) at high blood ethanol levels.

Population Genetics of ADH Genotypes and Relation to Risk of Alcoholism

The kinetics of the β2-ADH encoded by *ADH2*2* had originally suggested that this gene might be involved in the flush reaction, and we have preliminary data indicating that this is so. We studied Chinese living in Taiwan to see if there was an association between *ADH2* genotype and drinking behavior. We found that the *ADH2*2* allele was significantly more common in the nonalcoholic control group than in the alcoholics (Thomasson et al., 1991). Moreover, the *ADH3*1* allele, which encodes the γ1 ADH isozyme, was also more prevalent in the nonalcoholics than in the alcoholics. These results are consistent with the hypothesis that rapid alcohol metabolism results in elevated levels of acetaldehyde, which discourages drinking. The *ADH2*2* and *ADH3*1* alleles encode more active ADH isozymes that permit faster alcohol metabolism; hence, these genes could be postulated to be "protective" against heavy drinking and alcoholism in the sense that *ALDH2*2* is protective, but to a lesser degree. Interestingly, the alcoholic Atayal also had an increased frequency of *ADH2*1* relative to *ADH2*2*, in support of the preceding hypothesis (Thomasson et al., 1990b, and unpublished data).

Genotyping studies in other populations have been less informative, since there is virtually no variability at the *ADH2* and *ALDH2* loci in Caucasians. We did not see a difference in *ADH3* alleles between alcoholics and controls from the vicinity of Grodno, Byelorussia. The *ADH3*1* allele was significantly more common (although the absolute difference was small) in alcoholics with cirrhosis or chronic pancreatitis than in controls, in a group from the United Kingdom (Newcastle-upon-Tyne) (Day et al., 1991).

A similar result was found among a French cohort, although because of the sample size, the difference did not reach statistical significance (Poupon et al., 1992). When the British and French data are pooled, the difference in *ADH3*1* allele frequency between controls and cirrhotics approached conventional significance (Day et al., 1993). This suggests that higher rates of acetaldehyde production by the γ ADH encoded by *ADH3*1* may contribute to an increased risk of organ damage in heavy drinkers, as may occur in a subset of Japanese subjects with *ALDH2*2* (see earlier).

Variation in ADH expression

An area of study that has gained attention recently is the control of expression of the alcohol-metabolizing enzymes. As yet there is no evidence for between-individual differences in expression of either *ADH, CYP2E1,* or *ALDH2* genes in humans; however, it seems highly likely that sequence variations in the promoters of these genes will be found that alter the basal rates of transcription. In fact, a polymorphism in the first intron of the mouse *Adh1* gene was associated with variation in the mRNA levels and enzyme activity (Patterson et al., 1987; Zhang et al., 1987).

The activity and mRNA level of ADH in liver of rats is modified by diet (reduced by food restriction or fasting), endocrine states (decreased in males or androgen-treated females, and in hyperthyroidism; increased in females and hypothyroid animals), and time of day (circadian rhythms) (Crabb et al., 1987). These factors could alter the rate at which alcohol is metabolized, and thus the rate at which acetaldehyde is generated. Some of these factors might modify aversive reactions to alcohol by modifying alcohol elimination rate.

Conclusion

Many of the results discussed in this chapter have been obtained since the advent of PCR-based genotyping. More information will certainly be derived from studies of additional patient groups; studies of African-Americans will be particularly interesting because of the kinetic properties of *ADH2*3*. Aside from gaining knowledge about factors that alter risk of alcoholism, we can also hope to understand the between-individual differences in organ-specific complications, especially alcoholic liver disease.

Other mutations in the *ADH* and *ALDH2* genes may yet be discovered. It is particularly interesting to consider mutations that could alter expression of the genes; to date, virtually nothing is known about variation in gene expression in humans. Sensitivity to acetaldehyde is still poorly understood. We do not know the mediators of the flushing; therefore, we have no idea if additional variation at this level may exist between individuals. It seems likely that acetaldehyde has both aversive and rewarding properties, depending upon the particular setting.

Finally, there are undoubtedly additional mechanisms by which alcohol causes aversive reactions. Indeed, most drugs of abuse exhibit both rewarding effects, e.g., as seen in paradigms in which experimental animals work for the drug, as well as aversive effects, e.g., conditioned taste aversion. Recent studies on the P and NP rats have shown that both lines exhibit conditioned taste aversion to alcohol, but that the NP rats are innately more sensitive to this effect of alcohol (Froehlich, et al. 1988). Moreover, the P rats, when allowed to drink chronically, have an attenuated conditioned taste aversion to alcohol (Stewart et al., 1991). This indicates that additional genetic, but at present poorly understood, factors may control the aversive reaction to alcohol and protect against heavy drinking. The brain mechanisms underlying ethanol- or acetaldehyde-induced aversions are unknown. It has been reported that $5HT_{1A}$ agonists are proaversive, while $5\text{-}HT_{1B/1C}$ agonists appear to be antiaversive when tested in a periaqueductal gray stimulation paradigm (Jenck et al., 1989a). Conversely, nonspecific serotonin antagonists appeared to be proaversive, while $5\text{-}HT_2$-receptor antagonists decreased the aversive response to periaqueductal gray stimulation (Jenck et al., 1989b). These findings are interesting in light of the known differences in brain serotonin levels between the alcohol-preferring and nonpreferring lines (McBride et al., 1990) and point to future areas of exploration.

Acknowledgments: During the preparation of this review, we were supported by grants from the National Institute on Alcohol Abuse and Alcoholism (NIAAA) (AA 06434, DWC; AA02342 and AA07611, TKL; and AA 06040, HJE) and the Alcoholic Beverages Medical Research Foundation (DWC). We appreciate discussions with Katrina Dipple, Rebecca Mellencamp, and Mona Qulali.

References

Anonymous (1989). Nomenclature of mammalian aldehyde dehydrogenases. In *Progress in Clinical and Biological Research,* Vol. 290, H. Weiner and T. G. Flynn, eds. New York: Alan. R. Liss, pp. xix–xxi.

Asmussen, E., Hald, J., and Larsen, V. (1948). The pharmacological action of acetaldehyde on the human organism. *Acta. Pharm.* **4:**311–320.

Bosron, W. F., and Li, T. -K. (1987). Catalytic properties of human liver alcohol dehydrogenase isoenzymes. *Enzyme* **37:**19–28.

Bosron, W. F., Li, T. -K., Dafeldecker, W., and Vallee, B. L. (1979). Human liver pi-alcohol dehydrogenase: Kinetic and molecular properties. *Biochemistry* **18:**1101–1105.

Bosron, W. F., Li, T. -K., and Vallee, B. L. (1980). New molecular forms of human liver alcohol dehydrogenase: Isolation and characterization of ADH Indianapolis. *Proc. Natl. Acad. Sci. (USA)* **77:**5784–5788.

Burnell, J. C., and Bosron, W. F. (1989). Genetic polymorphism of human liver alcohol dehydrogenase and kinetic properties of the isoenzymes. In *Human Metabolism of Alcohol,* Vol. II, K. E. Crow and R. D. Batt, eds. Boca Raton, FL: CRC Press, pp. 65–75.

Carr, L. G., Mellencamp, R. J., Crabb, D. W., Weiner, H., Lumeng, L., and Li, T. -K. (1991). Polymorphism of the rat liver mitochondrial aldehyde dehydrogenase cDNA. *Alcohol.: Clin. Exp. Res.* **15:**753–756.

Cloninger, C. R., Bohman, M., and Sigvardsson, S. (1981). Inheritance of alcohol abuse. *Arch. Gen. Psychiatr.* **38:**861–868.

Cotton, N. S. (1979). The familial incidence of alcoholism: A review. *J. Stud. Alcohol* **40:**89–116.

Crabb, D. W., Bosron, W. F., and Li, T. -K. (1987). Ethanol metabolism. *Pharm. Ther.* **34:**59–73.

Crabb, D. W., Edenberg, H. J., Bosron, W. F., and Li, T. -K. (1989). Genotypes for aldehyde dehydrogenase deficiency and alcohol sensitivity. The inactive *ALDH2²* allele is dominant. *J. Clin. Invest.* **83**:314–316.

Day, C. P., Bashir, R., James, O. F. W., Bassendine, M. F., Crabb, D. W., Thomasson, H. R., Li, T. -K., and Edenberg, H. J. (1991). Investigation of the role of polymorphisms at the alcohol and aldehyde dehydrogenase loci in genetic predisposition to alcohol-related end-organ damage. *Hepatology* **14**:798–801.

Day, C. P., James, O. F. W., Bassendine, M. F., Crabb, D. W., and Li, T. -K. (1993). Alcohol dehydrogenase polymorphisms and predisposition to alcoholic cirrhosis. *Hepatology* **18**:230–231.

Dipple, K. M., and Crabb, D. W. (1993). The mitochondrial aldehyde dehydrogenase gene resides in an HTF island but is expressed in a tissue-specific manner. *Biochem. Biophys. Res. Commun.* **193**:420–427.

Ehrig, T., Bosron, W. F., and Li, T. -K. (1990). Alcohol and aldehyde dehydrogenase. *Alcohol Alcohol.* **25**:105–116.

Enomoto, N., Takase, S., Takada, N., and Takada, A. (1991a). Alcoholic liver disease in heterozygotes of mutant and normal aldehyde dehydrogenase-2 genes. *Hepatology* **13**:1071–1075.

Enomoto, N., Takase, S., Yasuhara, M., and Takada, A. (1991b). Acetaldehyde metabolism in different aldehyde dehydrogenase 2 genotypes. *Alcohol.: Clin. Exp. Res.* **15**:141–144.

Ferencz-Biro, K., and Pietruszko, R. (1984). Human aldehyde dehydrogenase: Catalytic activity in Oriental liver. *Biochem. Biophys. Res. Commun.* **118**:97–102.

Forte-McRobbie, C. M., and Peitruszko, R. (1986). Purification and characterization of human liver high Km aldehyde dehydrogenase and its identification as glutamic γ semialdehyde dehydrogenase. *J. Biol. Chem.* **261**:2154–2163.

Froehlich, J. C., Harts, J., Lumeng, L., and Li, T. -K. (1988). Differences in response to the aversive properties of ethanol in rats selectively bred for oral ethanol preference. *Pharmacol. Biochem. Behav.* **31**:215–222.

Goedde, H. W., and Agarwal, D. P. (1987). Polymorphism of aldehyde dehydrogenase and alcohol sensitivity. *Enzyme* **37**:29–44.

Goedde, H. W., Agarwal, D. P., and Harada, S. (1983a). The role of alcohol dehydrogenase and aldehyde dehydrogenase isozymes in alcohol metabolism, alcohol sensitivity, and alcoholism. *Isozymes Curr. Top. Biol. Med. Res.* **8**:175–193.

Goedde, H. W., Agarwal, D. P., Harada, S., Meier-Tachmann, D., Ruofu, D., Bienzle, U., Kroeger, A., and Hussenin, L. (1983b). Population genetic studies of aldehyde dehydrogenase isozyme deficiency and alcohol sensitivity. *Am. J. Hum. Genet.* **35**:769–772.

Goedde, H. W., Agarwal, D. P., Harada, S., Rothhammer, F., Whittaker, J. O., and Lisker, R. (1986). Aldehyde dehydrogenase polymorphism in North American, South American, and Mexican Indian populations. *Am. J. Hum. Genet.* **38**:395–399.

Goedde, H. W., Singh, S., Agarwal, D. P., Fritze, G., Stapel, K., and Paik, Y. K. (1989). Genotyping of mitochondrial aldehyde dehydrogenase in blood samples using allele-specific oligonucleotides: Comparison with phenotyping in hair roots. *Hum. Genet.* **81**:305–307.

Harada, S., Agarwal, D. P., Goedde, H. W., Tagaki, S., and Ishikawa, B. (1982). Possible protective role against alcoholism for aldehyde dehydrogenase isozyme deficiency in Japan. *Lancet* **ii.**:827.

Harada, S., Agarwal, D. P., Goedde, H. W., and Ishikawa, B. (1983). Aldehyde dehydrogenase isozyme variation and alcoholism in Japan. *Pharmacol. Biochem. Behav.* **18**:151–153.

Hayashi, S. -I., Watanabe, J., and Kawajiri, K. (1991). Genetic polymorphisms in 5'-flanking region change transcriptional regulation of the human cytochrome P450IIE1 gene. *J. Biochem.* **110**:559–565.

Heath, A. C., Meyer, J., Eaves, L. J., and Martin, H. G. (1991a). The inheritance of alcohol consumption patterns in a general population twin sample. I. Multidimensional scaling of quantity/frequency data. *J. Stud. Alcohol* **52**:345–352.

Heath, A. C., Meyer, J., Jardine, R., and Martin, N. G. (1991b). The inheritance of alcohol consumption patterns in a general population twin sample. II. Determinants of consumption frequency and quantity consumed. *J. Stud. Alcohol* **52**:425–433.

Ho, S. B., DeMaster, E. G., Shafer, R. B., Levine, A. S., Morley, J. E., Go, V. L. M., and Allen, J. I. (1988). Opiate antagonist nalmefene inhibits ethanol-induced flushing in Asians: A preliminary study. *Alcohol.: Clin. Exp. Res.* **12**:705–712.

Höög, J. O., von Bahr-Lindstrom, H., Heden, L. O., Holmquist, B., Larsson, K., Hempel, J. D., Vallee, B. L., and Jörnvall, H. (1987). Structure of the class II enzyme of human liver alcohol dehydrogenase: Combined cDNA and protein sequence determination of the pi subunit. *Biochemistry* **26**:1926–1932.

Hsu, L. C., and Chang, W. -C. (1991). Cloning and characterization of a new functional human aldehyde dehydrogenase gene. *J. Biol. Chem.* **266**:12257–12265.

Hsu, L. C., Bendel, R. E., and Yoshida, A. (1987). Direct detection of the usual and atypical alleles on the human aldehyde dehydrogenase—2 (ALDH2) locus. *Am. J. Hum. Genet.* **41**:996–1001.

Ijiri, I. (1974). Studies on the relationship between the concentrations of blood acetaldehyde and urinary catecholamine and the symptoms after drinking alcohol. *Jpn. J. Stud. Alcohol.* **9**:35–59.

Jenck, F., Broekkamp, C. L., and Van Delft, A. M. L. (1989a). Opposite control mediated by central 5-HT1A and non-5-HT1A (5-HT1B or 5-HT1C) receptors on periaqueductal gray aversion. *Eur. J. Pharmacol.* **161**:219–221.

Jenck, F., Broekkamp, C. L. E., and Van Delft, A. M. L. (1989b). Effects of serotonin antagonists on PAG stimulation induced aversion: Different contributions of 5HT1, 5HT2, and 5HT3 receptors. *Psychopharmacology* **97**:489–495.

Johnson, C. T., Bosron, W. F., Harden, C. A., and Li, T. -K. (1987). Purification of human liver aldehyde dehydrogenase by high-performance liquid chromatography and identification of isoenzymes by immunoblotting. *Alcohol.: Clin. Exp. Res.* **11**:60–65.

Koivusalo, M., Baumann, M., and Uotila, L. (1989). Evidence for the identity of glutathione-dependent formaldehyde dehydrogenase and class III alcohol dehydrogenase. *FEBS Lett.* **257**:105–109.

Korsten, M. A., Matsuzaki, S., Feinman, L., and Lieber, C. S. (1975). High blood acetaldehyde levels after ethanol administration: Differences between alcoholic and non-alcoholic subjects. *New Engl. J. Med.* **292**:386–389.

Li, T. K., Lumeng, L., Doolittle, D. P., McBride, W. J., Murphy, J. M., Froehlich, J. C., and Morzorati, S. (1988). Behavioral and neurochemical associations of alcohol-seeking behavior. In *Biomedical and Social Aspects of Alcohol and Alcoholism,* K. Kuriyama, A. Takada, and H. Ishii, eds. Amsterdam: Elsevier, pp. 435–438.

Lieber, C. S. (1987). Microsomal ethanol-oxidizing system. *Enzyme* **37**:45–56.

Lieber, C. S. (1990). Interaction of ethanol with drugs, hepatotoxic agents, carcinogens and vitamins. *Alcohol Alcohol.* **25**:157–176.

Lieber, C. S., and DeCarli, L. M. (1970). Hepatic microsomal ethanol oxidizing system: In vitro characteristics and adaptive properties in vivo. *J. Biol. Chem.* **245**:2505–2512.

Lindahl, R., and Hempel, J. (1990). Aldehyde dehydrogenases: What can be learned from a baker's dozen sequences? In *Enzymology and Molecular Biology of Carbonyl Metabolism,* 3, H. Weiner, B. Wermuth, and D. W. Crabb, eds. New York: Plenum Press, pp. 1–8.

McBride, W. J., Murphy, J. M., Lumeng, L., and Li, T.- K. (1990). Serotonin, dopamine, and GABA involvement in alcohol drinking of selectively bred rats. *Alcohol* **7**:199–205.

Malpas, S. C., Robinson, B. J., and Maling, T. J. B. (1990). Mechanism of ethanol-induced vasodilation. *J. Appl. Physiol.* **68**:731–743.

Miller, N. S., Goodwin, D. W., Jones, F. C., Pardon, M. P., Anand, M. M., Gabrielli, W. F., and Hall, T. B. (1987). Histamine receptor antagonism of intolerance to alcohol in the Orienta population. *J. Nerv. Ment. Dis.* **175**:661–667.

Mizoi, Y., Ijiri, W., Tatsuno, Y., Kijima, T., Fujiwara, S., Adachi, J., and Hishida, S. (1979). Relationship between facial flushing and blood acetaldehyde levels after alcohol intake. *Pharmacol. Biochem. Behav.* **10**:303–311.

Mizoi, Y., Tatsuno, Y., Adachi, J., Kogame, M., Fukunaga, T., Fujiwara, S., Hishida, S., and Ijiri, I. (1983). Alcohol sensitivity related to polymorphism of alcohol-metabolizing enzymes in Japanese. *Pharmacol. Biochem. Behav.* **181**:127–133.

Moreno, A., and Pares, X. (1991). Purification and characterization of a new alcohol dehydrogenase from human stomach. *J. Biol. Chem.* **266**:1128–1133.

Muramatsu, T., Higuchi, S., Shigemori, K., Saito, M., Sasao, M., Harada, S., Shigeta, Y., Yamada, K., Muraoka, H., Takagi, S., Maruyama, J., and Kono, H. (1989). Ethanol patch test—a simple and sensitive method for identifying ALDH phenotype. *Alcohol.: Clin. Exp. Res.* **13**: 229–231.

O'Dowd, B. F., Rothhammer, F., and Israel, Y. (1990). Genotyping of mitochondrial aldehyde dehydrogenase locus of native American Indians. *Alcohol.: Clin. Exp. Res.* **14**:531–533.

Pares, X., Moreno, A., Cederlund, E., Höög, J. -O., and Jörnvall, J. (1990). Class IV mammalian alcohol dehydrogenase. Structural data of the rat stomach enzyme reveal a new class well separated from those already characterized. *FEBS Lett.* **277**:115–118.

Patterson, L. S., Zhang, K., Edenberg, H. J., and Bosron, W. F. (1987). Genetic control of liver alcohol dehydrogenase expression in inbred mice. *Alcohol Alcohol.* **1**:157–159.

Poupon, R. E., Nalpas, B., Coutelle, C., Fleury, B., Couzigou, P., Higueret, D., and the French Group for Research on Alcohol and Liver. (1992). Polymorphism of the alcohol dehydrogenase, alcohol and aldehyde dehydrogenase activities: Implication in alcoholic cirrhosis in white patients. *Hepatology* **15**:1017–1022.

Rex, D. K., Bosron, W. F., Smialek, J. E., and Li, T. -K. (1985). Alcohol and aldehyde dehydrogenase isoenzymes in North American Indians. *Alcohol.: Clin. Exp. Res.* **9**:147–152.

Schwitters, S. Y., Johnson, R. C., Johnson, S. B., and Ahern, F. M. (1982). Familial resemblances in flushing following alcohol use. *Behav. Genet.* **12**:349–352.

Shibuya, A., and Yoshida, A. (1988). Frequency of the atypical aldehyde dehydrogenase-2 gene (ALDH2-2) in Japanese and Caucasians. *Am. J. Hum. Gen.* **43**:741–743.

Shibuya, A., and Yoshida, A. (1989). Genotypes of alcohol metabolizing enzymes in Japanese with alcoholic liver diseases: A strong correlation of the usual Caucasian type aldehyde dehydrogenase gene (ALDH2-1) with the disease. *Am. J. Hum. Genet.* **43**:744–748.

Shibuya, A., Yasunami, M., and Yoshida, A. (1989). Genotypes of alcohol dehydrogenase and aldehyde dehydrogenase loci in Japanese alcohol flushers and nonflushers. *Hum. Genet.* **82**:14–16.

Smith, M. (1986). Genetics of human alcohol and aldehyde dehydrogenases. *Adv. Hum. Genet.* **15**:249–290.

Stamatoyannopoulos, G., Chen, S. -H., and Fukui, M. (1975). Liver alcohol dehydrogenase in Japanese: High population frequency of atypical form and its possible role in alcohol sensitivity. *Am. J. Hum. Genet.* **27**:789–796.

Stewart, R. B., McBride, W. J., Lumeng, L., Li, T. -K., and Murphy, J. M. (1991). Chronic alcohol consumption in the alcohol-preferring P rats attenuates subsequent conditioned taste aversion produced by ethanol injections. *Psychopharmacology* **105**:530–534.

Thomasson, H. R., Li, T. -K., and Crabb, D. W. (1990a). Correlations between alcohol-induced flushing, genotypes for alcohol and aldehyde dehydrogenases, and alcohol elimination rates. *Hepatology* **12**:903 (abstract).

Thomasson, H. R., Yin, S. -J., Crabb, D. W., Edenberg, H. J., and Li, T. -K. (1990b). Associations between alcohol and aldehyde dehydrogenase genotypes and alcoholism in Chinese and Atayal. *Clin. Res.* **38**:862A (abstract).

Thomasson, H. R., Edenberg, H. J., Crabb, D. W., Mai, X. -L., Jerome, R. E., Li, T. -K., Wang, S. -P., Lin, Y. -T., Lu, R. -B., and Yin, S. -J. (1991). Alcohol and aldehyde dehydrogenase genotypes and alcoholism in Chinese men. *Am. J. Hum. Genet.* **48**:677–681.

Truitt, E. B., Rowe, C. S., and Meh, D. (1985). Aspirin alteration of alcohol-induced flushing and intoxication in Oriental and Occidental subjects. *Alcohol.: Clin. Exp. Res.* **9**:196.

Tsutsumi, M., Lasker, J. M., Shimizu, M., Rosman, A. S., and Lieber, C. S. (1989). The intralobular distribution of ethanol-inducible P450IIE1 in rat and human liver. *Hepatology* **10**:437–446.

Tu, G. C., and Weiner, H. (1987). Aldehyde dehydrogenase: a multifunctional enzyme. *Prog. Clin. Biol. Res.* **232**:67–75.

von Wartburg, J. P., Papenberg, J., and Aebi, H. (1964). An atypical alcohol dehydrogenase. *Can. J. Biochem.* **43**:889–898.

Wagner, F. W., Pares, X., Holmquist, B., and Vallee, B. L. (1984). Physical and enzymatic properties of a class III isozyme of human liver alcohol dehydrogenase: chi-ADH. *Biochemistry* **23**:2193–2199.

Williamson, R. et al. (1990). Report of the DNA committee and cataloques of cloned and mapped genes and DNA polymorphisms. *Cytogen. Cell Genet.* **55**:457–778.

Wilson, J. R., McClearn, G. E., and Johnson, R. C. (1978) Ethnic variation in the use and effects of alcohol. *Drug Alcohol Depend.* **3**:147–151.

Wolff, P. H. (1972). Ethnic differences in alcohol sensitivity. *Science* **175**:449–451.

Wolff, P. H. (1973). Vasomotor sensitivity to alcohol in diverse mongoloid populations. *Am. J. Hum. Genet.* **25**:193–199.

Yasunami, M., Chen, C. -S., and Yoshida, A. (1991). A human alcohol dehydrogenase gene (ADH6) encoding an additional class of isozyme. *Proc. Natl. Acad. Sci. (USA)* **88**:7610–7614.

Yin, S. -J., Bosron, W. F., Magnes, L. J., and Li, T. -K. (1984). Human liver alcohol dehydrogenase: Purification and kinetic characterization of the beta 2 beta 2, beta 2 beta 1, alpha beta 2, and beta 2 gamma 1 "Oriental" isoenzymes. *Biochemistry* **23**:5847–5853.

Yin, S. -J., Wang, M. -F., Liao, C. -S., Chen, C. -M., and Wu, C. -W. (1990). Identification of a human stomach alcohol dehydrogenase with distinctive kinetic properties. *Biochem. Int.* **22**:829–835.

Yoshida, A. (1983). A possible structural variant of aldehyde dehydrogenase with diminished enzyme activity. *Am. J. Hum. Genet.* **35**:1115–1116.

Yoshida, A., Huang, I., and Ikawa, M. (1984). Molecular abnormality of an inactive aldehyde dehydrogenase variant commonly found in Orientals. *Proc. Natl. Acad. Sci. (USA)* **81**:258–261.

Yoshida, A., Dave, V., Ward, R. J., and Peters, T. J. (1989). Cytosolic aldehyde dehydrogenase (ALDH1) variants found in alcohol flushers. *Ann. Hum. Genet. Lond.* **53**:1–7.

Zeiner, A. R., Paredes, A., and Christiansen, D. H. (1979). The role of acetaldehyde in mediating reactivity to an acute dose of ethanol among different racial groups. *Alcoholism* **3**:11–18.

Zhang, K., Bosron, W. F., and Edenberg, H. J. (1987). Structure of the mouse Adh-1 gene and identification of a deletion in a long alternating purine-pyrimidine sequence in the first intron of strains expressing low alcohol dehydrogenase activity. *Gene* **57**:27–36.

9

Genetic Influences on the Development of Physical Dependence and Withdrawal in Animals

ANN E. KOSOBUD AND
JOHN C. CRABBE

Alcohol withdrawal can be as benign as the common hangover experienced after a single episode of intoxication, or with continued excessive use it can evolve into the dramatic and life-threatening delirium tremens. Before the development of effective treatment, mortality rates among severe cases were as high as 15%. The exact mechanisms underlying withdrawal, and their relationship to the complex disorder of alcoholism, remain unknown. Is withdrawal merely a side effect of chronic alcohol abuse? Or are the processes that result in withdrawal fundamental to the process of addiction?

Among the many symptoms and consequences of alcohol abuse, the withdrawal syndrome is one of the most puzzling. Although withdrawal symptoms can appear in an intoxicated individual, it is generally agreed that the syndrome intensifies as ethanol (EtOH) levels fall. The syndrome may continue to worsen long after the direct effects of EtOH have become negligible, and the severest form of withdrawal in humans can appear as many as five days after the last drink (Victor and Adams, 1953).

In order to explain this seemingly indirect action of EtOH, the development of physical dependence is commonly invoked. Physical dependence refers to the presumed secondary process or processes, initiated by the presence of EtOH, which become manifest only as blood EtOH levels fall. As has been pointed out by Cicero (1980) and others, the term physical dependence is problematic and requires careful definition. First, there is currently no objective way to measure physical dependence except by measuring withdrawal. Thus the terms are redundant, and withdrawal is preferable, since physical dependence is no more than a theoretical construct at present. Second, the term itself carries an implication that alcohol has become a required biochemical factor. Since the processes underlying the withdrawal syndrome remain unknown, such an assumption is unwarranted.

The potential role for genetic factors in predisposing individuals to alcoholism has been increasingly appreciated in recent years (Goodwin, 1983), and evidence has begun to accumulate that susceptibility to certain subtypes of alcoholism is influenced by genes (Cloninger, 1987; Penick et al., 1987; Schuckit, 1988). The demonstration of genetic influence on susceptibility to alcoholism has altered the way alcoholism is viewed and has initiated a search for concrete, identifiable, inheritable traits associated with increased liability. Identification of these traits could lead to a better understanding of alcoholism and to more effective prevention and treatment programs.

The literature concerning the genetic influence on alcoholism generally supports complex interactions of multiple genes rather than a major action of a single gene. The actions of EtOH are extremely complex, and the interrelationships between different actions remain poorly understood. An individual's response to EtOH can be characterized in terms of behavioral, physiological, pharmacological, or biochemical measures. Further, these measures can be couched in terms of initial sensitivity, tolerance and sensitization (changes in response following repeated exposure), and physical dependence (demonstrated by the presence of the withdrawal syndrome). These measures can develop simultaneously or on independent time courses. Tolerance might develop to some effects, and sensitization to others. Initial sensitivity, tolerance, and physical dependence could represent alterations in unique processes, each regulated by independent sets of genes. Alternatively, these different phenomena could be manifestations of a single effect of EtOH, and by regulated, at least to some degree, by a similar gene set. The truth probably lies somewhere in the middle, with some actions of ethanol sharing common genetic variance, and other actions being genetically independent.

The influence of genetic factors on EtOH withdrawal severity in animals was first demonstrated by Goldstein (1973). She measured withdrawal in three generations of mice from the outbred Swiss Webster line. Parents for the succeeding generations were selected on the basis of having severe or mild withdrawal scores. Offspring of parents that had severe withdrawal scores displayed more severe withdrawal than offspring of mildly withdrawing parents. This finding suggested that genetic models, including inbred strains, recombinant inbred strains, and selectively bred lines, could be usefully employed to study physical dependence and withdrawal. It is the goal of this chapter to review the progress in studies that use the techniques of behavior genetics to reveal the structure beneath the complex and bewildering EtOH withdrawal syndrome. All of the nonhuman research presented in this chapter has involved rats or mice; to our knowledge, no genetic studies of EtOH withdrawal have been conducted in other species. A more detailed discussion of issues surrounding the appropriate application and interpretation of studies employing genetic animal models has been presented elsewhere (Crabbe et al., 1990b).

Withdrawal Severity in Genetic Animal Models
Studies of Alcohol Dependence and Withdrawal in Inbred Mouse Strains

An inbred strain is derived from 20 generations of matings between close relatives (usually brother/sister). The result is a population of animals that is essentially genetically identical (and homozygous at all gene loci). As a result, trait variation within an inbred strain can be attributed largely to environmental (i.e., nongenetic) causes. The mean value of a trait measured in members of an inbred strain therefore eliminates environment as a source of influence and reflects only genetic effects. Thus, differences among inbred strain means (if all strains are measured in a single environment) can be attributed largely to genetic causes, and covariance among traits suggests that the traits share common gene influence. Thus, screening a panel of inbred strains can reveal genetic relations between traits.

Studies with inbred mouse strains have confirmed the presence of genetic influences on severity of EtOH withdrawal. Crabbe et al., (1983c) demonstrated that in a panel of inbred strains, a wide range of variation was found in severity of EtOH withdrawal. Mice of the C57BL strain show consistently mild withdrawal reactions, while DBA/2 mice generally develop severe withdrawal (Goldstein and Kakihana, 1974; Griffiths and Littleton, 1977; Kakihana, 1979; Grieve et al., 1979). Genetic variation in withdrawal severity has also been demonstrated for acute withdrawal (Roberts et al., 1992). By testing several inbred strains simultaneously on a number of measures, genetic correlations between traits can be estimated. Crabbe et al. (1983c) correlated withdrawal scores from 20 inbred strains with 13 measures of responsiveness to EtOH, including acute hypothermia, activity, loss of righting reflex, and ataxia. Genetic variation in sensitivity was found for all traits measured (Crabbe et al. 1982; Crabbe, 1983). No strong correlations were detected between EtOH withdrawal severity and other measures (Crabbe et al., 1983c) although a moderate negative correlation was found between withdrawal severity and hypothermic response, as well as withdrawal severity and degree of tolerance developed to EtOH-induced hypothermia. This finding suggested that genes that contributed to a large initial hypothermic response and rapid development of hypothermic tolerance, would tend to make withdrawal less severe. On the whole, however, EtOH effects showed a surprising degree of genetic independence. In other words, sensitivity assessed using one measure proved, for the most part, a poor predictor of sensitivity using any other measure. The implication is that separate genes mediate different actions EtOH.

In contrast, acute withdrawal has been shown to occur following single injections of hypnotic doses of EtOH and pentobarbital, and can be precipitated by injection of flumazenil following a single dose of diazepam (McQuarrie and Fingl, 1958; Kosobud and Crabbe, 1986; Crabbe et al., 1991b). When 15 inbred strains were characterized for handling-induced convulsion severity following administration of each of these drugs, significant strain differences in withdrawal severity were found for each drug. EtOH and pentobarbital withdrawal severities were positively genetically correlated, indicating the influence of some of the same genes on both responses. A positive genetic correlation was also found between the severity of withdrawal from pentobarbital and diazepam; however, diazepam and EtOH withdrawal severities were not found to be genetically related. These experiments suggest that some genes influence severity of withdrawal from multiple depressant drugs (Metten and Crabbe, 1994).

Recombinant Inbred Mouse Strains

A recent development in pharmacogenetics has been the construction of specific sets of inbred strains derived from a pair of standard inbred strains. When two inbred strains are crossed to form an F_1 population, and the F_1 mice are themselves crossed to form an F_2 generation, the Mendelian phenomena of segregation and independent assortment are brought into play. This F_2 population has the special characteristic that each mouse bears alleles at each gene which must have derived only from one of the two parental strains. A brother–sister pair of F_2 mice is then mated, and their offspring inbred until a new inbred strain is formed. This Recombinant Inbred (RI) strain possesses a unique, randomly generated set of genetic recombinations of the parental genotypes, and a set of such RIs is highly useful for genetic mapping (Bailey, 1971).

Taylor (1978) crossed the C57BL/6J (C57) and DBA/2J (DBA) inbred strains and formed a panel of 24 RI strains, termed BXD-RIs. The C57 and DBA strains differ markedly in terms of their genomic similarity (Taylor, 1972), a distinct advantage for mapping strategies. Furthermore, they are known to differ markedly in response to virtually every effect of EtOH for which they have been tested (Belknap, 1980; Phillips and Crabbe, 1991). While studies of panels of RI strains are informative in much the same way as discussed earlier for standard inbreds, they have two specialized uses that make them a more powerful genetic tool.

Classic Recombinant Inbred Analysis. If a single gene (major gene) exerts a major influence on a trait (for example, if it determines 50% or more of the variance in the trait). RI strain analysis can be useful in locating that gene. We sought evidence for such a gene or genes in the BXD RIs by testing all strains for ethanol withdrawal severity using our standard inhalation paradigm. For the RI analysis to be successful, any such gene must be in different allelic states in the two parental strains, C57 and DBA. Initial evidence for such a substantial difference between parental strains was seen in an earlier study that found that DBAs were among the most severely withdrawing inbred strains, while C57s were among the least (Crabbe et al., 1983c). This is at least consistent with a major gene effect. More compelling evidence for such a gene was found in the BXD–RI results (Crabbe et al., 1983b). Strains tended to fall into one of two modes of withdrawal. That is, strains had extremely high or low, but not intermediate, withdrawal responses. Of the 16 BXD–RI strains tested in addition to C57 and DBA, 8 resembled the DBA parental strain, and 8 resembled the C57 strain. This pattern of results suggested that a single locus exerted an important influence on EtOH withdrawal severity, and that half the RI strains had inherited the C57 allele, while half had inherited the DBA allele.

The power of RI analysis lies in the existence of many strain distribution patterns (SDP) identifying the genetic map location of previously typed genes. In the mouse, there are over 800 such polymorphic markers, covering over 90% of the genome (Deitrich et al., 1992; Woodward et al., 1992). Table 9-1 summarizes such an analysis. We compared the pattern of BXD–RI strains for chronic EtOH withdrawal with the SDPs for all other known gene loci that had been typed in the strains. There were no

Table 9-1 Strain Distribution Patterns for Ethanol Withdrawal and
Car-2

BXD Strain Number	Ethanol Withdrawal Allele[a]	Car-2 Allele[b]	Concordance?
BXD-1	DBA	DBA	Yes
BXD-2	DBA	DBA	Yes
BXD-6	C57	C57	Yes
BXD-11	DBA	DBA	Yes
BXD-12	DBA	DBA	Yes
BXD-14	DBA	DBA	Yes
BXD-15	C57	C57	Yes
BXD-18	C57	DBA	No
BXD-21	C57	C57	Yes
BXD-23	C57	C57	Yes
BXD-24	DBA	C57	No
BXD-25	C57	C57	Yes
BXD-27	DBA	DBA	Yes
BXD-28	C57	C57	Yes
BXD-29	C57	DBA	No
BXD-30	DBA	DBA	Yes

[a]Data from Crabbe et al. (1983b).

[b]Data from Lyon and Searle (1989, table 18.2).

Note: DBA = resembles DBA/2J parental strain; C57 = resembles C57BL/6J parental
strain.

cases where a perfectly concordant fit was found between a mapped gene and the SDP
for EtOH withdrawal. However, a reasonably close fit was found with the *Car-2* locus
located near the centromere on chromosome 3: three of the sixteen RI strains were discordant. We were able to conclude that a major gene apparently influenced EtOH withdrawal severity. Furthermore, it was likely to reside on chromosome 3, near *Car-2*.
Car-2 determines carbonic anhydrase-2. Under acid conditions in red blood cells, electrophoretic variants for a slow form (as in C57 mice), and a fast form (as in DBA mice)
have been reported (Eicher et al., 1976). Since three RI strains were discordant, *Car-2*
could not itself be the major gene, for discordance is evidence that recombinations had
occurred between the EtOH withdrawal locus and *Car-2*. Since it was linked, however,
Car-2 could serve as a marker for EtOH withdrawal severity, since the two genes
would tend to be inherited together.

Quantitative Trait Loci Analyses. The previous example serves to illustrate the potential for RI strain analyses for finding genes of importance to a genetic susceptibility to
alcohol withdrawal. It also serves to illustrate the limitations of RI analyses as originally conceived. First, for many traits, most likely including alcohol withdrawal in
humans, there are probably no single genes that exert a major influence. Rather, many
genes, variously called *polygenes* or *quantitative trait loci* (QTLs), are likely to determine the trait, each gene contributing a relatively small amount to the trait variance.
The classic RI analysis just described is too insensitive to detect linkage for such minor
genes, even if in the aggregate they virtually completely control the trait. This is

because the method depends upon the necessity of detecting a bimodal pattern of RI strain differences. Second, the limited number of RI strains is a problem, since the technique is essentially correlational. The BXD–RI panel, with 24 strains, is the largest available, but 40 or more would be preferable. Third, an RI analysis could reveal a bimodal pattern of strain differences in the RIs that resembles no mapped SDP. In our early research examining several drug-related traits, this was a frequent and frustrating outcome. Although evidence for a single-gene effect was found, one was left with no idea where it was, which hampered further efforts at characterization.

Most of these problems have been addressed by the application of a recently developed agricultural genetic method to RI strain analysis. Thoday (1961) first developed a method for examining associations between mapped loci, such as the SDPs described earlier, and quantitatively varying traits. Lander and Botstein (1989) recently developed a statistical methodology for incorporating information about genetic map distance between markers in the analysis of QTLs. Plomin et al. (1991) realized that these techniques could be applied to the BXD–RI series to analyze behavioral and psychopharmacological traits where QTLs were presumptively controlling behavior. They used the existing datasets for the BXD–RI mice and compared the continuously varying data for behavioral and pharmacological responses with existing SDPs. The technique they developed has the capability of resolving linkages between previously mapped genes and QTLs controlling as little as 20% of the trait variance.

This represents a major advance in mapping technology, as well as a significant extension of the value of RI analyses. For example, in collaboration with Plomin and his colleagues, we reanalyzed the chronic EtOH withdrawal data collected in 1982 (Crabbe et al., 1983b). Using the QTL mapping technique, we again saw evidence for a linkage with *Car-2* (Gora-Masiak et al., 1991). The QTL linked to *Car-2* controlled approximately 29% of the variance in chronic alcohol withdrawal severity, a substantial proportion. This probably explains why the classic RI analysis previously discussed detected this linkage. In addition, in the QTL analysis, we found evidence for significant linkage with six other marker genes, among which were *Ly-9* on chromosome 12, *D12N6u2* on chromosome 12, and two closely linked loci on chromosome 13. Thus, the more powerful QTL approach was able to confirm the earlier locus on chromosome 3, and provided evidence for other genes of importance (Gora-Maslak et al., 1991).

Several other features of QTL analysis can also be applied to future genetic studies of withdrawal-related characters. For example, multiple regression analyses of the withdrawal data revealed that the aggregate set of markers could account for 62% of the variance in withdrawal severity. Furthermore, it was possible to estimate that the addition of genes above and beyond that marker contributing most to the multiple R added 27% to the variance controlled (Gora-Masiak et al., 1991).

An additional possibility for QTL analysis is the identification of gene loci that have pleiotropic effects: that is, affect multiple characters. The BXD–RI lines were also characterized for low-dose ethanol-induced locomotor activation, a trait that has been conceptually linked to drug dependence. Several QTLs contributing to this trait were also identified. Interestingly, one of the pairs of chromosome 13 markers associated (*r*

= .63) with withdrawal severity was also significantly associated (r = .42) with low-dose activation. This suggests how the cumulative power of QTL analysis in the BXD RIs could ultimately be used to link behavioral, neurochemical, and molecular genetic data controlling individual or multiple traits (Gora-Maslak et al., 1991). A number of methodological improvements to the QTL approach have been discussed elsewhere (Belknap et al., 1992), and in Chapter 13 this volume (McClearn and Plomin).

In a recent study, we first identified six candidate QTL possibly influencing the severity of acute ethanol withdrawal in BXD RI mice (Belknap et al., 1992). For one of these candidate sites, in the *Pmv-7* region on chromosome 2, we sought confirmation using F_2 mice derived from C57BL/6 and DBA/2 parental crosses (Crabbe et al., 1994b). If an influential gene were on chromosome 2, genetic markers from this region should predict withdrawal severity in individual mice. Furthermore, such an association should allow us to map the QTL more precisely and to identify potential candidate genes. The need for verification of the RI results follows from the differences between linkage analyses in inbred and genetically segregating populations. Individual F_2 mice were tested for EtOH withdrawal and then genotyped at 4 loci on chromosome 2 (*D2Mit9, D2Mit7, D2Mit61,* and *D2Mit12*). These markers are simple sequence length polymorphisms (SSLPs) associated with or flanking the candidate QTL, and polymorphic between the B6 and D2 inbred strains. Mice were genotyped using PCR amplification of each SSLP. We assessed the statistical significance of the association with *D2Mit9* by grouping the F_2 mice according to genotype and analyzing phenotypic (withdrawal) scores. Each F_2 animal was assigned a genotypic score of 0, 1, or 2 for each marker based on gene dosage, i.e., the number of DBA/2J alleles at that marker. Withdrawal severity was then regressed on gene dosage for each marker (Falconer, 1983).

Withdrawal severity was significantly associated with gene dosage only for *D2Mit9,* reflecting the location of a gene influencing alcohol withdrawal closer to *D2Mit9* than the other three markers. Forty of the 145 F_2 mice tested were DBA/2J homozygotes at *D2Mit9,* and they had withdrawal reactions significantly more intense and of longer duration than the 32 C57BL/6J homozygotes (Crabbe et al., 1994b). This finding confirmed our BXD findings and strongly suggested that there is a QTL in the *Pmv-7/D2Mit9* region of chromosome 2 accounting for about 40% of the total genotypic variance in acute withdrawal intensity.

After these first two steps, we also verified the association by examining allelic status of mouse lines selectively bred for severe (WSP) and mild (WSR) ethanol withdrawal. Results with the selected mouse lines were also consistent with different gene frequencies for a locus closely linked to *D2Mit9* (Buck et al., unpublished data).

Strikingly, markers in this region were also identified by QTL analyses in BXD RIs tested for ethanol withdrawal severity after chronic inhalation of ethanol vapor (*Brp-13*), nitrous oxide withdrawal seizures (*Neb, Pmv-7, Scn2a*), and hyperbaric pressure-induced convulsions (*Brp-13*) (McCall and Frierson, 1981; Crabbe et al., 1983). A gene in this region of chromosome 2 might well influence acute and chronic alcohol withdrawal, withdrawal from the gaseous anesthetic nitrous oxide, and the severity of convulsions resulting from hyperbaric pressure.

These data represent the first report where a gene not previously known to influence drug withdrawal has been detected by initial screening for QTL in the BXD RI strain panel and independently verified in a segregating genetic population. The data demonstrate that there is sufficient sensitivity to detect associations in an F_2 population, even though there is a much stronger influence of environmental factors in a segregating genetic population than in the original analysis with RI strains.

This region is syntenic with a large region of human genome and suggests the existence of a human equivalent to this QTL near 2q24-q37. Candidate genes near *D2Mit9* include *Gad-1,* coding for glutamic acid decarboxylase, the rate-limiting enzyme catalyzing synthesis of the inhibitory neurotransmitter γ-aminobutyric acid (GABA). It is noteworthy that diazepam, which enhances GABA action, is preferred clinically to prevent or ameliorate ethanol withdrawal seizures in alcoholics. Other candidate genes to consider include a cluster of genes (*Scnla, Scn2a,* and *Scn3a*) for the α (major) subunit of brain voltage-dependent sodium channels, responsible for the rapid rising phase of the action potential in a variety of excitable cells, including neurons.

These results emphasize the utility of QTL analysis as a powerful hypothesis-generating approach to identify genes influencing drug sensitivity, both in animal models and humans. Furthermore, identification of candidate genes may indicate their more general role in central nervous system excitability and seizure susceptibility.

Breeding for Alcohol Withdrawal Severity

Selective breeding can be used as a direct test of the role of genes in the expression of a given trait and its relation to other traits of interest. Typically, selection is bidirectional—one line is selected for maximal expression of a given trait, while the other is selected for minimal expression of that trait. After many generations, the genes that influence expression of the selected train will become fixed in a homozygous state, while unrelated genes continue to show normal variation. If differences emerge between such a pair of lines when measured on other traits, these differences can be attributed to the same set of genes responsible for the selected trait. Traits other than the selected trait in which differences arise are known as correlated responses to selection. Studies of selected lines offer an alternative method to using inbred strains means to detect shared genetic variance. In addition, selected lines provide a powerful tool for testing predicted genetic correlations, in part because both positive and negative findings can provide important information. If a pair of lines that have been selected for maximal divergence on a given trait do not diverge when measured on some second trait, it constitutes strong evidence that the two traits are *not* gentically correlated. Positive evidence of genetic correlations could result from random fixing of genes during selection, but can be detected if the selected lines are replicated. In addition, unselected control lines should be maintained, to provide a continued representation of the effect of the breeding strategy on the foundation population (Falconer, 1983).

Since the initial demonstration of feasibility provided by Goldstein (1973), three independent breeding projects have directly addressed the question of genetic influence on EtOH withdrawal severity. The Severe and Mild Ethanol Withdrawal (SEW and MEW: McClearn et al., 1982) and the High and Low Addictability (HA and LA: Berta and Wilson, 1989) mouse lines were developed at the Institute for Behavioral Genetics at the University of Colorado. The Withdrawal Seizure-Prone and -Resistant lines (WSP and WSR) were developed at the Department of Veteran's Affairs Medical Center in Portland, Oregon (Crabbe et al., 1983a, 1985). For their foundation populations, all three projects utilized mice from a genetically heterogeneous stock of known composition (HS/ibg), and proceeded generally by within-family, bidirectional selection with replicate and control lines. The projects differed in methods of chronic intoxication and assessment withdrawal severity. In the following section, we describe each of these selection projects in some detail, concentrating on the elements that differ. To begin, we describe the methods commonly used for chronic intoxication and measurement of withdrawal, and discuss the factors influencing choice of one or another. As in other sections of this chapter, most of the research discussed used rats or mice, and other factors may be important when other species are used.

Methods of Chronic Administration of Alcohol

A variety of methods have been used to induce dependence in animal models. The most common are (1) a liquid diet containing EtOH as the sole source of calories (Freund, 1969), (2) chronic inhalation of EtOH vapor (Goldstein, 1972), and (3) multiple daily dosing by injection or intubation (Majchrowicz, 1975).

Each of these methods has both advantages and disadvantages. The liquid diet is frequently advocated because the route of administration is similar to that employed by human alcoholics. However, it allows no control over individual patterns of consumption. An animal that drinks large amounts of an EtOH solution in a short period of time will achieve higher blood EtOH concentrations (BEC), and remain intoxicated longer, than an animal that drinks very small amounts spaced throughout the day. Thus, two animals that consume similar total daily amounts may in fact experience very different exposure. Furthermore, under voluntary consumption paradigms, a different pattern of consumption is observed between experimental animals (receiving ad libitum diet with EtOH) and paired controls (each of which received diet limited to match calories consumed by an experimental animal). Control animals inevitably drink all their diet at once, while experimental animals consume their diet much more slowly. This difficulty can be partially overcome by the use of an ingenious pair-feeding apparatus (Israel et al., 1984) in which a control animal's access to and amount of diet is yoked to an experimental animal's voluntary consumption. In general, both experimental and paired control animals lose weight, or gain less weight than free-feeding animals, suggesting that there is something aversive about the EtOH-adulterated diet. One possibility is that animals regulate their intake of EtOH to avoid some pharmacological action of EtOH. A second possibility is that animals dislike the taste of the EtOH. In either case, it appears that these animals are at least slightly food deprived, and this deprivation may be contributing to their consumption of a disliked food. Furthermore, they may be seeking to avoid the very effects of EtOH that alcoholics drink to obtain. These methodological concerns weaken any claim that this approach constitutes purely voluntary consumption, and it remains unknown whether the drinking of these subjects is controlled by factors similar to those controlling drinking in the alcoholic.

Intragastric or intraperitoneal administration allows control over administered dose and increases consistency of exposure between animals, but it is probably more acutely stressful to the subject and is clearly burdensome to the investigator. This method is particularly impractical for selection studies in which large numbers of animals must be simultaneously intoxicated. Chronic inhalation procedures allow large numbers of animals to be intoxicated while maintaining control of dose and timing of exposure. In addition, with concurrent administration of an ADH inhibitor such as pyrazole, rapid induction of dependence is obtained. Without ADH inhibition, longer exposure times may be required and much more variation in BEC is seen. Drawbacks of this procedure include the potential adverse effects of EtOH vapor on the lungs of the animals, and the possible toxic effects of pyrazole. Use of the inhalation method has been discussed in detail elsewhere (Goldstein, 1980; Terdal and Crabbe, 1994).

Measurement of Withdrawal

Signs of Withdrawal. The signs observed during withdrawal in animals are similar to those seen in humans, including tremor and other motoric dysfunctions, and autonomic overactivity indicated by sweating, salivation, piloerection, mydriasis, and photophobia (Barry, 1979; Friedman, 1980). Convulsions are seen in all species during severe withdrawal, while milder withdrawal can be demonstrated by lowered threshold to induced convulsions (McQuame and Fengl, 1958; Szabo et al., 1984). It is not known to what degree the different signs of withdrawal represent different manifestations of a single underlying abnormality, or whether the withdrawal syndrome includes a number of simultaneously occurring abnormalities. The latter seems more likely, given the diversity of action EtOH has on the central nervous system (CNS). A wide variety of measures have been used in assessing withdrawal in experimental animals. (For reviews, see Barry, 1979; Friedman, 1980.) These measures can be roughly grouped as follows.

1. *Activity measures.* Both hyperactivity (Cicero et al., 1971; Majchrowicz, 1975; Crawshaw et al., 1994) and hypoactivity (Hunter et al., 1975; Pohorecky, 1976) have been observed. Some specialized test chambers have been devised to induce certain types of activity. Mice showed reduced exploratory activity, and were slower to enter dark compartments in 4-compartment hole-in-wall apparatus (Hutchins et al., 1981; Crabbe et al., 1993). Mice tested on a vertical screen were less active (Hutchins et al., 1981), but showed increased climbing behavior in a mesh tube (Becker et al., 1987). It is likely that measure used, degree of dependence, and withdrawal test time all influence activity levels (Friedman, 1980).

2. *Disturbances in vegetative functions.* These indices include sleep disorders (Mendelson, 1978), irritability, and hyper- and hyporeactivity (Friedman, 1980). While the syndrome is usually described as autonomic overactivity, a recent study reported *decreased* respiration and startle amplitudes, as well as disrupted regulation of body temperature and heart rate (Gilliam and Collins, 1986). Usually hypothermia is

reported as a withdrawal sign but hyperthermia is also seen (Friedman, 1980). A recent study in mice withdrawing from 72-hr exposure to EtOH vapor found that the temperature at which the body was regulated was altered very little; however, much cooler temperatures were selected by withdrawing mice, suggesting a significantly greater capacity for heat dissipation (Crawshaw et al., 1994). A few studies have attempted to assess dose–response relationships in withdrawal hypothermia. Ritzmann and Tabakoff (1976) found that hypothermia increased with increasing duration of EtOH treatment. Consistent with this finding, withdrawing rats preferred a warmer environment than controls, and this preference increased with increasing treatment duration (Brick and Pohorecky, 1977).

3. *Stereotypic behaviors.* Stereotypies such as tail stiffening, tail rattling, and backward walking (Freund, 1969; Majchrowicz, 1975) are observed.

4. *Motor abnormalities.* Withdrawal-induced signs include tremor and broad-based gait (Freund, 1969), as well as wet shakes and teeth chattering (Majchrowicz, 1975).

5. *Seizureform signs.* Many signs are seen, including unprovoked bouts of squealing, sudden sprawling movements of the limbs (Freund, 1969), and reduced thresholds to convulsions induced by auditory (Noble et al., 1976), electrical (Geisler, 1978), chemical (McQuarrie and Fingl, 1958; Szabo *et al.,* 1984), or mechanical (Goldstein and Pal, 1971) stimulation. Spontaneous convulsions are seen during severe withdrawal, and appear to be of several types, including generalized tonic-clonic and wild-running convulsions (Freund, 1969). EEG abnormalities are seen, including synchronous activity and transient spikes (Hunter et al., 1973; Walker and Zornetzer, 1974) and enhanced evoked potentials (Begleiter and Porjesz, 1977).

Temporal Characteristics. Although alcoholism is by definition a chronic disorder, signs of physical dependence can be observed in mice following a single episode of intoxication. This phenomenon, which may be the equivalent of hangover in humans, is most readily demonstrated by increased susceptibility to induced convulsions, using chemical (McQuarrie and Fingl, 1958; Sanders, 1980), electrical (Mucha and Pinel, 1979), and handling (Goldstein, 1972; Vosobud and Crabbe, 1986) stimuli. With increasing dose and/or length of administration, the withdrawal syndrome becomes increasingly severe and prolonged (Goldstein, 1972).

In humans, the withdrawal syndrome appears to include at least three phases. Victor and Adams (1953) observed 101 patients undergoing withdrawal at Boston City Hospital. They identified three separate states that appeared in varying combinations and varying levels of severity. The earliest, present in 50 of the 101 cases, was characterized by tremulousness and transient hallucinations, and usually appeared within the first 24 hours of abstinence. Convulsions constituted the second state, occurring usually within the first 48 hours, and present in 60 of 101 cases. The third state, delirium tremens, consisted of motor and autonomic overactivity, confusion, and disordered sense perception. This state was observed in 44 of 101 cases, and usually appeared between 3 and 4 days after the last drink.

Most animal studies have focused on the early stage of EtOH withdrawal, usually limiting observations to the first 24 hours. However, in recent studies (Gonzalez et al., 1989; Gonzalez, 1993) susceptibility to spontaneous seizures and those induced by picrotoxin, audiogenic stimuli, were strychnine measured through 84 hours of withdrawal. Sensitivity to picrotoxin was assessed at different withdrawal times in independent groups of animals by measuring latencies to four different convulsant signs; myoclonus, partial seizures, tonic/clonic seizures, and tonic extension. Rats were made dependent by 21 days of exposure to EtOH vapor in inhalation chambers (without ADH inhibition). Control animals received similar treatment, but were not exposed to EtOH. These investigators were able to identify several apparently distinct phases of withdrawal. Audiogenic convulsions were most severe at about 10 hours, but very rare or absent after 16 hours. For spontaneous convulsions, the time of maximal appearance depended on the convulsion, with myoclonic jerks most frequent in the first 24 hours, jumping episodes and tonic/clonic seizures most frequent between 24 and 54 hours, and most tonic extensions occurring no earlier than 42 hours, and continuing to appear through hour 84 (Gonzalez et al., 1989). A recent study has suggested that different mechanisms may underlie sensitivity to different convulsion signs induced by picrotoxin as well as other drugs (Kosobud and Crabbe, 1990). Consistent with this finding, different measures of sensitivity to picrotoxin showed somewhat independent withdrawal time courses. Thus, reduced latency to picrotoxin-induced myoclonus and partial seizures was observed at 10 and 20 hours after withdrawal, while latency to tonic extension was reduced at 20 and 40 hours. Picrotoxin-induced tonic/clonic seizure latencies were reduced at 10, 20, and 40 hours, but significantly increased at 72 hours postwithdrawal (Gonzalez et al., 1989). In addition, sensitivity to strychnine seizures was unaltered during EtOH withdrawal (Gonzalez, 1993). Thus, in animals as well as humans, there is good evidence for distinct phases of the withdrawal syndrome, reflecting different underlying mechanisms.

Choice of Withdrawal Measures for Selective Breeding. To be a useful index for a selective breeding study, a measure must be quantifiable, reliable, and valid, accurately reflecting the withdrawal severity of each individual mouse. Thus, signs that appear unpredictably or infrequently are poor indices. Furthermore, signs that have a complex (i.e., nonlinear) dose dependence are problematical. The dose dependence of many of the measures described before has not been adequately studied. Measures that distinguish very clearly between a withdrawing mouse and a control mouse are not necessarily good discriminators for individual mice at different levels of withdrawal (Friedman, 1980). For example, while certain tests show that most withdrawing mice are hypoactive relative to controls, it is not clear that *within* a group of withdrawing mice, differences in activity reflect differences in withdrawal severity. Furthermore, the withdrawal syndrome waxes and wanes over a prolonged period of time. It is possible that two mice scored for handling-induced convulsions (HIC) at 6 hours postwithdrawal will have the same score, but in one animal this could represent the highest value this animal will attain, while the other animal may be in the earliest stages of withdrawal.

Many of the measures listed appear so infrequently that they are, in practice, useless for accurate comparisons of individual mice. Indeed, with measures such as backward walking and straub tail, we have obtained highly variable appearances of these signs, despite careful observation of all animals at several different times during withdrawal.

Tremor, which is one of the more reliable withdrawal measures seen in observations of mice, was observed in our previous study in only about 40% of the mice on the average, and even at its peak in only 80% of withdrawing mice (Kosobud and Crabbe, 1986). Furthermore, at best it can be visually scored on a three-point scale (absent, mild, severe), leaving little room for ranking of individual mice. To our knowledge, HICs are the best single measure that can be used to test large numbers of mice repeatedly throughout the time course of withdrawal, and that can be reliably scored at many levels of dependence, so that an accurate estimate of withdrawal severity can be made for each individual mouse at each time it is tested. Hypothermia may also be a good measure, but the dose–response relationship needs to be studied further, as well as the physiological bases for altered core temperature. An alternative approach is to use multiple measures to assess withdrawal. In principle, this strategy could allow for the peak emergence of different signs at different times during withdrawal, and result in selection for a more general withdrawal syndrome than any single measure. This is technically known as *index selection,* and is extensively used in agricultural genetics (Falconer, 1983). An example of this approach is discussed in the next section.

Results of Selection

The Severe and Mild Ethanol Withdrawal Mouse Lines. In the selection of the SEW and MEW lines, chronic intoxication was achieved with a liquid diet. Consumption was measured twice daily, at 0700 (7 A.M.) (lights on) and 1900 (7 P.M.) (lights out). The concentration of EtOH in the liquid diet was 10% EtOH-derived calories (EDC) on days 1 and 2, 20% EDC on days 3 and 4, and 35% EDC on days 5–9. An estimate of daily consumption in grams of ethanol per kilogram of body weight per day was derived from the two daily measures of consumption. Blood EtOH concentrations were not routinely measured. Withdrawal occurred on treatment day 10. Thus, in this study, the route of administration was the same as in alcoholic humans. However, no control over the amount any individual animal drank could be imposed, nor could the pattern of drinking, and the resulting peaks and valleys in BEC, be assessed.

Withdrawal testing occurred between 6 and 7 hours after the EtOH containing diet was removed. The withdrawal measure used in the selection of the SEW and MEW lines was a composite index (McCleam et al., 1982), using measures derived from an earlier study (Hutchins et al., 1981). EtOH withdrawn and untreated control animals were observed for a variety of withdrawal signs, and from these, several were identified that differentiated the groups. These signs included HICs assessed on a three-point scale, body temperature, measures of crossing, rearing and seizures in a hole-in-wall (HW) apparatus, crossings on a vertical screen (VS), and EtOH consumption (9-day total) (Hutchins et al., 1981). These measures were then applied to the EtOH-withdrawn foundation population (McClearn et al., 1982), and first-principal-component loadings were derived from principal-component analysis of the withdrawal scores. Because several measures showed a significant gender difference, the component loadings derived for females differed from those derived for males. This index provided a measure of severity based on multiple indicators of withdrawal severity. While it is clear that this index reliably distinguishes between withdrawing mice and EtOH-naive mice, it is not clear that it provides an accurate ranking within a group of withdrawing mice. One way to assess the accuracy within withdrawing mice would be to perform dose–response studies. Currently, the only measure in this index for which dose–response characteristics are known is HIC. Whether variation on the index as a whole accurately reflects dose-related differences in withdrawal severity remains untested.

After five generations (Allen et al., 1983), divergence was seen on the selection index in one replicate (SEW2/MEW2) but not in the other (SEW1/MEW1). Most of the response to selection was seen in the SEW lines rather than the MEW lines, which were similar to the unselected control lines. The possibility that the index may have changed during selection was evaluated, and the component structure was found not to have changed significantly in the first five generations (Allen et al., 1983). After 10 selected generations (Wilson et al., 1984), both replicates had diverged to greater than are standard deviation apart. Selection continued to be asymmetrical, with much greater response in the SEW lines. When individual components were examined, SEW mice were rated as significantly more severely withdrawing than MEW mice in seizure severity, body temperature, and HW rearings, and drank more EtOH during induction. Both HW crossings and VS crossings were significantly different in the second replicate, but not in the first. No difference was detected between SEW and MEW mice in HW seizures, but these did not occur very frequently.

In addition to the withdrawal measures, naive mice from the tenth selected generation were tested for loss of righting reflex, hypothermia, and blood alcohol concentration after an acute anesthetic dose of EtOH. Some evidence for more rapid elimination of ethanol in SEW mice relative to MEW mice was found. Also, MEW mice tended to regain righting reflex at slightly higher BAC than SEW mice, suggesting that they may be less sensitive to alcohol.

One unexpected outcome was that all six lines (SEW, MEW, and control mice of both replicates) dramatically increased their consumption of EtOH diet over generations. This 35–50% increase in EtOH consumption has been interpreted as the result of natural selection favoring mice that can tolerate larger doses of EtOH and thus maintain a better nutritional state through the intoxication procedure (Wilson et al., 1984). This increase has greatly exceeded the effect of artificial selection, which has resulted in the SEW mice drinking about 15% more EtOH than the MEW mice.

The multivariate analysis of withdrawal severity (McClearn et al., 1982) was based on correlations among individual mice of heterogenous stock, and thus represented phenotypic rather than genotypic correlations. As a result, the index may not have been ideal for a genetic selection; for any of the components, the phenotypic and genotypic correlations might have differed significantly in magnitude, or have been of different sign. For example, the phenotypic correlation between EtOH consumption and withdrawal severity is positive—the more EtOH consumed, the more severe the withdrawal. Some evidence suggests, however, that the genotypic correlation between EtOH consumption and withdrawal severity is negative. WSR mice, selected for mild withdrawal, tend to drink more EtOH than WSP mice, selected for severe withdrawal (Kosobud et al., 1988). Recently, the withdrawal index used in the selection of the SEW and MEW lines was evaluated using a multivariate diallele analysis, to allow assessment of genotypic correlations between measures of EtOH withdrawal (Corley and Allen, 1988). This study confirmed the negative genetic correlation between severity of EtOH withdrawal and amount of EtOH consumed. As a result, EtOH consumption was eliminated from the composite index, and an increase in response to selection in both the SEW and the MEW lines was observed (Corley and Allen, 1988). For the six remaining measures, the multivariate diallele analysis generally supported the weights used for male mice. For female mice, however, the composite index does not appear to take advantage of the additive genetic variance available in the remaining six measures. Consistent with this finding, response to selection was greater in male mice than in female mice of the SEW and MEW lines (Wilson et al., 1984). These lines are no longer undergoing selection, but are being maintained by inbreeding (Berta and Wilson, 1992).

The High and Low Addictability Mouse Lines. High addictability (HA) and low addictability (LA) mouse lines were selected by using a combination of techniques. A liquid diet protocol similar to that employed for the SEW/MEW selection was administered for 11 days. The concentration of EtOH in the liquid diet was 10% EDC on days 1 and 2, 20% EDC on days 3 and 4, 30% EDC on days 5 and 6, and 32% EDC on days 7–11. The liquid diet currently used is DYET #710266 (Dyets, Inc.). On day 12, the diet was withdrawn and handling-induced convulsions were scored using the Goldstein-Pal index at hours 0, 2, 4, 6, and 8 of withdrawal. Seizure scores were summed to index withdrawal severity (Berta and Wilson, 1989). Beginning with the second generation, mice of the two HA lines have shown significantly more severe withdrawal than the two LA lines (Berta and Wilson, 1990).

Results from the first seven generations of selection have recently been reported (Berta and Wilson, 1992). In both replications, response to selection gradually increased for the first 2 to 3 generations, while the magnitude of the (statistically significant) difference between HA and LA lines remained relatively stable through the seventh selected generation. Control lines are intermediate. After seven generations, mean HA seizure scores are approximately 5–8 of a maximum possible total of 20, and mean LA scores are approximately 2, with a minimum possible total of zero.

In early generations, HA lines consumed more ethanol than LA lines. These differences have declined in the last two generations, and were no longer significant in generation seven. The authors suggest that consumption differences may explain part of the early divergence between the lines in withdrawal seizure scores. The recent decline in consumption differences, paralleled by the stability of the difference in seizure scores between the lines in later generations, may represent, in effect, an increased divergence in susceptibility to withdrawal. The forced-consumption differences were not paralleled by differences in free-choice consumption. When naive mice from the third generation were tested for EtOH-preference drinking and sensitivity to EtOH-induced loss of righting reflex, lines did not differ (Berta and Wilson, 1990).

Use of a different liquid diet and alterations in the feeding protocol evidently have avoided some of the unexpected nonspecific increases in consumption in EtOH seen in the SEW/MEW study. Simplification of the withdrawal index to a single sign may also have contributed to the more rapid response to selection in the HA/LA lines.

The Withdrawal Seizure-Prone and -Resistant Mouse Lines. In the selection of the WSP and WSR lines, chronic intoxication was achieved using 72 hours of constant exposure to ethanol vapor. The EtOH vapor concentration was increased each day. On the first day, animals received an intraparitoneal injection of pyrazole (1 mM/kg) and 1.5 g/kg ethanol (20% v/v in saline). On the second and third days, the animals received injections of pyrazole only. On the fourth day, blood EtOH concentrations were obtained for all animals upon removal from the inhalation chambers and commencement of withdrawal. In initial stages of the selection, the WSP and WSR lines were placed together in a single inhalation chamber. In later generations (beginning with generation five) it was necessary to increase the EtOH vapor concentration for WSR mice, and decrease it for WSP mice, so the lines were intoxicated in separate chambers. We have seen no evidence of damage to the lungs of these animals from inhaling EtOH vapor. It does appear however, that mice of both the WSP and WSR lines tolerate the inhalation procedure better than many other strains of mice (unpublished observation).

The withdrawal measure used in the selection of the WSP and WSR mice was HIC. These were measured at time of removal from the inhalation chambers, hourly between hours 2 and 15, and again at 23 and 25 hours after withdrawal. Seizure severity scores ranged from 0 (no seizure) to 7 (spontaneous tonic/clonic seizure). In general, all but the most severely withdrawing animals returned to baseline scores by 25 hours postwithdrawal.

Throughout the selection of the WSP and WSR lines, we have monitored the divergence of these lines in both the primary selected trait, HIC, and in potential correlated responses. Thus, we have accumulated longitudinal data on a variety of measures. Periodically, these lines were subjected to a battery of tests, with three principal questions in mind. First, we were interested in the response of the lines to selection: Have the WSP and WSR lines reached a maximum level of divergence in HIC score? Second, we measured EtOH elimination: Are WSP and WSR lines still achieving similar blood EtOH concentrations during chronic EtOH administration? Third, we assessed the generality of selection: What other withdrawal signs distinguish the lines?

1. *Response to selection.* HIC scores were directly compared in withdrawing WSP and WSR mice of generations 0–5, and periodically thereafter through the twenty-fourth selected generation. For each of these comparisons, WSP and WSR mice were exposed to EtOH vapor for 72 hours in the same inhalation chamber, with daily pyrazole injections. In Fig. 9-1, 15-hour withdrawal scores are shown for female mice of the first and second replication of the WSP and WSR lines. The first point represents the unselected foundation stock from which all four lines were derived. Response to selection was very rapid, already apparent in the first generation of selection, and by the tenth generation, most of the response to selection appears to have occurred.

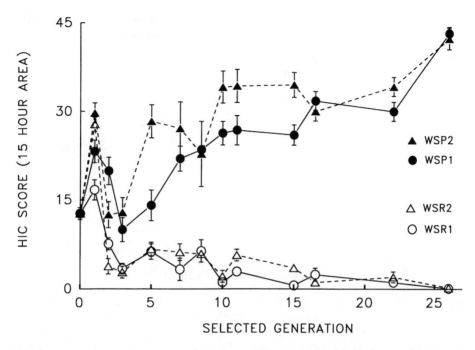

Fig. 9-1 Response to selection in female WSP and WSR mice from both replicates, for selected generations between 0 and 26. Pictured are HIC scores, calculated as area under the withdrawal curve for hours 0–15 of withdrawal. Data are shown as mean and SE (SE smaller than symbol size for some points). Following generation 21, relaxed selection (no withdrawal testing and random selection of parents within each line) occurred between some selected generations. Two generations of relaxed selection occurred prior to the test of selected generation 22. Eight additional generations of relaxed selection occurred prior to the test of selected generation 26.

Between the twenty-second and twenty-ninth generation, we relaxed selection for three of the seven generations. That is, parents were chosen randomly within each line and family. Since the twenty-ninth generation, we have continued relaxed selection, and are currently mating the forty-ninth generation. Current animals therefore represent the twenty-sixth selected generation. If significant genetic heterozygosity remained in the selected lines for genes important for expression of EtOH withdrawal, relaxed selection should long ago have led to regression of the selection response toward some intermediate mean value. Since this has not happened in the WSP and WSR lines, it suggests that the genes influencing withdrawal severity have become fixed in the homozygous state. In addition to maintaining the lines under relaxed selection, we are currently inbreeding each of the four selected lines. Three of the four have reached the nineteenth inbred generation, and may be considered to be inbred strains (Falcomer, 1983). These lines should be useful for molecular biological study requiring a homogeneous genetic background (e.g., representation difference analysis, cloning, development of subtractive libraries).

   2. *Elimination of alcohol.* In our previous study (Kosobud and Crabbe, 1986), EtOH

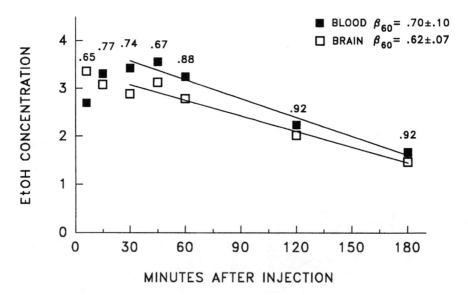

MINUTES AFTER INJECTION

Fig. 9-2 Comparison of blood and brain EtOH concentrations 6, 15, 30, 60, 120, and 180 minutes after an acute injection of ethanol (3g/kg, 20% v/v). Mean and SE (SE smaller than symbol size) for blood (filled squares) and brain (open squares) EtOH concentrations from groups of 20 female mice (5 each from the 21st and 22nd selected generation of the WSP1, WSR1, WSP2, and WSR2 selected lines) are plotted. Each mouse provided one brain and one blood sample at a single time. Relative to brain EtOH concentrations, blood EtOH concentrations were lower at 6 minutes, but higher at all other times. (Paired differences $T \geq$ 2.6, $p \leq 0.2$.) Correlation coefficients (plotted with each data pair for each time point) were calculated based on blood and brain concentrations obtained simultaneously in an individual mouse. The correlation between blood and brain concentrations increased over time, suggesting that blood concentrations provide better estimates of brain concentration at later times. Using data points after 15 minutes, regressions were calculated to estimate the elimination rate (β_{60}), expressed in milligrams/milliliter/hour. β_{60} were similar for blood and brain.

elimination was measured in WSP and WSR mice, following acute and chronic administration. In the fourth selected generation, no difference between the WSP and WSR lines was found in rate of EtOH elimination following an acute injection of EtOH (3g/kg, 20% v/v). Blood EtOH concentrations during and immediately following chronic administration were compared in mice from the seventh selected generation of the WSP and WSR lines. No difference was detected between WSR and WSP lines during chronic intoxication, either in BEC achieved or in rate of elimination. A difference was found between male and female mice, with males reaching higher BEC and displaying more severe withdrawal (Kosobud and Crabbe, 1986). Thus, in the early stages of the selection process, a clear difference in withdrawal severity emerged between the lines in the absence of any measurable difference in BEC during chronic administration.

In the data reported here, BEC were measured in female WSP1, WSR1, WSP2, and WSR2 mice from the twenty-first and twenty-second selected generation, following acute and chronic administration. Following an acute injection of EtOH (3g/kg, 20%

v/v), concentrations of EtOH were measured in whole brain and blood samples at 6, 15, 30, 45, 60, 120, and 180 minutes. Groups of five mice from each line and replicate were used for each time point, and each mouse provided one blood and brain sample. Figure 9-2 shows mean and SE for blood and brain EtOH concentrations, collapsed over line and replicate. Although blood concentrations were lower than brain concentrations at 6 minutes, and higher at all other times, the large positive correlations between blood and brain concentrations, and the similar elimination rate (β_{60}), suggest that blood EtOH concentration provides a good estimate of brain EtOH concentration, especially at longer intervals postinjection. (For analysis see the figure caption.) Figure 9-3 shows mean and SE for blood and brain EtOH concentrations for each replicate of the WSP and WSR lines. For brain EtOH concentration, a three-way ANOVA (time × line × replication) revealed no significant differences between WSP and WSR mice of either replicate at any time. For blood EtOH concentration, a significant three-way interaction compelled independent analysis of the replicates. Two-way ANOVA's (line × time) revealed that WSR1 mice had significantly higher BEC than WSP1 mice ($F(1, 56) = 4.96$, $p < .03$), but WSR2 and WSP2 mice did not differ. Thus, we have weak evidence of differences in acute EtOH elimination in WSP and WSR mice, albeit in a surprising direction.

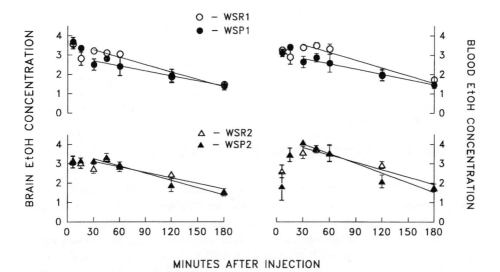

MINUTES AFTER INJECTION

Fig. 9-3 Ethanol concentrations measured in whole brain (left panel) and tail blood (right panel) following an acute injection of ethanol (3g/kg, 20% v/v). Groups of 5 female mice of the 21st and 22nd selected generation of the WSP1, WSR1, WSP2, and WSR2 selected lines were sampled at 6, 15, 30, 45, 60, 120, and 180 minutes postinjection. Each mouse provided one brain and blood sample at one time point. Data were initially analyzed using 3-way ANOVAs (time × line × replicate). For brain EtOH concentrations, no significant differences were found between lines or replicates. A significant main effect of time was found ($F(6, 110) = 33.9$, $p < .0001$). For blood EtOH concentrations, a significant interaction (time × line × replicate) was observed. Two-way ANOVAs (line × time) revealed that WSR1 mice had significantly higher BEC than WSP1 mice ($F(1, 56) = 4.96$, $p < .03$), but WSR2 and WSP2 mice did not differ. Regressions were plotted using data points after 15 minutes.

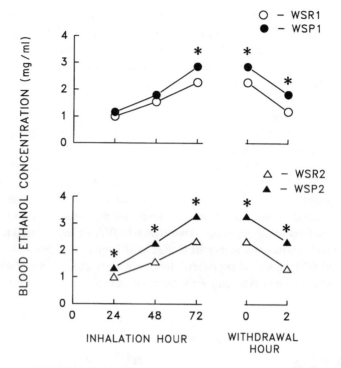

Fig. 9-4 Mean and SE for BEC for female mice of the 22nd generation of the WSP and WSR mouse lines (SE smaller than symbol size). BEC were measured at 24, 48, and 72 hours of chronic inhalation of ethanol vapor, and following 2 hours of withdrawal. Data presented for inhalation hour 72 is the same as that presented for withdrawal hour 0. Differences between WSP and WSR mouse lines were assessed by t-tests at each time point, independently for each replicate. BEC of WSP1 mice were significantly higher than BEC of WSR1 mice at withdrawal hours 0 and 2, while BEC of WSP2 mice were higher than BEC of WSR2 mice at all time points (all $t \geq 3.0$, $p < .006$).

In contrast to the earlier findings, WSP mice reached higher BEC than WSR mice during chronic administration (Fig. 9-4). Thus, the selection initially acted principally on genes influencing the primary trait, HIC, during EtOH withdrawal. However, by selected generation 22, additional genes had been selected resulting in relatively higher accumulation of EtOH in WSP mice than in WSR mice during chronic intoxication. Recently, we have investigated these phenomena more thoroughly in mice from selected generation 26 (filial generations 36–45) (Terdal and Crabbe, 1994). When different doses of pyrazole were given and WSP and WSR lines were exposed in the same vapor inhalation chamber, a dose of .75 mM/kg given to WSP mice yielded blood EtOH levels equivalent to those seen after 1.0 mM/kg pyrazole doses in WSR mice. In additional experiments, we gave a 1.5-g/kg loading injection of EtOH to both WSP and WSR mice, and exposed them to the same high EtOH vapor concentration (14 mg/l air) for 24 hours. Blood samples were taken after 2, 6, and 24 hours. No pyrazole was used. WSP mice showed slightly higher blood EtOH levels than WSR mice at 2 hours, and they remained at stable levels during the 24-hour exposure. In contrast, levels in WSR mice declined linearly over the exposure period, and were near zero 24 hours later. Since this difference in EtOH metabolism is not present during acute injections, it is possible that it arises through differences in inducible EtOH metabolizing enzymes.

Finally, we administered EtOH at different loading doses and exposed WSR mice to higher EtOH vapor concentrations than WSP mice. Under these conditions, with no pyrazole present, WSP mice showed significant withdrawal HIC after 48 or 72 hours, while WSR mice did not. Blood EtOH concentrations could be nearly matched between the genotypes, although this matching required selection of mice within each genotype based on blood EtOH level (Terdal and Crabbe, 1994).

3. *Generality of selection.* As an ongoing counterpart to the selection, we have assessed withdrawal in the WSP and WSR mouse lines using measures other than the selected trait, HIC. If multiple measures of withdrawal distinguish the lines, then the WSP and WSR mice could be said to model the general withdrawal syndrome as expressed in laboratory mice. Furthermore, it would imply that common genes influence HIC and other measures of withdrawal, and that the syndrome as a whole reflects a unitary disruption of function. However, if these lines do not differ in withdrawal severity on some measures, then the model is limited to a portion of the withdrawal syndrome, and furthermore, EtOH withdrawal itself must be seen as a syndrome involving several genetically independent processes.

The generality of the withdrawal syndrome in the WSP and WSR lines was first addressed in the eighth and ninth selected generation (Kosobud and Crabbe, 1986). Assessment of withdrawal included: (1) handling-induced convulsions; (2) observations on an open platform for tremor, straub tail, and backward walking; (3) activity on a vertical screen and in a four-compartment maze (hole-in-wall) similar to that used in the selection of the SEW and MEW lines. In the selection measure, HIC, withdrawing WSP mice showed severity scores roughly 5-fold greater than withdrawing WSR mice. Withdrawing WSP mice displayed more tremor, equal straub tail, and less backward walking than withdrawing WSR mice. No EtOH-naive animals showed these behaviors. Using the hole-in-wall and vertical screen tests, withdrawing mice were shown to be markedly less active than EtOH-naive mice on all measures, but no significant differences between withdrawing WSP and WSR mice were detected. However, WSP mice tended to score lower than WSR mice on measures of crossing and rearing in the hole-in-wall test, consistent with more severe withdrawal. Overall, WSP mice appeared to undergo more severe withdrawal than WSR mice for most measures, but the differences were small, especially relative to the large difference in HIC scores.

In addition, the basal expression of HIC has increased to an average of about a score of 2 in a naive WSP mice, and has decreased to virtually zero in WSR mice (Kosobud and Crabbe, 1986). Moreover, the form this convulsion takes in the two lines has changed, so that in WSR mice it is a very transient and subtle seizure, while in WSP mice the convulsion is very pronounced (unpublished observations). This makes strict comparisons of the lines on HIC-related traits difficult. Pyrazole treatment also appears to have a slightly greater effect on HIC in WSP mice (increasing scores by 0.5–1.0 on a 7-point scale), but this is also difficult to assess precisely because of the differences in the form of the seizure.

In more recent experiments using mice of the twenty-second selected generation, assessment of withdrawal included the following measures, scored at multiple times after removal from the EtOH vapor chamber: (1) HIC; (2) body temperature; (3) observations on an open platform for tremor, straub tail, and backward walking. HICs were measured at hours 0, 3, 7, 11, and 15 after removal from the EtOH vapor chambers (Fig. 9-5). For analysis of HIC, areas under the withdrawal curve were calculated. A two-way ANOVA yielded a significant main effect of line (WSP > WSR) and of replicate (replicate 2 > replicate 1), with no significant interaction. Body temperature was measured at 3, 7, 11, and 15 hours after withdrawal (Fig. 9-6). Overall, WSP mice were significantly more hypothemic than WSR mice, and this difference was larger in the second replicate. At hours 4, 8, and 12 after withdrawal, each mouse was placed on

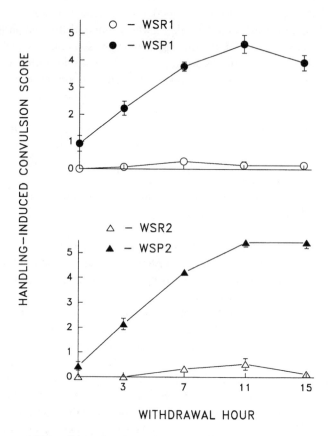

Fig. 9-5 Mean and SE handling-induced convulsion scores for female mice of the 22nd selected generation of both replicates of the WSP and WSR mouse lines (SE smaller than symbol size). HICs were scored on a scale of 0–7, with a score of 7 indicating maximum severity of withdrawal. For analysis, area under the withdrawal curve (AUC) was calculated for each subject. A 2-way ANOVA revealed significant effects of line (WSP > WSR; $F(1, 52) = 664$, $p < .0001$) and replicate ($2 > 1$; $F(1, 52) = 4.3$, $p < .04$). The mean AUC for WSP mice was 32.1, and for WSR mice was 1.6. Thus, WSP mice show HIC scores approximately 20-fold higher than WSR mice.

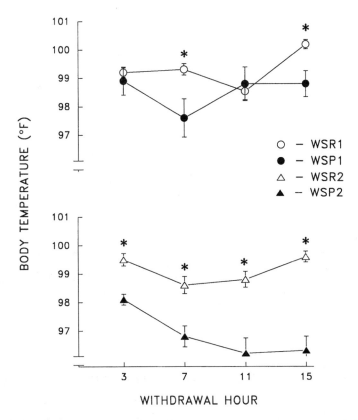

Fig. 9-6 Mean and SE for body temperature (°F) in female mice of the 22nd selected generation of the WSP and WSR selected mouse lines, measured at hours 3, 7, 11, and 15 hours of withdrawal. Differences between WSP and WSR mouse lines were assessed by t-tests at each time point, independently for each replicate. WSP1 mice were more hypothermic than WSR1 mice at 7 and 15 hours, while WSP2 mice were more hypothermic than WSR2 mice at all time points (all $t \le 2.5$, $p < .03$).

an open platform and observed for one minute for the presence of withdrawal signs including tremor, straub tail, and backward walking (Fig. 9-7). Fisher exact tests were used to assess significance at each time period. Backward walking did not occur frequently, and did not differ significantly in WSP and WSR mice. WSP2 mice displayed significantly more tremor than WSR2 mice at hour 8 and 12, but WSP1 and WSR1 mice did not differ. Straub tail occurred more frequently in WSP mice than WSR mice at all time points except hour 4, replicate 2. These observations are somewhat different from the results of the comparison of the eighth and ninth selected generation, in which WSP mice showed more severe tremor, equal straub tail, and reduced backward walking relative to WSR mice. These inconsistencies may arise due to variations in dependence level of the animals in the two different studies. Nonetheless, WSP mice are clearly more dependent than WSR mice on measures of withdrawal in addition to HIC (such as straub tail and hypothermia), although the difference between the lines in HIC scores remains the largest difference.

FREQUENCY OF APPEARANCE OF WITHDRAWAL SIGNS

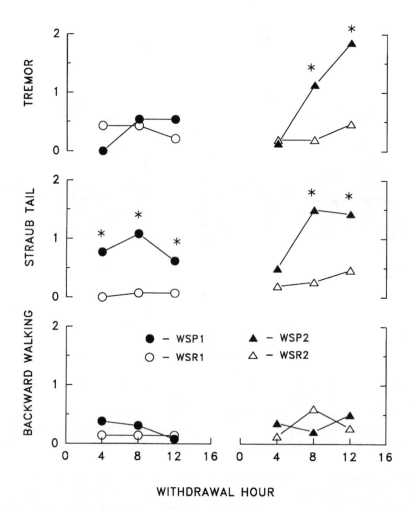

WITHDRAWAL HOUR

Fig. 9-7 Frequency of appearance of withdrawal signs in mice of the 22nd generation placed for 1 minute on a raised stainless steel platform. Differences were analyzed using a Fisher exact test. Straub tail was scored on a three-point scale in which 0 indicated no straub tail, 1 indicated a stiff tail held between 0° and 45° to the floor, and 2 indicated a stiffening and arching of the tail of greater than 45°. WSP mice showed significantly more straub tail than WSR mice (both replicates). Tremor was scored on a 3-point scale in which a score of 0 indicated no tremor, 1 indicated mild tremor involving part of the body only (usually head and neck), and 2 indicated whole body tremor. WSP2 mice displayed significantly more tremor than WSR2 mice ($p < .05$).

The withdrawal differences between WSP and WSR mice generalize in at least two other senses. First, WSP mice are more sensitive than WSR mice to acute EtOH-induced withdrawal indexed by HIC. When mice of the twelfth selected generation were given a single intraparitoneal dose of EtOH (4 g/kg), there was a significant suppression of HIC for 2–4 hours, followed by a rebound exacerbation of HIC peaking at 8–10 hours after injection (Kosobud and Crabbe, 1986). This phenomenon was characterized as representing an acute withdrawal response, and was not evident in WSR mice.

Second, EtOH and a number of drugs that exert hypnotic or sedative effects on the central nervous system are known to be cross-dependent. That is, a drug of this class will suppress symptoms associated with withdrawal from other such drugs. This phenomenon is the basis for the efficacy of benzodiazepines in suppressing EtOH withdrawal. WSP mice from the fifth selected generation had more severe precipitated withdrawal than WSR mice after chronic diazepam intoxication. These differences were greater in mice from the thirteenth generation (Belknap et al., 1989). Similarly, WSP mice have more severe withdrawal from chronic barbiturates (Belknap et al., 1988) and nitrous oxide (Belknap et al., 1987). Furthermore, we have recently shown that acute withdrawal is more severe in WSP than WSR mice after single injection of pentobarbital, diazepam, acetaldehyde, or tertiary butanol (Crabbe et al., 1991b). WSP mice also show acute withdrawal from the benzodiazepine-like compound, abecarnil (Cratte, 1993).

4. *Other findings.* WSP and WSR mice have generally been found to be similar in sensitivity to acute effects of EtOH, including EtOH stimulation in an open field test (Crabbe et al., 1988b), as well as hypothermic response, and brain concentration of EtOH at time of loss and regain of loss of righting reflex (Crabbe and Kosobud, 1986). Tolerance to the hypothermic response developed equally in the two lines as well. Because these results were found in both replicates of the selected line, they constitute strong evidence that the mechanisms underlying these measures of sensitivity, tolerance, and dependence are to a significant degree independent (Crabbe et al., 1990b). This is for the most part in agreement with inbred strain studies (Crabbe et al., 1982; Crabbe, 1983; Crabbe et al., 1983c), although the negative genetic correlation between acute hypothermic response and withdrawal severity, seen in inbred strains (discussed in the section titled "Methods of Chronic Administration of Alcohol"), was not detected in the WSP/WSR lines.

WSP and WSR mice have been useful in studies designed to ascertain the physiological basis for EtOH withdrawal. Several studies have implicated the GABA system in chronic EtOH responses. Although WSP and WSR mice do not differ in binding characteristics of GABA-benzodiazepine complex receptors in discrete brain areas (Feller et al., 1988), WSP mice are more sensitive than WSR mice to the effect of GABA antagonists to elevate HIC (Feller et al., 1988; Crabbe et al., 1991a). WSP mice are also equally or more sensitive to seizures induced by timed intravenous infusion of convulsant drugs acting through the GABA complex, such as bicuculline, DMCM, TBPS, picrotoxin, and PTZ (Kosobud and Crabbe, 1991; unpublished data). Recently, chronic EtOH was administered to WSP and WSR mice in a liquid diet. Expression of whole brain levels of mRNA specific for the α_1, α_3, α_6, gamma$_{2L}$, gamma$_{2s}$, and gamma$_3$ GABA receptor subunits was found to differ between the lines. Chronic EtOH reduced the content of α_1 mRNA in WSP but not WSR mice, and decreased the content of α_6 mRNA in WSR but not WSP mice. The content of gamma$_3$ mRNA was increased in both lines. Untreated WSP mice had lower content than untreated WSR mice of α_3 and α_6 mRNA. Thus, a decrease in brain message for a specific GABA receptor subunit, α_1, may be linked with the genetic predisposition to severe EtOH withdrawal (Buck et al., 1991).

The differences between WSP and WSR mice in susceptibility to convulsants are not limited to drugs acting through the GABA complex. WSP mice are more sensitive than WSR mice to the elevation of HIC induced by NMDA (N-methyl-D-aspartic acid), kainic acid, strychnine, nicotine, and BAY K 8644 (Crabbe et al., 1991b). WSP mice are more susceptible than WSR mice to seizures elicited by timed intravenous infusions of CHEB and 4-aminopyridine (Crabbe and Kosobud, 1990), and appear to be equally or more susceptible to seizures elicited by strychnine and kainic acid (unpublished data). Thus, in general, WSP mice appear to be more sensitive than WSR mice to any treatment that exacerbates HIC and to most treatments that induce other forms of convulsion. A notable exception, however, is that WSR mice are more susceptible than WSP mice to seizures elicited by timed intravenous infusion of NMDA (Kosobud and Crabbe, 1993).

Convulsants can also enhance HIC scores when given during the acute withdrawal from a single injection of EtOH. Studies comparing sensitivity during acute withdrawal with that of naive mice have found that WSP mice are more sensitive than WSR mice to the effects of excitatory amino acid receptor agonists and antagonists (e.g., NMDA, dizocilpire) during acute EtOH withdrawal (Crabbe et al., 1990a, 1993). This may be related to the finding that chronic EtOH treatment led to a much greater increase in the number of dihydropyridine-sensitive calcium channel binding sites in whole brain homogenate tissue from WSP mice than from WSR mice (Brennan et al., 1990). An additional finding of interest is that WSP mice have a 70% lower zinc content in dorsal hippocampal mossy fibers relative to WSR mice (Feller et al., 1990).

Comparison of WSP/WSR and SEW/MEW Lines

A direct comparison of withdrawal severity in all twelve lines [SEW, MEW, and Control (C) lines of both replicates (provided by James Wilson) and WSP, WSR, and WSC lines of both replicates] has been carried out. Groups of 7–11 mice from the SEW/MEW/C and WSP/WSR/WSC lines were treated with pyrazole (1 mM) and EtOH (1.5 g/kg) and placed together in an inhalation chamber for 72 hours of exposure to EtOH vapor. Additional injections of pyrazole were given at 24 and 48 hours. Blood EtOH concentrations were measured at 24, 48, and 72 hours. Withdrawal testing included measurement of HIC at 0, 3, 7, 11, 15, and 25 hours; body temperature at 3, 7, 11, 15, and 25 hours, climbing behavior in wire mesh cylinders at 4, 8, 12, and 25 hours, observations for activity levels, tremor, and straub tail in an open field at 8, 12, and 25 hours, and hole-in-wall activity tested once between 6 and 9 hours. Two weeks later, the same mice were tested in a modified protocol of withdrawal testing following 3 days of pyrazole injections with no exposure to EtOH, to provide an estimate of baseline scores.

Blood EtOH concentrations (BEC) differed significantly among the lines at time of

withdrawal (hour 0). The major difference was between the SEW/MEW/C lines, which
were at approximately three times higher BEC than the WSP/WSR/WSC lines. Thus, a
large difference in dose occurred despite the identical treatment of the lines.

For HIC, the expected order of withdrawal severity was found in the
WSP/WSR/WSC mice, WSP > WSC > WSR with both WSR lines showing near-zero
scores. SEW1 mice showed more severe HIC than MEW1 mice, but lines in the second replicate did not differ significantly: MEW2 mice had slightly higher HIC scores
than SEW2 mice. In body temperature, withdrawing mice were hypothermic at hour 3
(all mice) and hour 7 (SEW/MEW/C only). Differences between lines were not
observed. Climbing behavior, activity measures, straub tail, and tremor were not significantly altered in withdrawing mice, or were not altered in an interpretable manner.
Withdrawing mice showed consistently reduced activity in the hole-in-wall test,
but the differences among withdrawing groups were not significant in the
WSP/WSR/WSC mice, and significant but not interpretable among the SEW, MEW,
and C lines. The low BEC in WSP and WSR mice, and lack of significant withdrawal
straub tail, tremor, and hypothermia in WSP mice suggests that these mice were experiencing only a mild withdrawal syndrome.

The results of this comparison were somewhat disappointing for a comparison
between selection experiments. The large difference in BEC makes a direct comparison difficult, but could possibly be overcome by modifying the pyrazole treatment. It
would be interesting to compare the lines in a protocol similar to that used in the selection of the SEW and MEW lines, but because selective breeding has increased EtOH
consumption in the SEW/MEW lines, it is likely that the WSP/WSR lines will consume much less of the EtOH-adulterated liquid diet.

Comparison of HA/LA and WSP/WSR Lines

James Wilson kindly provided us with naive HA and LA mice from the seventh
selected generation. We tested these mice for ethanol withdrawal severity using the
same protocol as that used for the WSP/WSR selection. Ten to twelve male and female
mice from each of the four HA/LA lines, and 4–5 male and female mice from each
WSP/WSR line were tested in the same inhalation chamber. Selection control lines
were not tested. After an EtOH loading dose of 1.5 g/kg, mice were exposed for 3 days
to increasing EtOH vapor concentrations, with daily 1-mM/kg pyrazole doses. Mice
were removed from the chambers after 72 hours of vapor exposure, and a blood sample
was taken. Withdrawal HICs were tested hourly for 15 hours, and at hours 24 and 25.
The area under the HIC curve was taken as the index of withdrawal severity. For statistical analysis, the eight selected lines were compared in a single between-subjects factor ANOVA. Since sex differences in metabolism of EtOH were anticipated, the sexes
were considered in two separate ANOVAs. Post hoc comparisons were performed with
the Neuman-Keuls procedure at an α level of .05 (Winer, 1971).

The area under the 25-hr withdrawal curve is shown separately for females and
males in Figs. 9-8 and 9-9. Selected lines differed significantly in withdrawal severity
($Fs \geq 28$, $Ps < .0001$). For both sexes, both WSP lines had the highest withdrawal

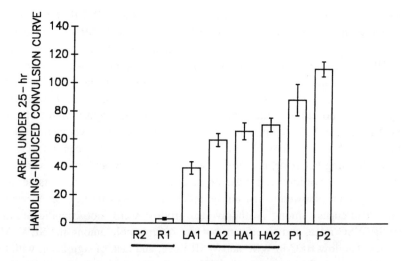

Fig. 9-8 Mean ± SE area under the HIC curve for female mice of 8 selected lines exposed to ethanol vapor in the same inhalation chamber for 3 days. R1, R2 = withdrawal seizure resistance; P1, P2 = withdrawal seizure prone; LA1, LA2 = low addictability; HA1, HA2 = high addictability. Genotypes connected by a solid line did not differ significantly.

severity and were significantly different from all other groups. Similarly, both WSR lines had significantly lower withdrawal scores than all other groups. For females, the LA1 line had significantly lower withdrawal than the other three HA/LA lines (which did not differ from each other), and significantly higher withdrawal than the two WSR lines. For females, the LA1 line had significantly *higher* withdrawal than the other

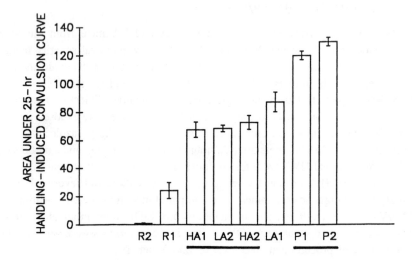

Fig. 9-9 Mean ± SE area under the HIC curve for male mice of 8 selected lines exposed to ethanol vapor in the same inhalation chamber for 3 days. R1, R2 = withdrawal seizure resistant; P1, P2 = withdrawal seizure prone; LA1, LA2 = low addictability; HA1, HA2 = high addictability. Genotypes connected by a solid line did not differ significantly.

three HA and LA lines (which did not differ from each other). All four HA/LA lines fell intermediate to the WSP and WSR lines, differing significantly from both WSP and both WSR pairs.

These results suggest that, in general, selection of mouse lines for withdrawal severity using two different methods of dependence induction did not lead to parallel results, even though the index of withdrawal severity was very similar in both studies. Although WSP mice have been found to develop greater withdrawal scores than WSR mice when administered a liquid diet containing EtOH (Harris et al., 1984), HA/LA lines did not differ markedly in withdrawal severity when tested with the pyrazole-assisted vapor inhalation method. This is a puzzling result. Analysis of blood EtOH concentrations at time of removal from the chambers, which provide an estimate of the total alcohol dose, did not appear to account for the pattern of selected line differences. There were no significant differences among the female genotypes ($F = 1.6$). Males, however, differed significantly among genotypes ($F = 6.9$, $P < .05$). WSR1 mice had significantly lower blood alcohol levels than all other genotypes except WSR2, and WSR2 mice had lower levels than all other genotypes, which did not differ from each other. However, WSR2 mice had unmeasurable withdrawal scores, while WSR1 mice had significant, albeit minimal, withdrawal scores. The correlations between withdrawal severity and BEC were $r = .25$ ($P = .05$) for all females and $r = .54$ ($P < .001$) for all males. Covariance analyses for each sex still resulted in significant genetic differences ($Fs \geq 28$, $Ps < .0001$). Thus, differences in metabolism of ethanol might have contributed to the generally lower scores of WSR male mice, but could not explain the higher scores of WSP male mice. Furthermore, differences in metabolism do not apparently account for the withdrawal severity differences among female genotypes, or for the contradictory response of the LA1 line.

A potential explanation is the drug history of the animals. WSP/WSR mice were naive at the time of testing, and HA/LA mice had been given two previous tests not reported here. Sixteen days before the start of inhalation testing, all mice received a single 4-g/kg EtOH injection and were scored for acute EtOH withdrawal. Eleven days before inhalation testing, the mice were similarly treated with 60 mg/kg pentobarbital. While it seems unlikely to us that these acute tests could have influenced chronic EtOH withdrawal two weeks later, it is not impossible.

Alcohol Dependence and Withdrawal in Lines Selected for Other Traits

Lines of rodents have been selectively bred for a variety of responses (reviewed in Phillips and Crabbe, 1991), and EtOH withdrawal has been measured in a number of these lines. The alcohol-preferring (P) and nonpreferring (NP) rats (Lumeng et al., 1977) differ in voluntary consumption of an EtOH-water solution. The P rats will eventually consume EtOH in quantities sufficient to result in a withdrawal syndrome (Waller et al., 1982). When EtOH was offered to hungry rats in a solution made palatable by the addition of saccharin and sodium chloride, the P line increased consumption from 7 to 14 g/kg/day, while the NP line increased EtOH consumption from 1 to 12 g/kg/day. When EtOH solutions were removed following 8 weeks of access, both lines displayed withdrawal symptoms (Waller et al., 1982). Unfortunately, it was not possible to evaluate relative severity of withdrawal in this study. The long-sleep (LS) and short-sleep (SS) mice (McClearn and Kakihana, 1981) were selected for differences in EtOH-induced loss of righting reflex. The SS mice displayed a more severe withdrawal syndrome than LS mice as assessed by HIC (Goldstein and Kakihana, 1975) and other measures (Gilliam and Collins, 1986). Recall, however, that WSP and WSR mice do not differ in sensitivity to loss of righting reflex (Crabbe and Kosobud, 1986). Duplicate HOT and COLD lines of mice were selected, respectively, for low or high initial sensitivity to hypothermia following acute administration of ethanol (Crabbe et al., 1987a). HOT2 mice displayed more severe withdrawal than COLD2 mice, consistent with the evidence from inbred strains presented earlier that there is a negative correlation between hypothermic response to EtOH and severity of withdrawal. However, HOT1 mice did not differ from COLD1 mice, consistent with the similar acute hypothermic response of WSP and WSR mice. FAST and SLOW mouse lines selected for differential sensitivity to the initial activating effects of EtOH (Crabbe et al., 1987b) were tested for EtOH withdrawal severity. SLOW2 mice had more severe withdrawal than FAST2 mice, but SLOW1 and FAST1 lines did not differ significantly (Crabbe et al., 1988a). This result is in contrast to the recent result of RI analysis suggesting that there is an association of at least one locus between the low-dose activating effect of EtOH and withdrawal severity (Gora-Maslak et al., 1991). Thus, these studies have largely supported the notion that EtOH actions are independent, in that selective breeding for one EtOH trait has in general not resulted in predictable divergence on other traits.

Conclusion: Contributions of Genetic Studies to the Understanding of Physical Dependence and Withdrawal

The most striking result of the genetic studies of EtOH withdrawal is the apparent independence of the various responses to EtOH. In general, the response of an animal to any given effect of EtOH has proved to indicate little about its likely response on another measure. This result is not so surprising when one considers that EtOH has broad effects throughout the central nervous system, and indeed throughout the body. It had been hoped, however, that one or more of the acute responses to ethanol would be identified as genetically related to withdrawal, leading to an indication of which system eventually results in the expression of the withdrawal syndrome. Unfortunately, the genetic studies have not yet revealed any clear way directly to measure physical dependence as it develops. This may be because the correct measurement has not yet been found. Alternatively, the development of physical dependence may turn out to be more complex and intricate, depending upon small changes in many systems, and thus require more subtle techniques for detection than are currently applied.

It seems likely that the withdrawal syndrome is not a unitary phenomenon. Although the WSP and WSR mice differ in some measures of withdrawal other than HIC, in no other measure does the difference approach the magnitude of the HIC difference. This suggests that only part of the genetic variance involved in measures such as withdrawal hypothermia, tremor, and straub tail has been affected through selection for differences in HIC. It is also interesting that the HA/LA selection, which used a withdrawal measure very similar to that used in selecting the WSP/WSR lines, appears to have proceeded at a slower rate of response. It may be that the difference in method of chronic administration of EtOH is responsible, possibly because of reduced selection pressure in the HA/LA mice (because it is more difficult to achieve high levels of dependence using liquid diet techniques). Another possibility is that the greater withdrawal difference in WSP/WSR mice is dependent upon an interactive effect of pyrazole. It is possible, however, that a fundamentally different withdrawal syndrome, with a different constellation of symptoms, will be found in these two selections. It will be very interesting to compare the results of these two studies as the HA/LA selection proceeds.

The WSP/WSR selection, which is essentially complete in that it has reached an apparently stable plateau of response to selection, is now beginning to yield some very promising results. For instance, the finding that levels of certain GABA subunits have different levels in WSP and WSR mice, and are differentially altered by chronic EtOH treatment, suggests that it may be possible to pursue behavioral differences to the level of the genome. The recent finding that a QTL influencing acute withdrawal severity may be linked to the gene encoding glutamic acid decarboxylase is potentially very important (Buck et al., unpublished data). Studies of the anatomical distribution of GABA receptors with the altered subunits could indicate which brain regions are critically involved in withdrawal. Furthermore, these mice may provide invaluable information about the functional consequences of alterations in the subunit composition of the GABA receptor.

The molecular workings of the brain are being elucidated at finer levels and in greater detail. The actions of EtOH continue to have dismayingly universal action on every CNS process studied (although recent results suggest that the NMDA system may be particularly sensitive to EtOH). The techniques of behavior genetics provide a link between the molecular actions of EtOH and the behavioral consequences for the organism as a whole. In so doing, they offer the potential of revealing the physiological mechanism underlying the myriad actions of EtOH.

References

Allen, D. L., Petersen, D. R., Wilson, J. R., McClearn, G. E., and Nishimoto, T. K. (1983). Selective breeding for a multivariate index of ethanol dependence in mice: Results from the first five generations. *Alcohol.: Clin. Exp. Res.* **7**(4):443–447.

Bailey, D. W. (1971). Recombinant inbred strains, an aid to finding identity linkage, and function of histocompatibility and other genes. *Transplantation* **11**:325–327.

Barry, III, H. (1979). Behavioral manifestations of ethanol intoxication and physical dependence. In *Biochemistry and Pharmacology of Ethanol,* Vol. 2, E. Majchrowicz and E. P. Noble, eds. New York: Plenum Press, pp. 511–531.

Becker, H. C., Anton, R. F., and Randall, C. L. (1987). Stereotypic wall climbing in mice during ethanol withdrawal: A new measure of physical dependence. *Alcohol* **4**:443–447.

Begleiter, H., and Porjesz, B. (1977). Persistence of brain hyperexcitability following chronic alcohol exposure in rats. In *Alcohol Intoxication and Withdrawal,* Vol. 3B, M. M. Gross, ed. New York: Plenum Press, pp. 209–222.

Belknap, J. (1980). Genetic factors in the effects of alcohol: Neurosensitivity, functional tolerance, and physical dependence. In *Alcohol Tolerance and Dependence*, H. Rigter and J. C. Crabbe, eds. Amsterdam: Elsevier/North Holland Biomedical Press, pp. 157–180.

Belknap, J. K., Laursen, S. E., and Crabbe, J. C. (1987). Ethanol and nitrous oxide produce withdrawal-induced convulsions by similar mechanisms in mice. *Life Sci.* **41:**2033–2040.

Belknap, J. K., Danielson, P. W., Lame, M., and Crabbe, J. C. (1988). Ethanol and barbiturate withdrawal convulsions are extensively codetermined in mice. *Alcohol* **5:**167–171.

Belknap, J. K., Laursen, S. E., and Crabbe, J. C. (1989). Mice bred to be either prone or resistant to ethanol withdrawal convulsions show closely parallel vulnerabilities with diazepam. *Life Sci.* **44:**2075–2080.

Belknap, J. K., Crabbe, J. C., Plomin, R., McClearn, G. E., Sampson, K. E., O'Toole, L. A., and Gora-Maslak, G. (1992). Single locus control of saccharin intake in BXD/Ty recombinant inbred mice: Some methodological implications for RI strain analysis. *Behav. Genet.* **22**(1):81–100.

Berta, J., and Wilson, J. R. (1989). Selection in mice for alcohol withdrawal seizures. *Behav. Genet.* **19:**745 (abstract).

Berta, J., and Wilson, J. R. (1990). Correlated responses to selection in mice for ethanol withdrawal seizures. *Behav. Genet.* **20:**703 (abstract).

Berta, J., and Wilson, J. R. (1992). Seven generations of genetic selection for ethanol dependence in mice. *Behav. Genet.* **22:**345–359.

Brennan, C. H., Crabbe, J. C., and Littleton, J. M. (1990). Genetic regulation of dihydropyridine-sensitive calcium channels in brain may determine susceptibility to alcohol physical dependence. *Neuropharmacology* **29:**429–432.

Brick, J., and Pohorecky, L. A. (1977). Ethanol withdrawal: Altered ambient temperature selection in rats. *Alcohol: Clin. Exp. Res.* **1:**207–211.

Buck, K. J., Hahner, L., Sikela, J., and Harris, R. A. (1991). Chronic ethanol treatment alters brain levels of γ-aminobutyric acid^A receptor subunit mRNAs: Relationship to genetic differences in ethanol withdrawal severity. *J. Neurochem.* **57:**1452–1453.

Cicero, T. J. (1980). Alcohol self-administration, tolerance and withdrawal in humans and animals: Theoretical and methodological issues. In *Alcohol Tolerance and Dependence*, H. Rigter and J. C. Crabbe, eds. Amsterdam: Elsevier/North Holland Biomedical Press, pp. 1–51.

Cicero, T. J., Snider, S. R., Perez, V. J., and Swanson, L. W. (1971). Physical dependence on and tolerance to alcohol in the rat. *Physiol. Behav.* **6:**191–198.

Cloninger, C. R. (1987). Neurogenetic adaptive mechanisms in alcoholism. *Science* **236:**410–415.

Corley, R., and Allen, D. (1988). Multivariate diallel analysis of ethanol withdrawal symptoms in mice. *Alcohol.: Clin. Exp. Res.* **12**(1):99–104.

Crabbe, J. C. (1983). Sensitivity to ethanol in inbred mice: Genotypic correlations among several behavioral responses. *Behav. Neurosci.* **97**(2):280–289.

Crabbe, J. C. (1992). Antagonism of ethanol withdrawal convulsions in WSP mice by diazepam and abecarnil. *Eur. J. Pharmacol.* **221:**85–90.

Crabbe, J. C., and Kosobud, A. (1986). Sensitivity and tolerance to ethanol in mice bred to be genetically prone or resistant to ethanol withdrawal seizures. *J. Pharmacol. Exp. Ther.* **239**(2):327–333.

Crabbe, J. C., and Kosobud, A. (1990). Alcohol withdrawal seizures: Genetic animal models. In *Alcohol and Seizures: Basic Mechanisms and Clinical Concepts*, R. J. Porter, R. H. Mattson, J. A. Cramer, and I. Diamond, eds. Philadelphia: F. A. Davis, pp. 126–139.

Crabbe, J. C., Janowsky, J. S., Young, E. R., Kosobud, A., Stack, J. S., and Rigter, H. (1982).

Tolerance to ethanol hypothermia in inbred mice: Genotypic correlations with behavioral responses. *Alcohol.: Clin. Exp. Res.* **6**:446–458.

Crabbe, J. C., Kosobud, A., and Young, E. R., (1983a). Genetic selection for ethanol withdrawal severity: Differences in replicate mouse lines. *Life Sci.* **33**:955–962.

Crabbe, J. C., Kosobud, A., Young, E. R., and Janowsky, J. S. (1983b). Polygenic and single-gene determination of responses to ethanol in BXD/Ty recombinant inbred mouse strains. *Neurobehav. Toxicol. Teratol.* **5**:181–187.

Crabbe J. C., Young E. R., and Kosobud A. (1983c). Genetic correlations with ethanol withdrawal severity. *Pharmacol. Biochem. Behav.* **18**(suppl 1):541–547.

Crabbe, J. C., Young, E. R., Kosobud, A., Tam, B. R., and McSwigan, J. D. (1985). Bidirectional selection for sensitivity to ethanol withdrawal seizures in Mus musculus. *Behav. Gene.* **15**(6):521–536.

Crabbe, J. C., Kosobud, A., Tam, B. R., Young, E. R., and Deutsch, C. M. (1987a). Genetic selection of mouse lines sensitive (COLD) and resistant (HOT) to acute ethanol hypothermia. *Alcohol Drug Res.* **7**:163–174.

Crabbe, J. C., Young, E. R., Deutsch, C. M., Tam, B. R., and Kosobud, A. (1987b). Mice genetically selected for differences in open-field activity after ethanol. *Pharmacol. Biochem. Behav.* **27**:577–581.

Crabbe, J. C., Deutsch, C. M., Tam, B. R., and Young, E. R. (1988a). Environmental variables differentially affect ethanol-stimulated activity in selectively bred mouse lines. *Psychopharmacology* **95**:103–108.

Crabbe, J. C., Kosobud, A. E., Feller, D. J., and Phillips, T. J. (1988b). Use of selectively bred mouse lines to study genetically correlated traits related to alcohol. In *Biomedical and Social Aspects of Alcohol and Alcoholism,* K. Kuriyama, A. Takada, and H. Ishii, eds. Amsterdam: Elsevier/North Holland Biomedical Press, pp. 427–430.

Crabbe, J. C., Merrill, C. D., Kim, D., and Belknap, J. K. (1990a). Alcohol dependence and withdrawal: A genetic animal model. *Annals Med.* **22**:259–263.

Crabbe, J. C., Phillips, T. J., Kosobud, A., and Belknap, J. K. (1990b). Estimation of genetic correlation: Interpretation of experiments using selectively bred and inbred animals. *Alcohol.: Clin. Exp. Res.* **14**:141–151.

Crabbe, J. C., Merrill, C. D., and Belknap, J. K. (1991a). Effects of convulsants on handling-induced convulsions in mice selected for ethanol withdrawal severity. *Brain Res.* **550**:1–6.

Crabbe, J. C., Merrill, C. D., and Belknap, J. K. (1991b). Acute dependence on depressant drugs is determined by common genes in mice. *J. Pharmacol. Exp. Ther.* **257**:663–667.

Crabbe, J. C., Merrill, C. D., and Belknap, J. K. (1993). Effect of acute alcohol withdrawal on sensitivity to pro- and anticonvulsant treatments in WSP mice. *Alcohol.: Clin. Exp. Res.* **17**: 1233–1239.

Crabbe, J. C., Young, E. R., and Dorow, J. (1994a). Effects of dizocilpine in Withdrawal Seizure-Prone and -Resistant mice. *Pharmacol. Biochem. Behav.* **47**: 443–450.

Crabbe, J. C., Belknap, J. K., and Buck, K. J. (1994b). Genetic animal models of alcohol and drug abuse. *Science* **264**:1715–1723.

Crawshaw, L. I., O'Connor, C. S., Crabbe, J. C., and Hayteas, D. L. (1994). Temperature regulation in mice during withdrawal from ethanol dependence. *Am. J. Physiol.,* **267**:R929–R934.

Dietrich, W., et al. (1992). A genetic map of the mouse suitable for typing intraspecific crosses. *Genetics* **131**:423–427.

Eicher, E. M., Stern, R. H., Womack, J. E., Davisson, M. T., Roderick, T. H., and Reynolds, S. C. (1976). Evolution of mammalian carbonic anhydrase loci by tandem duplication: Close linkage of *Car-1* and *Car-2* to the centromere region of chromosome 3 of the mouse. *Biochem. Genet.* **14**:651–660.

Falconer, D. S. (1983). *Introduction to Quantitative Genetics,* 2d ed. London and New York: Longman.

Feller, D. J., Harris, R. A., and Crabbe, J. C. (1988). Differences in GABA activity between ethanol withdrawal seizure prone and resistant mice. *Eur. J. Pharmacol.* **157:**147–154.

Feller, D. J., Tso-Olivas, D. Y., and Savage, D. D. (1990). Hippocampal mossy fiber zinc deficit in mice genetically selected for ethanol withdrawal seizure susceptibility. *Brain Res.* **545:**73–79.

Freund, G. (1969). Alcohol withdrawal syndrome in mice. *Arch. Neurol.* **21:**315–320.

Friedman, H. J. (1980). Assessment of physical dependence on and withdrawal from ethanol in animals. In *Alcohol Tolerance and Dependence,* H. Rigter and J. C. Crabbe, eds. Amsterdam: Elsevier/North Holland Biomedical Press, pp. 93–121.

Geisler, R. Y., Hunter, B. E., and Walker, D. W. (1978). Ethanol dependence in the rat: Temporary changes in neuroexcitability following withdrawal. *Psychopharmacology* **56:**287–292.

Gilliam, D. W., and Collins, A. C. (1986). Quantification of physiological and behavioral measures of alcohol withdrawal in long-sleep and short-sleep mice. *Alcohol.: Clin. Exp. Res.* **10:**672–678.

Goldstein, D. B. (1972). Relationship of alcohol dose to intensity of withdrawal signs in mice. *J. Pharmacol. Exp. Ther.* **180:**203–215.

Goldstein, D. B. (1973). Inherited differences in intensity of alcohol withdrawal reactions in mice. *Nature* **245:**154–156.

Goldstein, D. B. (1980). Inhalation of ethanol vapor. In *Alcohol Tolerance and Dependence,* H. Rigter and J. C. Crabbe, eds. Amsterdam: Elsevier/North Holland Biomedical Press, pp. 81–92.

Goldstein, D. B., and Kakihana, R. (1974). Alcohol withdrawal reactions and reserpine effects in inbred strains of mice. *Life Sci.* **15:**415–425.

Goldstein, D. B., and Kakihana, R. (1975). Alcohol withdrawal reactions in mouse strains selectively bred for long or short sleep times. *Life Sci.* **17:**981–986.

Goldstein, D. B., and Pal, N. (1971). Alcohol dependence produced in mice by inhalation of ethanol: Grading the withdrawal reaction. *Science* **172:**288–290.

Goodwin, D. W. (1983). Familial alcoholism: A separate entity? *Subst. Alcohol Actions/Misuse* **4:**129–136.

Gonzalez, L. P. (1993). Sensitivity to strychnine seizures is unaltered during ethanol withdrawal. *Alcohol.: Clin. Exp. Res.* **17:**1029–1034.

Gonzalez, L. P., Czachura, J. F., and Brewer, K. W. (1989). Spontaneous versus elicited seizures following ethanol withdrawal: Differential time course. *Alcohol* **6:**481–487.

Gora-Maslak, G., McClearn, G. E., Crabbe, J. C., Phillips, T. J., Belknap, J. K., and Plomin, R. (1991). Use of recombinant inbred strains to identify quantitative trait loci in psychopharmacology. *Psychopharmacology* **104:**413–424.

Grieve, S. J., Griffiths, P. J., and Littleton, J. M. (1979). Genetic influences on the rate of development of ethanol tolerance and the ethanol physical withdrawal syndrome in mice. *Drug Alcohol Depend.* **4:**77–86.

Griffiths, P. J., and Littleton, J. M. (1977). Concentrations of free amino acids in brains of mice of different strains during the physical syndrome of withdrawal from alcohol. *Br. J. Exp. Pathol.* **58:**391–399.

Harris, R. A. Crabbe, J. C., and McSwigan, J. D. (1984). Relationship of membrane physical properties to alcohol dependence in mice selected for genetic differences in alcohol withdrawal *Life Sci.* **35:**2601–2608.

Hunter, B. E., Boast, C. A., Walker, D. W., and Zornetzer, S. F. (1973). Alcohol withdrawal syndrome in rats: Neural and behavioral correlates. *Pharmacol. Biochem. Behav.* **1**:719–725.

Hunter, B. E., Riley, J. N., Walker, D. W., and Freund, G. (1975). Ethanol dependence in the rat: A parametric analysis. *Pharmacol. Biochem. Behav.* **3**:619–629.

Hutchins, J. R., Allen, D. L., Cole-Harding, S., and Wilson, J. R. (1981). Behavioral and physiological measures for studying ethanol dependence in mice. *Pharmacol. Biochem. Behav.* **15**(1):55–59.

Israel, Y., Oporto, B., and Mcdonald, A. D. (1984). Simultaneous pair-feeding system for the administration of alcohol-containing liquid diets. *Alcohol.: Clin. Exp. Res.* **8**:505–508.

Kakihana, R. (1979). Alcohol intoxication and withdrawal in inbred strains of mice: Behavioral and endocrine studies. *Behav. Neural Biol.* **26**:97–105.

Kosobud, A., Bodor, A. S., and Crabbe, J. C. (1988). Voluntary consumption of ethanol in WSP, WSC and WSR selectively bred mouse lines. *Pharmacol. Biochem. Behav.* **29**:601–607.

Kosobud, A., and Crabbe, J. C. (1986). Ethanol withdrawal in mice bred to be genetically prone or resistant to ethanol withdrawal seizures. *J. Pharmacol. Exp. Ther.* **238**:170–177.

Kosobud, A. E., and Crabbe, J. C. (1990). Genetic correlations among inbred strain sensitivities to convulsions induced by 9 convulsant drugs. *Brain Res.* **526**:8–16.

Kosobud, A. E., and Crabbe, J. C. (1993). Sensitivity to N-methyl-D-aspartic acid-induced convulsions is genetically associated with resistance to ethanol withdrawal seizures. *Brain Research* **610**:176–179.

Lander, E. S., and Botstein, D. (1989). Mapping Mendelian factors underlying quantitative traits using RFLP linkage maps. *Genetics* **121**:185–199.

Lumeng, L., Hawkins, T. D., and Li, T. -K. (1977). New strains of rats with alcohol preference and nonpreference. In *Alcohol and Aldehyde Metabolizing Systems,* Vol. 3, R. G. Thurman, J. R. Williamson, H. Drott, and B. Chance, eds. New York: Academic Press, pp. 537–544.

Lyon, M. F., and Searle, A. G., eds. (1989). *Genetic Variants and Strains of the Laboratory Mouse.* Oxford, Great Britain: Oxford University Press.

McCall, R. D., and Frierson, D. (1981). Evidence that two loci predominantly determine the difference in susceptibility to the high-pressure neurological syndrome type I seizure in mice. *Genetics* **99**:285–307.

McClearn, G. E., and Kakihana, R. (1981). Selective breeding for ethanol sensitivity: Short-sleep and long-sleep mice. In *Development of Animal Models as Pharmacogenetic Tools* G. E. McClearn, R. A., Deitrich and V. G. Erwin, eds. Washington DC: U.S. Government Printing Office (USDHHS-NIAA Research Monograph No. 6), pp. 147–159.

McClearn, G. P., Wilson, J. R., Petersen, D. R., and Allen, D. L. (1982). Selective breeding in mice for severity of the ethanol withdrawal syndrome. *Subst. Alcohol Actions/Misuse* **3**:135–143.

McQuarrie, D. G., and Fingl, E. (1958). Effects of single doses and chronic administration of ethanol on experimental seizures in mice. *J. Pharmacol. Exp. Ther.* **124**:264–271.

Majchrowicz, E. (1975). Induction of physical dependence upon ethanol an the associated behavioral changes in rats. *Psychopharmacologia* **43**:245–254.

Mendelson, W. B., Majchrowicz, E., Mirirani, N., Dawson, S., Gillin, J. L., and Wyatt, R. J. (1978). Sleep during chronic ethanol administration and withdrawal in rats. *J. Stud Alcohol* **39**:1213–1223.

Metten, P., and Crabbe, J. C. (1994). Common genetic determinants of severity of withdrawal from ethanol, pentobarbital and diazepam in inbred mice. *Behav. Pharmacol.,* **5**:533–547.

Mucha, R. F., and Pinel, J. P. J. (1979). Increased susceptibility to kindled seizures in rats following a single injection of alcohol. *J. Stud. Alcohol* **40**:258–271.

256 **Selective Breeding Studies**

Noble, E. P., Gillies, R., Vigran, R., and Mandel, P. (1976). The modification of the ethanol withdrawal syndrome in rats by di-n-propylacetate. *Psychopharmacologia* **46:**127–131.

Penick, E. C., Powell, B. J., Bingham, S. F., Liskow, B. I., Miller, N. S., and Read, M. R. (1987). A comparative study of familial alcoholism. *J. Stud Alcohol* **48:**136–146.

Phillips, T. J., and Crabbe, J. C. (1991). Behavioral studies of genetic differences in alcohol action. In *The Genetic Basis of Alcohol and Drug Actions,* J. C. Crabbe and R. A. Harris, eds. New York: Plenum Press, pp. 25–104.

Plomin, R., McClearn, G. E., and Gora-Maslak, G. (1991). Use of recombinant inbred strains to detect quantitative trait loci associated with behavior. *Behav. Genet.* **21:**99–116.

Pohorecky, L. A. (1976). Withdrawal from ethanol: Simple quantitative behavioral tests for its evaluation. *Psychopharmacology* **50:**125–129.

Ritzmann, R. F., and Tabakoff, B. (1976). Body temperature in mice: A quantitative measure of alcohol tolerance and physical dependence. *J. Pharmacol. Exp. Ther.* **199:**158–170.

Roberts, A. J., Crabbe, J. C., and L. D. Keith. (1992). Genetic differences in hypothalamic-pituitary-adrenal axis responsiveness to acute ethanol and acute ethanol withdrawal. *Brain Res.* **577:**296–302.

Sanders, B. (1980). Withdrawal-like signs induced by a single administration of ethanol in mice that differ in ethanol sensitivity. *Psychopharmacology* **68:**109–113.

Schuckit, M. A. (1988). Reactions to alcohol in sons of alcoholics and controls. *Alcohol.: Clin. Exp. Res.* **12:**465–470.

Szabo, G., Kovacs, G. L., and Telegdy, G. (1984). Increased sensitivity to picrotoxin as an index of physical dependence on alcohol in the mouse. *Drug Alcohol Depend.* **14:**187–195.

Taylor, B. A. (1972). Genetic relationships between inbred strains of mice. *J. Heredity* **63:**83–86.

Taylor, B. A. (1978). Development of recombinant inbred lines of mice. *Behav. Genet.* **6:**118 (abstract).

Terdal, E. S., and Crabbe, J. C. (1994). Indexing withdrawal in mice: Matching genotypes for exposure in studies using ethanol vapor inhalation. *Alcohol.: Clin. Exp. Res.,* **18:**542–547.

Thoday, J. M. (1961). Location of polygenes. *Nature* **191:**368–370.

Unwin, J. W., and Taberner, P. V. (1980). Sex and strain differences in GABA receptor binding after chronic ethanol drinking in mice. *Neuropharmacology* **19:**1257–1259.

Victor, M., and Adams, R. D. (1953). The effect of alcohol on the nervous system. In *Metabolic and Toxic Disease of the Nervous System,* vol. 32, H. H. Merrit and C. L. Hare, eds. Baltimore: Association for Research in Nervous and Mental Disease, pp. 526–573.

Walker, D. W., and Zornetzer, S. F. (1974). Alcohol withdrawal in mice: Electroencephalographic and behavioral correlates. *Electroencephalogr. Clin Neurophysiol.* **36:**233–244.

Waller, M. B., McBride, W. J., Lumeng, L., and Li, T. -K. (1982). Induction of dependence on ethanol by free-choice drinking in alcohol-preferring rats. *Pharmacol. Biochem. Behav.* **16:**501–507.

Wilson, J. R., Erwin, V. G., DeFries, J. C., Petersen, D. R., and Cole-Harding, S. (1984). Ethanol dependence in mice: Direct and correlated responses to ten generations of selective breeding. *Behav. Genet.* **14**(3):235–255.

Winer, B. J. (1971). *Statistical Principles in Experimental Design.* New York: McGraw-Hill.

Woodward, S., Sudweeks, J., and Teuscher, C. (1992). Random sequence oligonucleotide primers detect polymorphic DNA products which segregate in inbred strains of mice. *Mammal. Genome* **3:**73–78.

III

Phenotypic Studies

10

Biochemical Phenotypic Markers in Genetic Alcoholism

IVAN DIAMOND AND
ADRIENNE GORDON

There is extensive evidence that genetic factors play a role in alcoholism (Begleiter and Porjesz, 1988; Kiianmaa et al., 1989; Cloninger, 1991) and in the development of alcoholic medical disorders (Devore et al., 1988). Moreover, Cloninger (1987) has shown by adoption studies that a "male-limited" type of alcoholism in the biologic father is a much greater predictor for alcohol abuse in the son that the environment in which the boy is raised. However, these observations do not suggest pathophysiologic mechanisms. Instead, clinical and experimental work with alcohol intoxication, tolerance, and dependence may provide clues to candidate phenotypes in alcoholism. For example, we know that ethanol alters many specific membrane-dependent events in the cell that may account for ethanol-induced changes in neural function. In addition, membrane functions affected by ethanol are under precise regulation and might be abnormally regulated in genetically vulnerable patients. Since alcoholics exhibit alcoholism only when drinking, it is also possible that critically regulated functions in the brain are abnormal only when challenged by ethanol, and that these altered functions are responsible for intoxication, tolerance, and dependence. Therefore, ethanol-induced changes in the regulation of cellular and molecular mechanisms that underlie alcohol intoxication, tolerance, and the symptoms of withdrawal may be excellent candidate phenotypes for exploring the genetics of alcoholism.

Ethanol crosses the blood–brain barrier and enters the brain quickly. Shortly after alcohol consumption, the blood alcohol level is directly proportional to the concentration of ethanol in brain tissue. Despite increasing blood ethanol levels, tolerance to ethanol can develop during a single bout of drinking (Victor and Adams, 1953; Goldstein, 1983). This is characterized by a reduced intoxicating response to ethanol; subjects can become sober at blood alcohol levels higher than those at which intoxication first developed (Mirsky et al., 1941). This well-recognized phenomenon of *acute tolerance* is most likely due to adaptive changes in the central nervous system (CNS) that probably involve complex regulatory mechanisms.

Chronic tolerance also occurs in alcoholics. These patients show increased resistance to the intoxicating effects of ethanol and are often sober at blood alcohol levels that might be fatal in naive individuals (Urso et al., 1981). For example, a serum ethanol level of 1510 mg/dl was reported in a chronic alcoholic who had stopped drinking three days before walking into the hospital (Lindblad and Olsson, 1976). This striking degree of tolerance suggests that the magnitude of biochemical adaptation to alcohol can vary extensively between different individuals. Thus, adaptive biochemical mechanisms could be quite different in patients at risk of developing alcoholism because of genetic factors. Consistent with this possibility, it is well known that genetic variability in response to ethanol has been demonstrated in many experimental animal studies (Kiianmaa et al., 1989). Moreover, Crabbe and colleagues (Crabbe and Kosobud, 1986) have shown that the magnitude and occurrence of alcohol withdrawal seizures is under genetic control in experimental animals. Thus, there is considerable experimental evidence to suggest variable genetic regulation of the proteins that mediate the acute or chronic effects of ethanol. Ethanol-induced changes in such proteins could underlie genetic vulnerability to alcoholism.

Candidate Mechanisms for Genetic Vulnerability

Many studies indicate that biochemical and molecular changes in the properties and function of membrane-dependent events are related to acute intoxication, tolerance, and physical dependence. Ethanol diffuses into cell membranes (Rottenburg, 1986) and increases membrane fluidity (Goldstein and Chin, 1981). After chronic exposure to ethanol, cellular membranes become resistant to the fluidizing effect of ethanol (Goldstein, 1986). In addition, there are also acute and chronic ethanol-induced changes in many membrane components and functions. Therefore, candidate genetic markers of ethanol-induced changes in membrane function that could be studied in human cells include alterations in membrane lipids (Sun and Sun, 1985) and phosphatidylinositol (Taraschi et al., 1986), receptors (Charness et al., 1986; Mhatre and Ticku, 1989; Valverius et al., 1989; Reynolds et al., 1990), second messengers (Gordon et al., 1986; Hoffman et al., 1986; Richelson et al., 1986; Stenstrom et al., 1986; Diamond et al., 1987), GTP binding proteins (Saito et al., 1987; Charness et al., 1988, Mochly-Rosen et al., 1988), neuromodulators (Nagy et al., 1989; Nagy et al., 1990), ion channels, transporters, and proteins whose gene expression is altered by ethanol (Miles et al., 1991). Many of these membrane components are acutely affected by ethanol and later exhibit tolerance to ethanol when rechallenged. Such adaptive membrane components are excellent phenotypic marker candidates for a genetic predisposition to alcoholism, and many can be studied in cultured lymphocytes. Once a phenotypic biochemical marker for genetic alcoholism is identified, it will be possible to identify a gene(s) that is (are) responsible for this phenotype and transmit a risk for alcoholism in genetically vulnerable individuals.

Recently, several specific systems, often regulated by protein kinases, are beginning to attract increasing attention. The benzodiazepine/GABA receptor complex appears to be a major target for ethanol, exhibiting cross-tolerance with benzodiazepines and barbiturates (Mehta and Ticku, 1988; Glowa et al., 1989; Harris and Allan, 1989; McQuilkin and Harris, 1990). Differences in $GABA_A$-activated Cl^- channel function have recently been found in $GABA_A$ receptors expressed in *Xenopus* oocytes using mRNA from brains of long-sleep (LS) or short-sleep (SL) mice (Wafford et al., 1990), animals with differential genetic sensitivity to the hypnotic effect of ethanol (Harris and Allan, 1989). These differences in $GABA_A$ receptor function between LS and SS mice could be due to changes in receptor subunit phosphorylation (Wafford et al., 1991).

The excitatory NMDA receptor in the hippocampus appears to play a role in learning and memory, and is exquisitely sensitive to ethanol (Hoffman et al., 1989; Lovinger et al., 1989; Lovinger et al., 1990). The voltage-dependent calcium channel is also a major target for the acute and chronic effects of ethanol. The increased number of voltage-dependent calcium channels found after chronic exposure to ethanol (Messing et al., 1986; Dolin et al., 1987; Skattebol and Rabin, 1987) involves regulation by protein kinase C (Messing et al., 1990) and may play a role in alcohol withdrawal seizures (Little et al., 1986; Koppi et al., 1987). Indeed, mice genetically prone to develop ethanol withdrawal seizures exhibit an increase in voltage-dependent calcium channels (Brennan et al., 1990). Abnormal sensitivity to ethanol or altered regulation of these membrane-dependent events by ethanol could play a role in a genetic predisposition to alcoholism.

cAMP signal transduction is a second messenger system that undergoes acute and chronic adaptive responses to ethanol. Our laboratory has been interested in adenosine-dependent cAMP signal transduction because adenosine appears to mediate many acute and chronic effects of ethanol in the nervous system (Dar et al., 1983; Proctor and Dunwiddie, 1984; Dar et al., 1987; Nagy et al., 1989; Nagy et al., 1990; Gordon et al., 1990). Adenosine is an inhibitory modulator affecting many receptors, ion channels, and second messengers in several cellular systems, including the brain (Daly et al., 1981; Dunwiddie, 1985; Snyder, 1985; Ribeiro and Sebastiao, 1986). There is also pursuasive evidence that adenosine mediates many of the hepatic effects of ethanol (Carmichael et al., 1988). Ethanol potentiates adenosine A_2 receptor stimulation of cAMP signal transduction in many cells, presumably by increasing the coupling of $G\alpha_s$, the stimulatory GTP-binding protein, to adenylyl cyclase (Rabin and Molinoff, 1981; Gordon et al., 1986; Diamond et al., 1987; Nagy et al., 1988). In addition, ethanol inhibits adenosine uptake into cells via a nucleoside transporter (Nagy et al., 1990; Gordon et al., 1990). As a result of this ethanol inhibition, there is an accumulation of extracellular adenosine, leading to activation of adenosine A_2 receptors and stimulation of cAMP production. However, other ethanol-dependent mechanisms could also stimulate cAMP production.

As in most cellular systems under homeostatic control, acute increases in cAMP levels are followed by desensitization of this response (Sibley and Lefkowitz, 1985). Indeed, when neural cells experience prolonged exposure to ethanol, the cells adapt by a "heterologous desensitization" of receptors coupled positively to adenylyl cyclase via $G\alpha_s$. Thus, receptor-stimulated cAMP production is decreased when measured in the absence of ethanol (Gordon et al., 1986; Mochly-Rosen et al., 1988; Rabin, 1990). However, when ethanol is added back to the cultures, cAMP levels return to normal (Gordon et al., 1986). This is an example of ethanol dependence at a cellular level brought about by cellular adaptation to the initial inhibition of adenosine uptake by acute ethanol. Moreover, since heterologous densitization involves many receptors coupled to adenylyl cyclase, relatively specific effects of ethanol on adenosine uptake appear to account for many diverse effects of ethanol in the nervous system and elsewhere.

Recent evidence suggests that ethanol-induced heterologous desensitization is due to selective changes in G protein function. Prolonged exposure of NG108-15 cells to ethanol causes a decrease in mRNA and protein for $G\alpha_s$ (Mochly-Rosen et al., 1988; Charness et al., 1988). In turn, this leads to a reduction in functional activity of G_s (Mochly-Rosen et al., 1988), thereby accounting for the ethanol-induced decrease in receptor-dependent cAMP production. The implication of these findings is that a selective effect of ethanol on adenosine uptake ultimately leads to specific changes in $G\alpha_s$ that underlie many of the pleiotropic effects of ethanol. Therefore, genetic differences in the regulation of such adenosine-dependent pathways might account for genetic variability and vulnerability in selected patients.

Studies on Circulating Cells

Since it is not possible to study brain samples in living patients, a number of investigators have begun to search for biologic and genetic markers in circulating cells from alcoholics. Recently, we have measured adenosine receptor-activated cAMP production in freshly isolated lymphocytes. Cells from alcoholics showed a 76% reduction in basal and adenosine receptor-stimulated cAMP levels when compared to either age- and sex-matched controls or patients with nonalcoholic liver disease (Diamond et al., 1987). Consistent with these findings, subsequent studies in platelet membranes from alcoholics showed a small but significant reduction in stimulated adenylyl cyclase activity (Tabakoff et al., 1988). Differences in monamine oxidase activity were also observed (Faraj et al., 1987; Tabakoff et al., 1988).

Freshly isolated human lymphocytes have also been used to search for abnormal ethanol metabolism in alcoholics. Ethanol can be an exogenous substrate for phospholipase D, leading to the accumulation of an abnormal product, phophatidylethanol (Alling et al., 1984; Kobayashi and Kanfer, 1987; Mueller et al., 1988), rather than the normal product, phosphatidylethanolamine. Lymphocytes from alcoholics show increased synthesis of phosphatidylethanol, leading Mueller and colleagues (1988) to suggest that this might be a potential genetic marker for alcoholism. However, it is difficult to establish genetic linkage to alcoholism by studying freshly isolated lymphocytes or platelets from actively drinking alcoholics. Acute and chronic exposure to alcohol *in vivo* can alter cellular physiology and produce long-lasting nutritional, metabolic, and hormonal variables that are difficult to control. In order to avoid this methodologic limitation, investigators are beginning to examine preparations that are not affected directly by alcohol consumption.

Advantages of Cultured Lymphocytes

We have found that cultured lymphocytes offer many advantages in the search for a biochemical marker for genetic alcoholism. Studies of homogeneous cells in culture avoids many of the variables encountered in studying cells and fluids taken from actively drinking alcoholics. The nutrient and growth conditions for the cells can be precisely controlled and the amount of ethanol added and time of exposure can be manipulated with great precision. Homogeneous preparations of lymphocytes can be rapidly prepared from freshly drawn blood. The cells are quite tolerant to laboratory bench manipulations and are easily grown in culture to generate adequate amounts of cellular material for study. Many growth factors are spontaneously released by the dividing cells and commercially available growth factors such as interleukin 2 can be added to promote proliferation. Most important, cell division in lymphocytes takes about 24 hours, so that a new generation of cells is produced nearly every day. This valuable characteristic of cultured lymphocytes enables the investigator to study cellular offspring that have not been exposed to ethanol. Thus, cells cultured for many generations allow the investigator to distinguish between secondary toxic effects of ethanol and genetic differences passed from one generation to another in the absence of ethanol. Therefore, studies with cultured lymphocytes provide an exceptional advantage over studies with nondividing erythrocytes and platelets.

Similar to experiments with cultured cell lines that have been useful in identifying ethanol-induced changes in cellular regulatory mechanisms, studies of cultured lymphocytes can also be carried out after acute and chronic exposure to ethanol. Because all of the cells in culture are lymphocytes, a homogeneous response can be studied and the signal-to-noise ratio in biochemical assays is usually quite favorable. Therefore, responses to ethanol can be measured with considerable accuracy. These features make it possible to search for differences in cells from alcoholics and to recognize abnormal biochemical responses to ethanol in cultured lymphocytes from alcoholics when compared to cells from nonalcoholics. Indeed, some biochemical differences may only be demonstrable when cells from alcoholics are challenged by exposure to ethanol in culture. Such a phenotypic biochemical feature of genetic alcoholism might be expected since subjects predisposed to develop alcoholism because of genetic factors appear to be normal when not drinking.

Finally, it is also possible to create established cell lines from cultured lymphocytes by transformation with Epstein-Barr virus (EBV) (Anderson and Gusella, 1984). Such transformed cells are immortal and provide an unlimited source of genetic material for analysis. It should be pointed out however, that EBV transformed lymphocytes might shed chromosomes and exhibit altered biochemical properties as a consequence of transformation. This could limit the identification of biochemical markers in alcoholism. Nevertheless, DNA preparations from EBV transformed lymphocytes have been exceedingly useful in screening for RFLPs in many inherited disorders.

Cellular Phenotypes for Alcoholism

Because of accumulating evidence that specific functional changes or altered regulation of function might be characteristic biochemical features of alcoholism, cultured lymphocytes are a useful preparation for identifying abnormal cellular and molecular phenotypes. This approach of examining candidate phenotypes in cultured lymphocytes to guide the search for specific genetic defects may prove to be more fruitful than random exploration of the human genome for RFLPs linked to alcoholism. Indeed, even if a specific probe for a proven linked gene to alcoholism was used in linkage studies in families, it still might not be possible to achieve a significant lod score because of the heterogeneity of alcoholism and the difficulty of identifying individuals carrying the altered genes. Therefore, it is necessary to search first for phenotypic biochemical markers of genetic alcoholism that would allow identification of genetic carriers. Subsequently, RFLP analyses can be used to identify which gene(s) is (are) responsible for the altered biochemical phenotype. To date, the only published candidates for biochemical markers in cultured cells are adenosine-mediated cAMP signal transduction (Nagy et al., 1988; Smith and Palmour, 1991), adenosine uptake (Gordon et al., 1991), and transketolase (Mukherjee et al., 1987).

Inheritance of the Alcoholic Phenotype

When a specific biochemical or functional abnormality in cultured lymphocytes from alcoholics is passed from one generation to the next, the results suggest that the product of an altered gene may have been identified in cell culture. In order to investigate this possibility, the next step is to examine whether this phenotype is inherited by nondrinking offspring of drinking parents. In addition, it will be important to demonstrate that this phenotypic abnormality occurs with greater frequency in high-risk individuals. Detailed studies of alcoholic families should establish whether an observed phenotypic abnormality in cultured lymphocytes segregates with alcoholism and is linked to a genetic vulnerability for alcoholism. Finally, studies with cultured lymphocytes from abstinent alcoholics will also be informative since any genetic abnormality should persist in their cultured cells.

Cloning the Gene(s) for Alcoholism

Cultured lymphocytes will prove useful in cloning the gene(s) responsible for the cellular phenotype. Once the genes for the specific candidate proteins responsible for the phenotype are cloned, e.g., adenylyl cyclase, $G\alpha_s$, and the nucleoside transporter, they can be used for RFLP analyses in families with alcoholism. Even without a candidate gene, reverse genetics can be used once a biochemical marker is recognized that identifies individuals carrying the altered gene. After genetic linkage is established and the specific gene identified, the gene(s) from alcoholics can be cloned and sequenced, thereby characterizing the genetic defect in alcoholism.

Acknowledgement: We wish to thank Ms. R. C. Webb for assistance in preparing this manuscript.

This work was supported in part by grants from the National Institute of Alcohol Abuse and Alcoholism (NIAAA), the March of Dimes Birth Defects Foundation, and the Alcoholic Beverage Medical Research Foundation.

References

Alling, C., Gustavsson, L., Mansson, J -E., Benthin, G., and Anggard, E. (1984). Phosphatidylethanol formation in rat organs after ethanol treatment. *Biochim. Biophys. Acta* **793:**119–122. 1984.

Anderson, M. A., and Gusella, J. F. (1984). Use of cyclosporin A in establishing Epstein-Barr virus-transformed human lymphoblastoid cell lines. *In Vitro* **20:**856–858.

Begleiter, H., and Porjesz, B. (1988). Potential biological markers in individuals at high risk for developing alcoholism. *Alcohol.: Clin. Exp. Res.* **12:**488–493.

Brennan, C. H., Crabbe, J., and Littleton, J. M. (1990). Genetic regulation of dihydropyridine-sensitive calcium channels in brain may determine susceptibility to physical dependence on alcohol. *Neuropharmacology* **29:**429–432.

Carmichael, F. J., Saldivia, V., Varghese, G. A., Israel, Y., and Orrego, H. (1988). Ethanol-induced increase in portal blood flow: Role of acetate and A_1- and A_2-adenosine receptors. *Amer. J. Physiol.* **255:**417–423.

Charness, M. E., Querimit, L. A., and Diamond, I. (1986). Ethanol increases the expression of functional δ-opioid receptors in neuroblastoma x glioma NG108-15 hybrid cells. *J. Biol. Chem.* **261:**3164–3169.

Charness, M. E., Querimit, L. A., and Henteleff, M. (1988). Ethanol differentially regulates G proteins in neural cells. *Biochem. Biophys. Res. Commun.* **155:**138–143.

Cloninger, C. R. (1987). Neurogenetic adaptive mechanisms in alcoholism. *Science* **236:**410–416.

Cloninger, C. R. (1991). D_2 dopamine receptor gene is associated but not linked with alcoholism. *JAMA* **266:**1833–1834.

Crabbe, J. C., and Kosobud, A. (1986). Sensitivity and tolerance to ethanol in mice bred to be genetically prone or resistant to ethanol withdrawal seizures. *J. Pharmacol. Exp. Ther.* **239:**327–333.

Daly, J. W., Bruns, R. F., and Snyder, S. H. (1981). Adenosine receptors in the central nervous system: Relationship to the central actions of methylxanthines. *Life Sci.* **28:**2083–2097.

Dar, M. S., Mustafa, S. J., and Wooles, W. R. (1983). Possible role of adenosine in the CNS effects of ethanol. *Life Sci.* **33:**1363–1374.

Dar, M. S., Jones, M., Close, G., Mustafa, S. J., and Wooles, W. R. (1987). Behavioral interactions of ethanol and methylxanthines. *Psychopharmacology* **91:**1–4.

Devor, E. J., Reich, T., and Cloninger, C. R. (1988). Genetics of alcoholism and related end-organ damage. *Seminars Liver Dis.* **8:**1–11.

Diamond, I., Wrubel, B., Estrin, E., and Gordon, A. S. (1987). Basal and adenosine-receptor stimulated levels of cAMP are reduced in lymphocytes from alcoholic patients. *Proc. Natl. Acad. Sci. (USA)* **84:**1413–1416.

Diamond, I., Nagy, L., Mochly-Rosen, D., and Gordon, A. (1991). The role of adenosine and adenosine transport in ethanol-induced cellular tolerance and dependence. *Ann. NY Acad. Sci.* **625:**473–478.

Dolin, S., Little, H., Hudspith, M., Pagonis, C., and Littlejohn, J. (1987). Increased dihydropyridine-sensitive calcium channels in rat brain may underlie ethanol physical dependence. *Neuropharmacology* **26:**275–279.

Dunwiddie, T. V. (1985). The physiological role of adenosine in the central nervous system. *Int. Rev. Neurobiol.* **27:**63–139.

Faraj, B. A., Lenton, J. D., Kutner, M., Camp, V. M., Stammers, T. W., Lee, S. R., Lolies, P. A., and Chandora, D. (1987). Prevalence of low monoamine oxidase function in alcoholism. *Alcohol.: Clin. Exp. Res.* **11:**464–467.

Glowa, J. R., Crawley, J., Suzdak, P. D., and Paul, S. M. (1989). Ethanol and the GABA receptor complex: Studies with the partial inverse benzodiazepine receptor agonist Ro 15-4513. *Pharmacol. Biochem. Behav.* **31:**767–772.

Goldstein, D. B. (1983). *Pharmacology of Alcohol.* New York: Oxford University Press, p. 179.

Goldstein, D. B. (1986). Ethanol-induced adaptation in biological membranes. *Ann. NY Acad. Sci.* **492:**103–111.

Goldstein, D. B., and Chin, J. H. (1981). Interaction of ethanol with biological membranes. *Fed. Proc.* **40:**2073–2076.

Gordon, A. S., Collier, K, and Diamond, I. (1986). Ethanol regulation of adenosine receptor-dependent cAMP levels in a clonal neural cell line: An in vitro model of cellular tolerance to ethanol. *Proc. Natl. Acad. Sci. (USA)* **83:**2105–2108.

Gordon, A. S., Nagy, L. E., Mochly-Rosen, D., Diamond, I. (1990). Chronic ethanol-induced heterologous desensitization is mediated by changes in adenosine transport. In *G Proteins and Signal Transduction,* Symposium No. 56, G. Milligan, M. J. O. Wakelam, and J. Kay, eds. London: London Biochemical Society.

Gordon, A. S., Krauss, S. W., Nagy, L., and Diamond, I. (1991). Nucleoside transport in lymphocytes from alcoholics and nonalcoholics. In *Purine and Pyrimidine Metabolism in Man VII,* Part A, R. A., Harkness, et al. eds. New York: Plenum, pp. 387–390.

Harris, R. A., and Allan, A. M. (1989). Genetic differences in coupling of benzodiazepine receptors to chloride channels. *Brain Res.* **490:**26–32.

Hoffman, B. B., Chang, H., Dall'Aglio, E., and Reaven, G. M. (1986). Desensitization of adenosine receptor-mediated inhibition of lipolysis: The mechanism involves the development of enhanced cyclic adenosine monophosphate accumulation in tolerant adipocytes. *J. Clin. Invest.* **78:**185–190.

Hoffman, P. L., Rabe, C. S., Moses, F., and Tabakoff, B. (1989). N-methyl-D-aspartate receptors and ethanol: Inhibition of calcium flux and cyclic GMP production. *J. Neurochem.* **52:**1937–1940.

Kiianmaa, K., Tabakoff, B., and Saito, T., eds. (1989). *Genetic Aspects of Alcoholism,* Vol. 37. Finnish Helsinki: Foundation for Alcohol Studies.

Kobayashi, M., and Kanfer, J. N. (1987). Phosphatidylethanol formation via transphosphatidylation by rat brain synaptosomal phospholipase D. *J. Neurochem.* **48:**1597–1603.

Koppi, S., Eberhardt, G., Haller, R., and Konig, P. (1987). Calcium-channel-blocking agent in the treatment of acute alcohol withdrawal—caroverine versus meprobamate in a randomized double-blind study. *Neuropsychobiology* **17:**49–52.

Lindblad, B., and Olsson, R. (1976). Unusually high levels of blood alcohol? *JAMA* **236:**1600–1602.

Little, H. J., Dolin, S. J., and Halsey, M. J. (1986). Calcium channel antagonists decrease the ethanol withdrawal syndrome. *Life Sci.* **39:**2059–2065.

Lovinger, D. M., White, G., and Weight, F. F. (1989). Ethanol inhibits NMDA-activated ion current in hippocampal neurons. *Science* **243**:1721–1724.

Lovinger, D. M., White, G., and Weight F. F. (1990). NMDA receptor-mediated synaptic excitation selectively inhibited by ethanol in hippocampal slice from adult rat. *J. Neurosci.* **10**:1372–1379.

McQuilkin, S. J., and Harris, R. A. (1990). Factors affecting actions of ethanol on GABA-activated chloride channels. *Life Sci.* **46**:527–541.

Mehta, A. K., and Ticku, M. K. (1988). Ethanol potentiation of GABAergic transmission in cultured spinal cord neurons involves γ-aminobutyric acid$_A$-gated chloride channels. *J. Pharmacol. Exp. Ther.* **246**:558–564.

Messing, R. O., Carpenter, C. L., Diamond, I., and Greenberg, D. A. (1986). Ethanol regulates calcium channels in clonal neural cells. *Proc. Natl. Acad. Sci. (USA)* **83**:6213–6215.

Messing, R. O., Sneade, A. B., and Saridge B. (1990). Protein kinase C participates in up-regulation of dihydropyridine-sensitive calcium channels by ethanol. *J. Neurochem.* **55**:1383–1389.

Mhatre, M., and Ticku, M. K., (1989). Chronic treatment selectively increases the binding of inverse agonists for benzodiazepine binding sites in cultured spinal cord neurons. *J. Pharmacol. Exp. Ther.* **251**:164–168.

Miles, M. F., Diaz, J. E., DeGuzman, V. S. (1991). Mechanisms of neuronal adaptation to ethanol. *J. Biol. Chem.* **266**:2409–2414.

Mirsky, I. A., Piker, P., Rosenbaum, M., and Lederer, H. (1941). "Adaptation" of the central nervous system to varying concentrations of alcohol in the blood. *Q. J. Stud. Alcohol* **2**:35–45.

Mochly-Rosen, D., Chang, F-U., Cheever, L., Kim, M., Diamond, I., and Gordon, A. S. (1988). Chronic ethanol causes heterologous desensitization by reducing α_s mRNA. *Nature* **333**:848–850.

Mueller, G. C., Fleming, M. F., LeMahieu, M. A., Lybrand, G. S., and Barry, K. J. (1988). Synthesis of phosphatidylethanol—a potential marker for adult males at risk for alcoholism. *Proc. Natl. Acad. Sci. (USA)* **85**:9778–9782.

Mukherjee, A. B., Svoronos, S., Ghazanfari, A., Marin, P. R., Fisher, A., Roecklein, B., Rodbard, D., Staton, R., Behar, D., Berg, C. J., and Manjunath, R. (1987). Transketolase abnormality in cultured fibroblasts from familial chronic alcoholic men and their male offspring. *J. Clin. Invest.* **79**:1039–1043.

Nagy, L. E., Diamond, I., and Gordon, A. S. (1988). Cultured lymphocytes from alcoholics have altered cAMP signal transduction. *Proc. Natl. Acad. Sci. (USA)* **85**:6973–6976.

Nagy, L. E., Diamond, I., Collier, K., Lopez, L., Ullman, B., and Gordon, A. S. (1989). Adenosine is required for ethanol-induced heterologous desensitization. *Mol. Pharmacol.* **36**:744–748.

Nagy, L. E., Diamond, I., Casso, D. J., Franklin, C., and Gordon, A. S. (1990). Ethanol increases extracellular adenosine by inhibiting adenosine uptake via the nucleoside transporter. *J. Biol. Chem.* **265**:1946–1951.

Nagy, L. E., Diamond, I., Gordon, A. S. (1991). cAMP-dependent protein kinase regulates inhibition of adenosine transport by ethanol. *Mol. Pharmacol.* **40**:812–817.

Proctor, W. R., and Dunwiddie, T. V. (1984). Behavioral sensitivity to purinergic drugs parallels ethanol sensitivity in selectively bred mice. *Science* **224**:519–521.

Rabin, R. A. (1990). Direct effect of chronic ethanol exposure on β-adrenergic and adenosine-sensitive adenylate cyclase activities and cyclic AMP content in primary cerebellar cultures. *J. Neurochem.* **55**:122–128.

Rabin, R. A., and Molinoff, P. B. (1981). Activation of adenylate cyclase by ethanol in mouse striatal tissue. *J. Pharmacol. Exp. Ther.* **216**:129–134.

Reynolds, J. N., Wu, P. H., Khanna, J. M., Carlen, P. L. (1990). Ethanol tolerance in hippocampal neurons: Adaptive changes in cellular responses to ethanol measure in vitro. *J. Pharmacol. Exp. Ther.* **252:**265–271.

Ribeiro, J. A., and Sebastiao, A. M. (1986). Adenosine receptors and calcium: Basis for proposing a third (A_3) adenosine receptor. *Prog. Neurobiol.* **26:**179–209.

Richelson, E., Stenstrom, S., Forray, C., Enloe, L., and Pfenning, M. (1986). Effects of chronic exposure to ethanol on the prostaglandin E_1 receptor-mediated response and binding in a murine neuroblastoma clone (N1E-115). *J. Pharmacol. Exp. Ther.* **239:**687–692.

Rottenberg. H. (1986). Membrane solubility of ethanol in chronic alcoholism: The effect of ethanol feeding and its withdrawal on the protection by alcohol of rat red blood cells from hypnotic hemolysis. *Biochim. Biophys. Acta* **855:**211–222.

Saito, T. L., Lee, J. M., Hoffman, P. L., and Tabakoff, B. (1987). Effects of chronic ethanol treatment on the β-adrenergic receptor-coupled adenylate cyclase system of mouse cerebral cortex. *J. Neurochem.* **48:**1817–1822.

Sibley, D. R., and Lefkowitz, R. J. (1985). Molecular mechanisms of receptor desensitization using the β-adrenergic receptor-coupled adenylate cyclase system as a model. *Nature* **317:**124–129.

Skattebol, A., and Rabin, R. A. (1987). Effects of ethanol on $^{45}Ca^{2+}$ uptake in synaptosomes and in PC12 cells. *Biochem. Pharmacol.* **36:**2227–2229.

Smith, A. J. K., and Palmour, R. M. (1991). Lymphocyte adenosine A_2 receptors in abstinent alcoholics. Normal controls and families with multigenerational alcoholism. *Am. J. Hum. Genet.* **49:**517. 1991.

Snyder, S. H. (1985). Adenosine as a neuromodulator. *Ann. Rev. Neurosci.* **8:**103–124.

Stenstrom, S., Enloe, L., Pfenning, M., and Richelson, E. (1986). Acute effects of ethanol and other short-chain alcohols on the guanylate cyclase system of murine neuroblastoma cells (clone N1E-115). *J. Pharmacol. Exp. Ther.* **236:**458–463.

Sun, G. Y., and Sun, A. Y. (1985). Ethanol and membrane lipids. *Alcohol.: Clin. Exp. Res.* **9:**164–180.

Tabakoff, B., Hoffman, P. L., Lee, J. M., Saito, T., Willard, B., and DeLeon-Jones, F. (1988). Differences in platelet enzyme activity between alcoholics and nonalcoholics. *New Engl. J. Med.* **318:**134–139.

Taraschi, T. F., Ellingson, J. S., Wu, A., Zimmerman, R., and Rubin, E. (1986). Phosphatidylinositol from ethanol-fed rats confers membrane tolerance to ethanol. *Proc. Natl. Acad. Sci. (USA)* **83:**9398–9402.

Urso, T., Gavaler, J. S., and Van Thiel, D. H. (1981). Blood ethanol levels in sober alcohol users seen in an emergency room. *Life Sci.* **28:**1053–1056.

Valverius, P., Borg, S., Valverius, M. R., Hoffman, P. L., and Tabakoff, B. (1989). β-adrenergic receptor binding in brain of alcoholics. *Exp. Neurol.* **105:**280–286.

Victor, M., and Adams, R. D. (1953). The effect of ethanol on the nervous system. *Assoc. Res. Nerv. Ment. Dis.* **32:**526–573.

Wafford, K. A., Burnett, D. M., Dunwiddie, T. V., and Harris, R. A. (1990). Genetic differences in the ethanol sensitivity of GABA$_A$ receptors expressed in *Xenopus* oocytes. *Science* **249:**291–293.

Wafford, K. A., Burnett, D. M., Leidenheimer, N. G., Burt, D. R., Want, J. B., Kofuji, P., Dunwiddie, T. V., Harris, R. A., and Sikela, J. M. (1991). Ethanol sensitivity of the GABA$_A$ receptor expressed in *Xenopus* oocytes requires eight amino acids contained in the γ_{2L} subunit of the receptor complex. *Neuron* **7:**27–33.

11

Neurophysiological Phenotypic Factors in the Development of Alcoholism

HENRI BEGLEITER AND BERNICE PORJESZ

Alcoholism is clearly a genetically influenced disorder, but in many respects it is different from other disorders that follow a more traditional Mendelian mode of inheritance. In contrast to such disorders as cystic fibrosis, Huntington's chorea, and sickle-cell anemia, the development of alcoholism (at least in some individuals) depends on the interaction of genetically determined predisposing factors with environmentally determined precipitating factors. The search for genes is rather complicated because alcoholism is a common disorder with a number of features characteristic of complex diseases:

1. Clinical heterogeneity. Alcoholism has a variable age of onset and can involve a number of different symptoms. Because it might develop late in life, a person's status as an alcoholic could remain uncertain for a long period of time.
2. Reduced penetrance. Because of unknown genetic or environmental effects, not every individual who inherits the genes will develop the disorder.
3. Genetic heterogeneity. Single mutations at different genetic loci may result in clinically indistinguishable disease states.
4. Polygenic inheritance. The disorder might not be caused by any single gene, but could develop from additive effects of multiple genes.
5. Epistatic effects. The disorder might reflect the complex interactions between alleles at several loci.
6. Phenocopies. A substantial number of individuals without a disease genotype manifest alcoholism resulting from nongenetic causes.

The prospect for identifying genes involved in the predisposition toward alcoholism is clouded by these characteristics. Nevertheless, modern molecular genetic and data-analytic techniques make the search for genes underlying complex disorders quite feasible (Chapter 14 Wilson and Elston, this volume, Chapter 14; Ott, 1993). The quest for genetic factors in alcoholism would be greatly aided if it were possible to identify trait markers of a vulnerability for alcoholism.

While alcoholic patients are known to differ from nonalcoholics in many biological ways, such differences cannot be regarded as unique factors in the development of alcoholism. Indeed, any differences between alcoholic and nonalcoholic individuals do not just reflect potential antecedent factors, but are seriously confounded by such deleterious effects of drinking as tolerance, physical dependence, possible malnutrition, organ damage, and cognitive impairment. For these compelling reasons, the study of biologic factors leading to the development of alcoholism cannot be properly conducted in alcoholic patients.

Because of the solid evidence for genetic factors in the development of alcoholism, the study of offspring of alcoholic patients should provide an important sample of individuals known to be at risk for its development. Moreover, the selection of young males (Cloninger, 1987) from families with a history of alcoholism (Hill et al., 1988; Pihl et al., 1990), and studied long before the development of alcoholism, should provide an optimal sample of individuals at high risk. Such a sample may be ideal for studying antecedent factors in alcoholism. The longitudinal study of nonalcoholic individuals at high risk for developing alcoholism appears to provide the best cost/benefit ratio for identifying possible trait markers of vulnerability. Indeed, identification of either markers or risk factors should be quite valuable in the development of specific prevention and treatment initiatives.

The search for potential predisposing genetic markers in alcoholism must not only be conducted in individuals at high risk for developing alcoholism, but must meet a specific set of criteria critical for the identification of a genetically influenced marker as follows:

1. Individuals from the general population should demonstrate that the trait:
    (a) Can be reliably measured and is stable over time.
    (b) Is genetically transmitted.
    (c) The so-called "abnormal" trait has a low base rate in the general population.
    (d) The trait in question can identify individuals at risk with a significant degree of accuracy and reliability.
2. Studies in patients should demonstrate that the trait:
    (a) Is prevalent in the patient population.
    (b) Is present during symptom remission, and is not just a state marker.
    (c) Occurs among first-degree relatives of the proband at a rate higher than that of the normal population.
    d) Segregates with the illness in affected relatives of the proband.

Electroencephalography and Event-Related Brain Potentials

To date, several potentially critical risk markers have been investigated. Possibly the most intriguing data have come from a variety of studies investigating the electrical activity of the brain in both those at risk and controls. Some investigators have focused specifically on the spontaneous electrical activity of the brain, the electroencephalogram (EEG); others have examined the event-related brain potentials with the use of information-processing paradigms.

It is now well established that abstinent alcoholics manifest a number of EEG abnormalities, such as decreased alpha activity and increased delta, theta, and beta activity (for a review see Begleiter and Platz, 1972). Because these studies were conducted in abstinent alcoholics, it is difficult to determine if the EEG findings reflect the consequent deleterious effects of chronic alcohol intake or antecede the development of alcoholism. Indeed, many biological or behavioral anomalies observed in alcoholics reflect alterations in physiological and psychological systems constructed over many years of substantial ethanol intake.

Electroencephalogram Studies

In 1982 Gabrielli and his colleagues tested the hypothesis that young children (11–13 years of age) of alcoholic fathers manifest a higher percentage of fast EEG activity than children of nonalcoholic fathers. A number of EEG frequency bands were studied. However, only frequencies of 18–26 Hz and above showed absolute increases in activity. This EEG observation was characteristic of young males at high risk (HR) for alcoholism, although absolute increases in activity were also obtained for lower EEG amplitudes in each frequency band examined. It should be noted that the EEG amplitude findings in HR males were opposite to those observed in HR females. Although these investigators did not record the incidence and severity of other psychiatric disorders in the parents of the offsprings, they concluded that an excess of fast EEG activity may precede the development of alcohol abuse or alcoholism. Moreover, they suggest that this EEG pattern is heritable, and thus represents genetically influenced factors.

In a different study conducted by the same group of investigators, Pollock et al. (1983) examined several EEG frequencies including theta (3.51–7.03 Hz), slow alpha (7.42–9.46 Hz), fast alpha (9.75–12.10 Hz) energy, and mean alpha frequency in a sample of 19- to 21-year-old males at high and low risk for alcoholism. Risk for alcoholism was established by determining that each individual subject was the offspring of a father who had been in attendance at a psychiatric or alcoholism clinic. Drinking history was assessed for both HR and LR subjects, and was found not to differ significantly. In this study all subjects were administered a challenge dose of alcohol (0.5 g/kg). After alcohol ingestion HR individuals demonstrated greater decreases in fast alpha activity and greater increases in slow alpha activity. The decreases were obtained at 120 minutes postethanol, and the increases were observed at both 90 and 120 minutes postethanol.

Moreover, HR individuals manifested greater decreases in alpha frequency than did LR individuals at 30, 60, and 120 minutes post ethanol. In contrast to earlier findings by the same group (Gabrielli et al., 1982) reporting that HR subjects manifest increased beta activity before alcohol challenge, Pollock et al. (1983) did not find any EEG differences between HR and LR subjects before ethanol challenge. In a separate report, Pollock et al. (1984) did not replicate the findings earlier reported by Gabrielli et al. (1982). While the HR subjects did not differ from the LR subjects in terms of alcohol consumption, they reported a significant subjective tolerance effect compared to the LR subjects. These findings suggest the HR subjects are more sensitive to the physiological effects of alcohol, including decreased subjective alcohol effects.

At the University of Connecticut, investigators have also been examining possible EEG differences between HR and LR subjects. Kaplan et al. (1988) recorded EEG frequencies between 2 Hz and 20 Hz; delta, theta, alpha, and beta. The male subjects ranged in age between 20 and 28 years, and were all social drinkers. Subjects classified as HR had a father diagnosed as alcohol dependent (DSM III) with additional first- and/or second-degree relatives with a similar diagnosis. Subjects with an alcohol-abusing mother were excluded from both groups. The authors found no statistically significant EEG difference between the two groups.

Another group of investigators at the University of California at San Diego studied similar potential EEG differences (Ehlers and Schuckit, 1990a). They recruited males (21 to 25 years old) using a questionnaire to assess the presence or absence of alcoholism in their families. An HR subject was identified as an individual who indicated the presence of some symptoms of alcoholism in his father. Both HR and LR were carefully matched on a myriad of important variables. The authors examined EEG frequencies in the 9- to 12-Hz range and the 12- to 20-Hz range. They observed that HR subjects manifested more energy in the 9- to 12-Hz range than did the LR individuals.

In a second study the same authors (Ehlers and Schuckit, 1990b) found no difference between the two groups in the 12- to 20-Hz range. It is somewhat puzzling that differences were not found, since this particular study was designed to replicate the previous result, which indicated that significant differences between the two were present in the 18- to 26-Hz band. It appears as if the differences in this frequency range were not examined by the investigators. As part of the same investigation, the authors reported that LR subjects classified as moderate drinkers had significantly more power in the 12- to 20-Hz range than did those individuals classified as low drinkers. This interesting relationship was not evident in the HR subjects. In conclusion, the authors stated that both genetic factors and drinking history contribute to an individual's EEG characteristics.

It should be pointed out that both the Pollock and the Ehlers laboratories have investigated fast frequency alpha in subjects at high risk for alcoholism. However, the results appear to be quite different. For example, Ehlers and Schuckit (1990b) report less physiological responsiveness and sensitivity to ethanol in the HR group compared to the LR group, whereas Pollock and her coworkers (1983) report more responsiveness and more sensitivity. In spite of these physiological differences it should be noted that both groups find that HR subjects report feeling less intoxicated than LR subjects after a single dose of alcohol (Schuckit, 1980, 1984; Pollock et al., 1983).

The relationship between prechallenge baseline EEG and postethanol effects is particularly significant in assessing the effects of alcohol. Propping (1983) observed that subjects manifesting poor alpha activity prior to ethanol are the ones who demonstrate the most synchronization following ethanol ingestion. Individuals with average preethanol alpha activity exhibit minimal change after an alcohol challenge. Lukas et al. (1986) have demonstrated that the magnitude of ethanol-induced frequency decrease varies as a function of the baseline frequency.

The Genetic Influences. It is now well established that some aspects of the spontaneous EEG are under genetic influence. For example, Vogel (1970) has reported different genetic EEG variants. He has proposed that low-voltage and regular alpha follow an autosomal-dominant model of transmission, whereas poor alpha and diffuse beta are under polygenic control. Recent studies from Germany indicate that a specific variant of the EEG is represented by a major gene located on chromosome 20 (Steinlein et al., 1991).

In order to test possible differences in baseline EEG between HR and LR individuals we (Cohen et al., 1991) examined a wide range of EEG frequencies. Baseline EEG activity was recorded in a group of 19- to 24-year old individuals at risk for developing alcoholism as well as another group of well-matched LR individuals. The HR subjects were all individuals whose fathers were currently undergoing treatment for alcohol dependency (DSM 111-R criteria). Moreover, inclusion in the HR group required a high density of alcoholism in the family. In this group the average number of alcoholic relatives was 3.5 individuals. However, alcoholism in one's mother was cause for exclusion from the study. Candidates for the LR group were excluded if any first-or second-degree relatives was diagnosed as alcoholic. Any subject with major medical problems, taking medication, or with a history of psychiatric problems or drug abuse was excluded. A 128-second EEG record was obtained for each subject at each of the 21 electrodes in the 10–20 International System. A fast Fourier transform (FFT) was performed on the first 12, artifact-free, 4-second intervals. The resulting power spectral densities were summed and averaged at 0.25-Hz intervals over a range from 0.25 to 63.75 Hz. The integrals of power densities over frequency were calculated for the following frequency bands: slow alpha (SA: 7.5–10 Hz), fast alpha (FA: 10.25–12.75 Hz), slow beta (SB: 13–19.5 Hz), fast beta (FB-19.75-26 Hz). In this study, only EEG activity at electrodes P4, P3, O2, and O1 was examined. The initial selection of these electrode sites was dictated by the fact that they were common to most of the previous studies.

This study demonstrates that at the selected electrode sites, over a wide range of frequencies investigated, the EEG in HR individuals does not differ significantly from the EEG recorded from LR individuals.

While baseline EEG findings indicate significant interlaboratory discrepancies, we have recently completed a study (Cohen et al., 1993) in which, for the first time, the effects of two doses of alcohol were studied on both the ascending and descending limb of the blood alcohol curve. We hypothesized that HR individuals would manifest greater sensitivity to the reinforcing properties of alcohol on the ascending limb of the blood alcohol curve (Newlin and Thomson, 1990). Moreover, we also hypothesized that on the descending limb, the HR individuals would manifest greater acute tolerance compared to the LR individuals (Schuckit et al., 1987). In keeping with findings in the literature (Schuckit, 1985), we found no statistically significant differences in the blood alcohol levels for the LR versus HR individuals under both the low- and high-dose conditions. We observed significant group differences in slow alpha activity between the HR and LR groups under alcohol only. During the ascending phase of the blood alcohol curve (BAC), the slow alpha activity increased under both low- and high-dose conditions. This increase is in agreement with the findings by Lukas and his collaborators (1986), who asserted that the production of slow alpha suggests greater reinforcing properties. Our results demonstrate that the magnitude of the increases were significantly greater in the HR than the LR subjects during the ascending BAC. These novel findings suggest that the HR individuals are more sensitive to the reinforcing effects of alcohol than are the LR individuals. During the descending phase of the blood alcohol curve for the low-dose condition, both groups showed decreases in slow alpha activity, though the magnitude of this decrease was significantly greater in HR than in LR individuals. Similarly, under the high-dose condition, LR subjects continued to show slow alpha increases, while the HR subjects manifested decreases. These findings suggest that HR individuals might manifest greater acute tolerance to the effects of alcohol.

While the aforementioned data from our laboratory provide a novel set of observations regarding the effects of alcohol on the ascending and descending limbs of the blood alcohol curve, the interpretation of the findings is complicated by the fact that the HR and LR individuals were all social drinkers. It is not possible, with the data at hand, to conclude that the observed effects are the direct consequence of differential genetic sensitivity and acute tolerance between HR and LR individuals. Indeed, while the effects of alcohol on EEG are different between HR and LR subjects, depending on the phase of the blood alcohol curve, they could well reflect an interaction between innate sensitivity and tolerance, and an individual's experience with alcohol. The issue of differential innate sensitivity and tolerance between HR and LR subjects can best be tested in individuals without experience with alcohol.

The obvious disparity among baseline EEG findings from different laboratories as well as, in some cases, within laboratories might be explained by a number of factors. The ascertainment procedures for the recruitment of HR individuals varies greatly across laboratories. In some cases, college students (Ehlers and Schuckit, 1990a, 1990b) were selected and the presence of alcoholism in one relative determined with the use of a questionnaire. In other studies, the HR individuals were recruited through fathers attending treatment facilities for alcoholism, and the presence of multiple affected relatives was necessary (Cohen et al., 1991; Kaplan et al., 1988). These are indubitably the most disparate recruitment procedures, yet other investigators adopted still different procedures (Pollock et al., 1983). Possibly one of the most compelling explanations for divergent baseline EEG findings in HR subjects is the fact that the EEG is typically obtained under conditions in which the subject's task is poorly defined. As a result, the investigator has no control over the subject's mental activity, including attentional and motivational factors. While recording the EEG affords an opportunity of examining the spontaneous activity of the brain, the uncontrolled mentation could produce excessive variability in the derived EEG variables.

Event Related Potentials

The event-related potentials (ERPs) represent a set of neurophysiologic techniques generally sensitive to the functional integrity of the brain. In addition to being sensitive to sensory aspects of information processing, ERPs are quite useful in indexing neurophysiological concomitants of complex cognitive tasks (Hillyard et al., 1978; Donchin, 1979). ERPs consist of an amalgam of characteristic components that typically occur within 100 ms for basic sensory processes reflecting the physical attributes of a sensory stimulus. Components occurring after 100 ms are more influenced by psychological factors and the information-processing demands of the task. One of the major advantage of ERPs is that they can easily be recorded in conjunction with, or without, any behavioral response, as well as with both attended and unattended stimuli.

In recent years a great deal of attention has focused on the P3 component of the ERP. This is a positive component that occurs between 300 and 600 ms after stimulus, and is also related to stimulus significance. For the past two decades we have investigated the P3 component of the ERP in abstinent alcoholics using a variety of different paradigms. We have repeatedly observed that they manifest a significantly reduced P3 component compared to matched normal control subjects (Porjesz and Begleiter, 1985). These findings have been replicated by a number of different investigators (Patterson et al., 1987; Emmerson et al., 1987; Pfefferbaum et al., 1987; 1991; Branchey et al., 1988). It should be noted, however, that while other components of the ERP show significant differences between abstinent alcoholics and controls, the P3 component does not change much over long abstinence periods (Porjesz and Begleiter, 1985).

Because of the protracted anomaly of the P3 component in abstinent alcoholics, we hypothesized that a decrease in its voltage did not necessarily reflect the deleterious effects of chronic alcohol abuse. Instead, we examined the possibility that this anomaly anteceded the development of alcoholism in young males at risk. Starting in 1980, we initiated a series of neurophysiological studies in various groups of HR individuals. In our first study, we studied young boys between the ages of 7 and 13 who had no prior exposure to alcohol or any illicit drugs (Begleiter et al., 1984). We selected boys whose fathers had received a diagnosis of alcohol dependence (DSM lll) and were in treatment for alcoholism. Indeed it is important to note that all the HR subjects were recruited from treatment facilities. We excluded boys whose mothers had either ingested alcohol during pregnancy or who drank excessively after birth. The LR group consisted of healthy, normal boys matched to the HR subjects for age, socioeconomic status, and school grade. They were included in the study only if they had no prior experience with alcohol or other substances of abuse, and if they had no first- or second-degree relatives with a family history of alcoholism or other psychiatric disorder. With the exception of latter factor, the same exclusion criteria were used in both the LR and HR groups.

In this study a complex visual paradigm was developed. The target stimulus was an infrequently occurring aerial view of a head with the nose and either the left or right ear included, and rotated in one of two possible positions. This paradigm yielded four different targets, namely, nose up and right ear, nose up and left ear, nose down and right ear, and nose down and left ear. These target stimuli were randomly interspersed among nontargets (ovals). Subjects were required to press one of two microswitches to the targets, as quickly and accurately as possible, indicating whether the right or left ear stimulus was presented. The easy condition included all target stimuli with the nose up, and the difficult condition included all targets with the nose down.

The results of this experiment represent a novel set of observations in which we noted that the P3 amplitude was significantly smaller in the HR compared to the LR groups for all target stimuli. This group difference was most significant at the parietal electrode.

The study was the first to indicate that P3 amplitude is significantly reduced in young boys at high risk for alcoholism, without exposure to alcohol. This finding is quite interesting because it is so strikingly similar to ERP results obtained in abstinent alcoholics. Since our initial observation in HR subjects, a number of laboratories have replicated our observations. At the University of Connecticut, O'Connor and colleagues used the same visual stimuli and task, and reported that in a group of young adult males at risk for alcoholism the P3 amplitude was significantly reduced compared to a matched control group (O'Connor et al., 1986). Whipple et al. (1988) used a complex visual task in a group of young male subjects similar to subjects examined in our laboratory (Begleiter et al., 1984), and noted a significantly reduced P3 amplitude in the HR group compared to the LR group. In a subsequent study, Whipple et al. (1991) once again reported a decrease in P3 amplitude in young HR subjects, and noted that this finding can only be observed if a sufficiently challenging cognitive task is used in the ERP paradigm.

In yet another study by O'Connor et al. (1987) the authors reported a decrease in the amplitude of the P3 component of the ERP obtained in HR subjects. The investigators recorded the ERP in HR and LR males using two different visual tasks. In both conditions the P3 amplitude was significantly smaller in HR compared to LR individuals.

Begleiter et al. (1987) studied another group of sons of alcoholics to determine whether the reduced P3 amplitudes observed in past studies was modality or task specific. A modified auditory oddball task was used in which subjects pressed a button in response to rarely occurring tones presented at a random rate. Twenty-three matched pairs of HR and LR males between the ages of 7 and 16 were studied; all subjects were carefully interviewed to ascertain that they had no exposure to alcohol or illicit drugs. The HR subjects were all sons of alcoholic men who manifested early onset alcoholism, a high rate of recidivism, and were from families in which there was a multigenerational incidence of alcoholism. As in the previous visual study, the HR males manifested significantly reduced P3 amplitudes compared to the LR subjects. These findings suggest that the reduced P3 voltage typically observed in HR subjects may not be task or modality specific.

Most recently in another auditory target selection task, we noted that adolescent HR males manifest lower amplitude P3 voltage compared to LR individuals. In this paradigm (modified after Hillyard et al., 1978), rare or frequent tones were randomly presented rapidly (600–800 ms ISI) to either the right or the left ear. The rare tones to a specific ear were designated as targets, and the subjects pressed a button as quickly as possible. The same rare tones to the opposite ear were to be ignored. In the absence of other ERP differences between groups, HR subjects manifested reduced P3 amplitude components to target stimuli when compared to LR subjects. The amplitude to both the rare attended (P3b) and unattended (P3a) stimuli were of lower voltage in HR subjects, suggesting that HR individuals manifest greater difficulties in probability matching than LR subjects.

More recently we (Porjesz and Begleiter, 1990) attempted to again replicate our P3 findings in males between 19 and 24 years of age. The sample consisted of the offspring of carefully diagnosed (DSMlll-R/RDC) male alcoholics selected from high-density families (mean number of alcoholic family members = 4). While this procedure is not foolproof, it provides a modicum of safety against selecting children of male alcoholics considered to be sporadic cases. Individuals with mothers who abused alcohol before, during, or after pregnancy were excluded. Controls were matched to the sons of male alcoholics on the basis of age, education, and socioeconomic status. They were selected from families in which there was no history of alcohol abuse or alcoholism in any first- or second-degree relatives. The HR and LR subjects were carefully matched on drinking history, including duration and quantity–frequency information.

In this experiment we used a visual task that consisted of an easy and difficult line orientation discrimination. We have in the past demonstrated that abstinent alcoholics manifest significantly reduced P3 with the use of this paradigm. The stimuli consisted of a nontarget (vertical line) and two different targets: an easy discrimination target that deviated from the vertical by 90° (horizontal line), and a difficult discrimination target that deviated from the vertical by only 3°. The subject performed a reaction time task (RT), responding as quickly as possible to all nonvertical stimuli. In this study, we replicated our previous findings (Begleiter et al., 1984, 1987) of significantly decreased P3 voltage in HR individuals compared to LR subjects. This finding was obtained in an older group of HR and LR subjects and replicates the work of O'Connor and his colleagues (1986, 1987). The largest difference in P3 voltage was obtained from the easily discriminable target, and is identical to our results with abstinent alcoholics (Porjesz et al., 1987). This P3 voltage difference was most significant at the Pz and Cz electrodes where P3 amplitude is typically maximum. Taken together these data indicate that with the use of a moderately challenging visual task the P3 voltage is significantly reduced in HR individuals compared to LR subjects.

Taken together, the ERP findings discussed so far indicate that P3 amplitude of the ERP is significantly reduced in HR compared to LR subjects. These results relate to both attended (P3b) and unattended (P3a) stimuli, and may be present in visual and auditory studies.

Some Conflicting Studies

Despite the general consensus that P3 amplitude is of lower voltage in HR than in LR subjects, there are some studies that have failed to replicate these findings. In various studies conducted by investigators in California, conflicting ERP results have been reported. One early study by Elmasian et al. (1982) examined the P3 and slow-wave components of the ERP in HR and LR male college students (age 20–25) under placebo, low, and high doses of alcohol. It should be noted that different groups, each consisting of only five pairs of subjects, were used for each dose. After alcohol or placebo administration, significantly lower P3 amplitudes were observed in the HR as compared to the LR subjects. The authors explained their results in terms of differential expectancies for alcohol characterized by different neuroelectric events. Moreover, the investigators suggested that the findings could be due to the higher than normal alcohol intake in the mothers of the HR subjects.

Investigating ERPs in male college students with and without family histories of alcoholism, Polich and Bloom (1987, 1988) and Schuckit et al. (1988) did not find P3 amplitude differences between groups. Further, using a simple auditory oddball paradigm, Schuckit et al. (1988) did not find any ERP differences between HR and LR individuals before or after placebo and ethanol. Following a high dose of ethanol (1.1 ml/kg), P3 latency delays returned to baseline values more rapidly in the HR subjects. It should be noted that the initial placebo effects observed in HR subjects by Elmasian et al. (1982) could not be replicated by this group (Polich and Bloom, 1988). However, the ERP results of all these studies were all obtained with relatively small samples.

An inverse relationship between the amount of alcohol consumption and the amplitude of P3 was reported by Polich and Bloom (1987) without the administration of ethanol in the laboratory. However, this relationship was only apparent for a difficult intensity discrimination task in the HR subjects. The authors conclude that the HR subjects are more sensitive to the effects of ethanol than the LR subjects. When a similar intensity discrimination study was carried out in the visual modality, no correlation between P3 characteristics and amount of alcohol consumed was found (Polich et al., 1988). Furthermore, in yet another study designed to replicate Elmasian et al. (1982), Polich and Bloom (1988) not only did not replicate their previous findings of a placebo effect in the HR group, but in addition they noted a correlation between P3 latency and amount of alcohol consumed. Taken together, these findings relating alcohol consumption to P3 characteristics do not appear to be robust.

In the same laboratory, using samples drawn from the same population at the University of California San Diego, the ERP findings are not readily replicable. Previous alcohol consumption has been found to correlate with P3 amplitude only, particularly in HR subjects (Polich and Bloom, 1987), to correlate with P3 latency only (Polich and Bloom, 1988), and to be uncorrelated with any previous drinking variables (Polich et al, 1988). The relationship between P3 characteristics and drinking history has also produced contradictory findings in other laboratories. O'Connor et al (1986) reported no relationship between any P3 characteristics and drinking history, while Steinhauer et al. (1987) found such a correlation. In addition to correlations between P3 characteristics and drinking history, Schmidt and Neville (1985) have reported a correlation between the N430 latency and the number of drinks ingested per occasion in HR subjects only.

Baribeau et al. (1987) examined HR and LR subjects, who were further subdivided according to the amount of alcohol consumed (heavy vs. light drinkers). They used an auditory selective attention paradigm in which rare and frequent tones were randomly presented to either the right or left ear at an irregular rate. Subjects were instructed to count the targets in one designated ear and ignore those in the other ear. Although the light drinkers did not exhibit reduced P3 amplitude, they did manifest somewhat smaller P3 voltages in the inattention condition. High-risk subjects manifested significantly larger N100 components than LR subjects in the attention condition, which suggests that the HR subjects may have found the tone discrimination task to be difficult, and hence needed to muster greater resources. It appears that the subject sample used in this study is somewhat atypical since it represents an older group of HR individuals, with an age range of (19–35) and a mean age of 27 (HR: heavy drinking), 22 (HR: light drinking, 24 (LR: heavy-drinking), and 25 (LR: light-drinking). It is certainly reasonable to assume that this older group of HR subjects has already passed the age when alcoholism develops, and thus represents an atypical sample of HR, perhaps endowed not with risk factors but with protective mechanisms. In fact, the increase in the N100 component above that obtained for the LR subjects suggests the presence of atypical factors. A study by Hill et al. (1988) reports increased cognitive efficiency in nonaffected siblings of alcoholics. These investigators observed shorter P3 latencies in the nonaffected siblings of alcoholics, and suggest that this phenomenon may indicate the presence of protective factors against the development of alcoholism.

More recently, we (Porjesz and Begleiter, 1992) investigated the effects of alcohol on visual ERPs in HR and LR subjects. Twenty-four pairs of male HR and LR subjects (19–24 years of age) were administered a placebo, a low dose of alcohol (0.5 ml/kg), and a high dose (0.8 ml/kg) mixed with three parts of ginger ale on three separate randomly determined occasions. A visual ERP paradigm involving easy and difficult line orientation discrimination was used. ERPs and subjective measures of intoxication were recorded preethanol and after 20, 60, 90, and 130 minutes following alcohol ingestion. Blood alcohol levels were recorded at 10 minute intervals throughout the entire experiment, but no significant differences were obtained between groups in terms of blood alcohol curves.

As mentioned earlier, before alcohol ingestion the amplitude of P3 to all target stimuli was significantly smaller in the HR compared to the LR subjects. Alcohol ingestion did not affect the difference in P3 amplitude initially observed between the two groups. While there was a tendency for alcohol to decrease the amplitude of the P3 component of the ERP in both groups, this finding did not reach statistical significance. During the ascending phase of the blood alcohol level, however, the HR group manifested a significantly larger percent decrement in P3 amplitude to all targets, compared to the LR group. This interesting finding perhaps indicates greater sensitization to alcohol in the HR subjects on the ascending limb of the blood alcohol curve (Newlin and Thomson, 1990).

We have obtained similar findings with slow alpha EEG activity in our laboratory (Cohen et al., 1993), where we found more of an increase in the HR group following an alcohol challenge. It should be noted that while no significant difference in P3 latency occurred between groups prior to alcohol ingestion, the high dose of alcohol significantly increased the latency of P3 to the difficult target in both groups of subjects. This effect was maximal between 60 and 90 minutes postethanol, namely at peak and early descending phase of the blood alcohol curve. The HR group recovered more rapidly to prealcohol levels in contrast to the LR subjects, who manifested a delay that lasted the length of the postethanol experiment. These findings replicate the results of Schuckit et al. (1988), who noted that HR subjects recover more quickly from ethanol-induced P3 delays. This result suggests that on the descending limb of the blood alcohol curve, HR subjects manifest a faster recovery (tolerance) to the effects of alcohol.

In this experiment, the N1 amplitude of the ERP was significantly decreased by alcohol starting at 20 minutes, particularly to the nontarget stimulus. This result was more pronounced at occipital sites for the LR compared to the HR group. While the N1 amplitude to nontargets remained depressed in the LR group throughout the experiment, it recovered by 90 minutes for the HR group. Once again, these results suggest that the HR subjects manifest more tolerance to alcohol compared to the LR group. The N1 amplitude did not decrease to the difficult target, and was only somewhat decreased to the easy target. These results are in agreement with the findings by Roth et al. (1977), indicating that attentional factors can vitiate the actions of alcohol on the N1 amplitude of the ERP. These findings also support the observations of Campbell and Lowick (1987) that indicate that the largest alcohol effects are typically obtained when attention is mobilized the least (to nontargets). The differential effects of alcohol on N1 amplitude between HR and LR groups are quite similar to the behavioral effects reported by Schuckit (1984), which suggest that the HR subjects exhibit more acute tolerance to alcohol than the LR group. It is quite obvious for the aforementioned data that ERP measures provide very sensitive indices of state and trait variables related to alcohol ingestion and alcoholism. Different ERP characteristics are sensitive to different aspects of this multifaceted problem.

Because of the striking similarity in P3 findings between abstinent alcoholics and sons of alcoholics, we decided to investigate the integrity of the brainstem potentials in young boys at risk for alcoholism. We had in the past observed brainstem anomalies in abstinent alcoholics (Begleiter et al., 1981). For our experiment, we recorded the auditory brainstem potentials in 23 sons of alcoholics (7–13 years old) and 23 control boys matched for age, socioeconomic status, and school grade. In contrast to the P3 amplitude findings, no significant difference in the brainstem potentials were noted between HR and LR boys. These results suggest that the brainstem abnormalities represent a potential state marker, that is, the consequence of alcohol abuse. In contrast, the significantly low-voltage P3 in both abstinent alcoholics and HR subjects seemingly antecedes the development of alcoholism, and may be considered a potential trait marker.

Conclusion

A review of the ERP data in individuals at risk for developing alcoholism indicates that the P3 component is characterized by low voltage. Except in a few studies noted earlier, this finding is quite robust. Indeed, in a recent meta-analysis of all ERP studies in HR and LR subjects, Polich et al. (1994) conclude that the amplitude of the P3 component of the ERP reliably discriminates between HR and LR subjects. Recently, Pfefferbaum et al. (1991) conducted a path analysis using family history of alcoholism and drinking history to predict the amplitude of P3 in abstinent alcoholics, concluding that family history is in fact the only significant predictor. These interesting data provide an important link between P3 studies of alcoholics and subjects at risk for alcoholism, indicating that P3 characteristics are genetically influenced and supporting the notion that low P3 voltages in HR individuals represent a trait rather than a characteristic state. There is substantial evidence indicating that several neurophysiological characteristics (EEG, ERP) are under genetic control. The P3 component has been demonstrated to be significantly more similar in MZ twins than in control subjects (Polich and Burns, 1987). In addition, ERP's deficits have been reported to be similar in abstinent alcoholic fathers and their young sons (Whipple et al. 1988). The aforementioned data suggest that the reduced P3 voltage may provide a phenotypic marker for alcoholism. It remains to be determined with longitudinal studies, however, whether HR subjects manifesting low P3 voltages are in fact those who in subsequent years develop alcoholism, drug abuse, or other psychiatric conditions.

Behavioral Reaction to Alcohol

Another promising area of research that has produced interesting findings deals with the subjective behavioral reaction of subjects at high risk to a challenge dose of alcohol. Much of this research has been carried out by Schuckit and his colleagues at the University of California at San Diego. Schuckit (1980) was the first to note that HR men reported significantly lower levels of subjective feelings of intoxication after drinking. In his studies, carried out since 1978, a questionnaire has been used to identify male students and staff at the university at elevated risk for alcoholism. The questionnaire uses a highly structured format to collect information on demographic variables as well as pattern of alcohol and drug intake. In addition, personal, medical and psychiatric information, and family history of major psychiatric disorders are all collected. From these completed questionnaires, those sons of alcoholics, who were drinkers but had not experienced major life problems from alcohol, drugs, or other psychiatric problems were selected as subjects at high risk for developing alcoholism. It should be noted that all HR subjects were carefully matched with LR subjects on several important variables including age, sex, race, educational level, quantity and frequency of drinking, substance intake history, height-to-weight ratio, and smoking history.

All individuals selected for this series of studies were tested on three separate occasions with a placebo, 0.75 ml/kg of ethanol, and 1.1 ml/kg of ethanol. The ethanol was given as a 20% by volume solution in a sugar-free, noncaffeinated beverage, which was consumed over a 10-minute period. Before any liquid was administered, all subjects were tested on a variety of cognitive and psychomotor tasks, mood, and anxiety scales, to establish baseline levels of functioning. After ingesting each beverage all subjects were tested for a period of 4 hours in order to note their subjective reactions to the placebo or the two doses of alcohol. Before challenges, both the HR and LR subjects reported similar expectations to the effects of alcohol. After ethanol ingestion, both groups manifested similar blood alcohol curves. Nevertheless, after drinking 0.75 ml/kg of ethanol, approximately 40% of the HR subjects reported feeling less intoxicated than did the LR subjects.

In addition to a decreased level of subjective intoxication in HR subjects compared to LR subjects, similar findings were obtained with a measure of body sway. While there were no differences in body sway before or after placebo administration between HR and LR subjects, significant differences emerged subsequent to the ethanol challenge. The LR subjects manifested a significantly greater increase in body sway after drinking the 0.75ml/kg dose of ethanol than did the HR group (Schuckit, 1985).

Most of the work investigating subjective intoxication after a challenge dose of ethanol in HR and LR individuals has been conducted by Schuckit and his colleagues (Schuckit et al., 1991a; 1991b; Schuckit, 1992). A number of studies by other investigators have been reviewed by Pollock (1992) and Newlin and Thomson (1990). It should be noted that the metaanalysis by Pollock (1992) reviews all the published studies that utilize a challenge dose of alcohol in HR and LR subjects. The author concludes that data from several studies support a less intense alcohol reaction in the group of males at risk of developing alcoholism.

In order to determine the pharmacological specificity of this effect, Schuckit and his colleagues compared the challenge effects of ethanol and diazepam (0.1 and 0.2 mg/kg of diazepam) in a large group of HR and LR subjects. In contrast to the results with the alcohol challenge, the diazepam challenge did not differentiate the two groups at high and low risk for developing alcoholism. This suggested to the authors that the postchallenge effects between HR and LR are indeed specific to alcohol. The authors further speculated that a decreased intensity of reaction to low doses of alcohol would make it more difficult for HR individuals to identify an oncoming state of intoxication. A deficient ability to detect a state of intoxication in oneself could seriously jeapordize one's ability to stop drinking and lead to drunkeness followed by stupor. With the currently available data it is not possible to determine if HR subjects manifest more innate tolerance to the effects of alcohol or are indeed more insensitive to its pharmacological effects. All the subjects recruited in these studies are at least in their 20s and all are social drinkers so it is quite likely that the presence of innate tolerance in HR subjects is interacting with varying degrees of exposure to alcohol.

Now, some 8 to 12 years after the initial study, Schuckit and his colleagues are carrying out a follow-up study to interview the majority of subjects tested. Although this study is currently in progress, some intriguing preliminary results are already available. For example, a decreased intensity of reaction to alcohol, as initially assessed, appears to be a reliable predictor of alcohol abuse. Moreover, the current data also indicate a potential trend toward subsequent cocaine and marijuana problems.

Neuropsychological Deficits

A number of studies have suggested that sons of alcoholics have difficulty attributing meaning to potentially relevant stimuli, resulting in a characteristic pattern of hyperactivity. Alcohol consumption serves a salutory function by significantly reducing this pattern.

For several decades investigators have reported that sons of alcoholics are characterized by excessive impulsivity (Cadoret et al., 1980; Tarter et al., 1984b; Knop et al., 1985), while others have described sons of alcoholics as hyperactive (Cantwell, 1972; Morrison and Stewart, 1973; Goodwin et al., 1975; Rydelius, 1981; 1983; Alterman et al., 1982; Tarter et al., 1984). In general, these studies depict sons of alcoholics as individuals who are unable to alter their behavior in ways commensurate with social expectations and mores. More recently Cloninger (1987) has identified a number of behavioral characteristics typical of sons of alcoholics, describing them as low in reward-dependence, high in novelty-seeking, and low in harm-avoidance. These traits imply that they are socially detached, impulsive, and overly confident. Moreover, Cloninger (1987) asserts that these traits are genetically influenced, and render sons of alcoholics particularly susceptible to the development of alcoholism.

A number of investigators have argued that the behavioral characteristics that have been identified in sons of alcoholics are the result of deviations in temperamental traits (Tarter et al., 1985; Zucker and Lisansky-Gomberg, 1986; Johnson and Rolf, 1990). These authors have proposed a developmental approach, and suggested that some of these temperamental traits are genetically determined (Plomin, 1983).

A group of investigators at McGill University have conducted a series of studies to assess the information-processing characteristics of sons of alcoholics. With the use of psychophysiological measures the Montreal investigators have found that sons of alcoholics manifest significant hyperactivity to external stimulation. Finn and Pihl (1987, 1988) reported that young nonalcoholic sons of alcoholics with extensive multigenerational family histories of alcoholism were characterized by increased heart rate and decreased digital blood volume amplitude (DBVA) when anticipating and receiving mild electric shock. In a subsequent study, Finn et al. (1990) observed the same pattern of cardiovascular hyperreactivity among HR subjects before and after receiving avoidable and unavoidable signaled electric shock. Moreover, these subjects manifested larger electrodermal orienting responses, shorter latency responses, and slower rates of habituation to novel nonaversive stimuli. In addition to these abnormalities in cued psychophysiological responses, HR individuals manifest an increased sensitivity to the stress-response dampening effects of alcohol intake.

The first study assessing the effects of alcohol on psychophysiological measures was conducted by Sher and Levenson (1982). The authors found that HR subjects were characterized by increased baseline heart rate after administration of alcohol and by decreased heart acceleration in response to stressors. In a subsequent study, Levenson et al. (1987) observed that alcohol ingestion reduced some aspects of cardiovascular reactivity as well as general somatic activity to self-disclosing speech and electric shock in HR individuals.

Alcohol has been consistently shown to normalize the exaggerated stress response typically manifested by HR subjects. A number of investigators have reported that alcohol intoxication dampens the psychophysiological responses of HR to aversive stimulation (Finn and Pihl, 1987; 1988; Finn et al., 1990; Peterson et al., 1990). It should be noted that abstinent alcoholics manifest significant reduction in electrodermal reactivity (Coopersmith and Woodrow, 1967; Garfield and McBreaty, 1970) after alcohol ingestion. Taken together, the findings in abstinent alcoholics and HR subjects suggest that alcohol has a major salutory effect in that it significantly reduces the effects of various stressors. In the short term, the consumption of alcohol by HR individuals may be perceived as an adaptive means to cope with unpleasant situations. The alcohol effects just described indicate that HR subjects may find alcohol more reinforcing than LR individuals. This is quite consistent with findings by Cohen et al. (1993) and by Porjesz and Begleiter (1993), who reported that HR individuals manifest sensitization on the ascending limb of the blood alcohol curve and tolerance on the descending limb of the blood alcohol curve.

The neuropsychological findings summarized earlier have resulted in a rather consistent set of inferences that attempt to relate the behavioral characteristics of HR subjects to potential brain processes. Several authors, such as Tarter et al. (1984a; 1988), Pihl et al. (1987), Gorenstein (1987), Peterson and Pihl (1990), have postulated that the pattern of behavioral deficits typically manifested by HR subjects is quite analogous to that displayed by individuals with dysfunction of the prefrontal cortex. This notion has of late received substantial support from an elegant study by Peterson et al. (in press), who have reported a significant relationship between the performance of HR subjects on two tests of prefrontal cortex function [Self-ordered Pointing test (Petrides and Milner, 1987) and Wisconsin Card Sort Test (Milner, 1964)], and their cardiovascular hyperreactivity to anticipation and receipt of electric shock.

Individuals who manifest dysfunction of prefrontal cortex typically manifest impulsivity, hyperactivity, antisocial behavior, and a strong tendency to avoid stimuli with delayed gratification (Luria, 1980; Damasio, 1986). Such individuals have difficulties with moderate to long attention span, and are quite prone to conduct disorder. Zucker and Lisansky-Gomberg (1986) and Sher (1992) have noted that individuals who develop serious difficulties with alcohol typically demonstrate poor school performance, more truancy, and completion of fewer school years.

Conclusion

As of now, a review of the literature on males at risk of developing alcoholism indicates that two specific set of features are characteristically observed in those individuals without the use of alcohol.

1. Specifically, in the absence of alcohol, HR males manifest neurophysiological characteristics, such as a significantly reduced amplitude of the P3 component of the ERP. This finding reflects an inability of HR subjects to differentiate relevant from irrelevant stimuli. While this robust finding has been replicated in many different laboratories with different experimental paradigms, the lack of unanimity among them can in part be attributed to differences in subject populations (see metanalysis by Polich et al., 1994). The clinical criteria for diagnosis of alcoholism in the father and the general method of diagnostic assessment contribute considerably to differences in the samples studied. For example, some studies require only one symptom of alcoholism for the father to quality for inclusion in the HR group. The number of affected relatives varies

greatly across studies. Some investigators select HR individuals from families where only a single individual manifests symptoms of alcoholism, while others select only HR subjects from multigenerational or high-density families. The selection of HR subjects from families where only one individual is affected increases the risk of selecting an individual from a family where alcoholism is not genetically influenced, but represents a sporadic case or phenocopy.

The issue of comorbidity for other psychiatric problems is also treated quite differently by various investigators. Some assert that alcoholism is a single, unique disorder that must be studied in the absence of other potentially confounding psychiatric disorders, while others maintain that it may not be a single and unique entity devoid of influence by other psychiatric disorders such as antisocial personality and anxiety disorders. As a result, some studies include HR individuals who manifest antisocial behavior or other psychiatric symptoms, while others clearly exclude such individuals. Because alcoholism is such a heterogeneous disease, the inclusion or exclusion of individuals in HR studies is quite likely to vary significantly across studies, and thus have a significant effect on outcome findings.

Another variable that is highly likely to influence study outcome is the age range of the selected population. In a study of traits potentially relevant to the development of alcoholism, it is critical to select subjects before they pass through the age of maximal risk. The selection of somewhat older individuals (25–40 years of age) is likely to yield a sample comprising subjects who may manifest protective factors instead of risk factors. Several investigators have published data obtained in a sample of older individuals. In addition, there are a number of demographic and environmental variables, such as education, scholastic achievement, socioeconomic status, nutritional deficiencies, and home environment, that could potentially influence the search for risk factors. It is quite obvious that subject selection remains a major problem in the conduct of research designed to identify markers for the development of alcoholism in HR individuals. Nevertheless, it is quite remarkable that in light of all of the aforementioned problems, there exists a substantial body of neurophysiological research indicating that HR individuals may be reliably differentiated from LR individuals.

2. Several psychophysiological characteristics differentiate HR from LR individuals. As reviewed earlier, a number of studies have demonstrated that HR subjects show increased heart rate and decreased digital blood volume amplitude when anticipating or faced with unpleasant stimuli. This pattern of cardiovascular hyperreactivity is indicative of impaired autonomic regulation. These data are seemingly consistent with the neurophysiological findings and indicate that HR subjects have difficulty placing potentially relevant stimuli into a meaningful context. This inability (reduced P3) leads to inappropriate autonomic reactivity (cardiovascular hypperreactivity). The affective/motivational response of HR subjects to internal and external stimuli is not commensurate with the significance of such stimuli. Some authors have elected to interpret this emotional instability to be concommitant with the development of temperamental traits that may be genetically influenced. It has been postulated that the hyperactivity, disinhibition, and emotional lability observed in HR subjects reflect a dysfunction of neural systems in the prefrontal region of the brain.

The second set of characteristics that differentiate HR from LR individuals is observed in response to a challenge dose of alcohol. Several studies indicate that after such a dose HR subjects report a less intense subjective reaction on the descending limb of the blood alcohol curve when compared to LR individuals. This finding implies that HR subjects may be more tolerant or more insensitive to the negative effects of alcohol. Because social drinkers are typically used in these studies, it is difficult to attribute the results to the potential presence of innate tolerance. Nevertheless, these results imply that this decreased subjective feeling of intoxication could lead to an inability to cease drinking alcohol.

Another group of studies indicates that HR individuals are particularly sensitive to the stress-dampening effects of alcohol. Indeed, for HR subjects alcohol reduces stress and normalizes their autonomic responses. For this group of individuals, alcohol appears to have an adaptive if not salutory effect. While studies that assess the subjective reaction to alcohol find a decreased effect in HR subjects, those studies that measure its stress-dampening effects find increased sensitization in HR subjects.

This seeming discrepancy can be explained by the differential time of measurement between these studies. For example, some studies record the dependent variables on the ascending limb of the blood alcohol curve, while others obtain their measures on the descending limb. It is important to note that recent neurophysiological studies indicate that subsequent to a dose of alcohol, HR subjects manifest increased sensitization on the ascending limb of the blood alcohol curve. Since this sensitization is only seen on the ascending limb, it might be speculated that HR subjects find the effects of alcohol more positively reinforcing than do the LR subjects. This would naturally lead to increased alcohol ingestion. On the descending limb of the blood alcohol curve the alcohol effects that differentiate the HR from the LR subjects are quite different from those on the ascending limb. Indeed, on the descending limb, the HR subjects manifest more tolerance or insensitivity to the effects of alcohol, which indicates that they are less sensitive to the detrimental or negative effects of alcohol.

In general, the behavioral, psychophysiological, and neurophysiological findings in HR subjects in response to a challenge dose of alcohol are interesting. The potential discrepancy between those studies that purport to find tolerance and those that indicate greater sensitization may easily be resolved by studying all individuals on both the ascending and descending limbs of the blood alcohol curve.

At present, the neurophysiological and psychophysiological data obtained in the absence of alcohol, and the behavioral, psychophysiological, and neurophysiological data obtained in response to a challenge dose of alcohol best differentiates HR from LR subjects. Taken together these data strongly support the conclusion that objective quantifiable measures differentiate reliably between them.

While the aforementioned findings may have identified a number of putative markers, several questions remain unanswered. With the exception of the neurophysiological variables, the heritability of the measures reviewed previously is not established. Therefore, these measures (i.e., subjective reaction to alcohol and stress-dampening effects of alcohol) do not meet the criteria for a genetic marker as defined at the beginning of this chapter.

This issue does not vitiate the potential use of these measures in predicting subsequent alcoholism or drug abuse. It does, however, limit the use of these measures in searching for the genes involved in the predisposition toward alcoholism. The most efficacious search for the genetic predisposition toward alcoholism must of necessity involve reliable and highly heritable markers. However, it is critical to remember that heritable biological factors will most likely not elucidate all of the etiological factors involved in alcoholism. The final development of alcoholism most probably represents the interaction between biological and environmental factors.

While the group of putative markers reviewed earlier does differentiate HR from LR subjects reliably, it remains to be determined whether these putative markers are related to one another, and the potential nature of this relationship. To date, not a single study has attempted to study all of the potential markers in one set of subjects. It should be noted, however, that different groups of investigators select HR and LR subjects using different ascertainment and assessment procedures. To the extent that alcoholism is a clinically heterogeneous condition, it may well be that various investigators are studying different subgroups of this disorder. Nevertheless, it would be of great importance to study all of the putative markers in one group to assess their relationships, and to better delineate the potential characteristics of different subgroups of individuals at risk to develop alcoholism.

Despite the diversity of ascertainment and assessment procedures, the use of various dependent variables, and the different time of testing on the ascending and descending limb of the blood alcohol curve, an interesting pattern of results is emerging from the myriad of studies reviewed here. In general, sons of alcoholics (HR) manifest impaired neurophysiological, autonomic, and behavioral regulation. They demonstrate an inability to differentiate relevant from irrelevant stimuli, are insensitive to interoceptive cues, and are hyperreactive to seemingly threatening or noxious stimuli. Alcohol consumption significantly reduces the negative consequences of this impaired regulation, and in that sense, appears to have greater rewarding properties for the HR as compared to the LR individuals. These greater reinforcing properties may thus lead to increased drinking on the part of the HR individuals. For example, the behavioral studies suggest that HR subjects are more insensitive or tolerant to the negative effects of alcohol intake on the descending limb of the blood alcohol curve. This decreased intensity of reaction to alcohol in HR subjects would prevent them from experiencing both the short- and long-term negative consequences of drinking. This inability to fully experience the negative consequences of alcohol could also lead to increased alcohol intake.

The notion of increased sensitization on the ascending limb of the blood alcohol curve and decreased reaction on the descending limb of the blood alcohol curve (Newlin and Thomson, 1990) is supported by recent neurophysiological studies in HR subjects. In that sense, sons of alcoholics are at high risk of developing alcoholism because they are quite susceptible to the immediate short-term reinforcing properties of alcohol, and are impervious to the negative consequences of alcohol intoxication. This impairment of behavioral regulation leads the HR individual to seek short-term gratification at the expense of long-term detriment. As drinking progresses and dependence develops, behavioral dysregulation becomes exacerbated, resulting in the progressive loss of control.

Some authors (Tarter et al., 1984) have suggested a developmental deficit in temperament based on a disturbance in arousal, while others (Cloninger, 1987) have proposed that HR individuals possess a number of specific heritable personality traits. While behavioral dysregulation is characteristic of alcoholism, it is not specific to this disorder. Indeed, behavioral dysregulation is typical of all of the addictive disorders. It has been proposed (Miller and Brown, 1992) that risk for alcohol and other drug abuse occurs in conjunction with behavioral problems characteristic of impairment in self-regulatory control. These authors suggested that risk markers for self-regulatory problems might include poor academic work, impulsive–aggressive behavior accompanied by disciplinary problems, and a variety of reckless driving offenses as young adults. It is of fundamental significance to note that poor attention span, impulsivity, insensitivity to interoceptive cues, hyperreactivity to potentially noxious stimuli, and risk-taking are typically found in HR individuals. All of these signs suggest a pattern of regulatory processes that are seemingly impaired in individuals at risk to develop alcoholism. Moreover, it is critical to note that for HR subjects, alcohol or drug use may well serve adaptive functions, which tend to normalize various processes (Kissin and Hankoff, 1959). For individuals at risk of developing alcoholism, the use of alcohol may have short-term salutory effects.

In reviewing the literature on HR individuals we have attempted to cull findings from research areas that provide the largest and most consistent body of data. To be sure, we have excluded some findings not as a result of bias, but primarily because several findings are quite preliminary, or are represented by just a few isolated results that could not be properly assessed at this time. As can be seen from this review, most of the data in this area of research have been published in the last decade. Indeed, it is quite remarkable how productive this research area has been in just ten years. As mentioned earlier, several findings appear to be quite reliable and promising. As a result, there is currently some cause for cautious optimism.

A number of interesting parallels are beginning to emerge between the HR findings and the results obtained with genetically bred strains of rodents. HR individuals manifest sensitization to alcohol on the ascending limb of the blood alcohol curve and tolerance on the descending limb of the blood alcohol curve; an identical set of findings obtains with rats genetically bred to manifest preference for alcohol (Lumeng et al., this volume). We have reviewed the neurophysiological deficits in HR individuals. There are a number of neurophysiological deficits that have been noted in genetically bred rats preferring alcohol when compared to nonpreferring rats (Marzoratti et al., 1988; Ehlers et al., 1991). While it is not currently possible to equate or even compare the human and animal neurophysiological data, the presence of anomalies in both species is potentially important.

It is interesting to note that rats preferring alcohol manifest increased motoric activity to a novel environment compared to nonpreferring rats, since hyperactivity has been noted in subjects at risk to develop alcoholism. While some interesting similarities are beginning to emerge between the human and animal research, it would be quite premature, if not inappropriate, to assume identity. While much remains to be done before valid similarities can be established, these interesting data provide an unprecented window of opportunity that is likely to guide research for the next decade.

The identification of valid and reliable genetic markers of risk to develop alcoholism has begun in earnest, and is critical to the search for the genes that influence the development of alcohol dependence. Several putative markers have been evaluated in cross-sectional studies. The value of any potential marker, however, will be significantly increased by testing its predictive power in the conduct of longitudinal studies. Moreover, we need to assess the relationship of all the putative markers in several different populations of individuals at risk of developing alcoholism. While the current epidemiological data indicate that males are at higher risk than females, it is critical to implement similar studies in females. It is important to determine if similar putative markers exist in them, as well as assessing the predictive value of such markers for the development of alcoholism or other psychiatric conditions.

The identification of genetic trait markers that are correlated with a predisposition to develop alcoholism will not only be critical for identifying potential genes but will be equally important in elucidating the etiological factors involved in the development of alcoholism. A better understanding of the causes of alcoholism will naturally result in the development of more rational and effective treatment procedures and the implementation of efficacious primary prevention initiatives.

References

Alterman, I., Petrarulo, E., Tarter, R., and McCowan, J. (1982). Hyperactivity and alcoholism: Familial and behavioral correlates. *Addict. Behav.* **7**:413–421.

Baribeau, J. C., Eier, M., and Braun, C. M. J. (1987). Neurophysiological assessment of selective attention in males at risk for alcoholism. In *Current Trends Event-Related Potential Research* (EEG suppl. 40), R. Johnson, Jr, J. W. Rohrbaugh, and R. Parasuraman, eds. Elsevier Science Publishers (Biomedical Div), pp. 651–656.

Begleiter, H., and Platz, A. (1972). The effects of alcohol on the central nervous system. In *The Biology of Alcoholism,* Vol. 2, B. Kissin and H. Begleiter, eds. New York: Plenum Press, pp. 293–343.

Begleiter, H., Porjesz, B., and Chou, C. L. (1981). Auditory brainstem potentials in chronic alcoholics. *Science* **211**:1064–1066.

Begleiter, H., Porjesz, B., Bihari, B., and Kissin, B. (1984). Event-related potentials in boys at high risk for alcoholism. *Science* **225**:1493–1496.

Begleiter, H., Porjesz, B., Rawlings, R., and Eckardt, M. (1987). Auditory recovery function and P3 in boys at high risk for alcoholism. *Alcohol* **4**:314–321.

Branchey, M., Buydens-Branchey, L., and Lieber, C. (1988). P3 in alcoholics with disordered regulation of aggression. *Psychiatr. Res.* **25**(1):49–58.

Cadoret, R. J., and Gath, A. (1978). Inheritance of alcoholism in adoptees. *Br. J. Psychiatr.* **132**:252–258.

Cadoret, R. J., Cain, C., and Grove, W. M. (1980). Development of alcoholism in adoptees raised apart from alcoholic biologic relatives. *Arch. Gen. Psychiatry.* **37**:561–563.

Campbell, K. B., and Lowick, B. M. (1987). Ethanol and event-related potentials: The influence of distractor stimuli. *Alcohol* **4**(4):257–263.

Cantwell, D. (1972). Psychiatric illness in the families of hyperactive children. *Arch. Gen. Psychiatr.* **27**:414–417.

Cloninger, C. R. (1987). Neurogenetic adaptive mechanisms in alcoholism. *Science* **236**:410–416.

Cohen, H. L., Porjesz, B., and Begleiter, H. (1991). EEG characteristics in males at risk for alcoholism. *Alcohol.: Clin. Exp. Res.* **15**(5):858–861.

Cohen, H. L., Porjesz, B., and Begleiter, H. (1993). The effects of ethanol on EEG activity in males at risk for alcoholism. *Electroencephalogr. Clin. Neurophysiol.* **86**:368–376.

Coopersmith, S., and Woodrow, K. (1967). Basal conductance levels of normals and alcoholics. *Q. J. Stud. Alcohol* **28**:27–32.

Damasio, A. R. (1986). The frontal lobes. In *Clinical Neuropsychology,* K. Heilman and E. Valenstein, eds. Oxford: Oxford University Press, pp. 89–96.

Donchin, E. (1979). Event-related brain potentials: A tool in the study of human information processing. In *Evoked Brain Potentials and Behavior,* H. Begleiter, ed. New York: Plenum Press, pp. 13–88.

Ehlers, C. L., and Schuckit, M. A. (1990a). EEG fast frequency activity in the sons (a/b) of alcoholics. *Biol. Psychiatr.* **24**(3):631–641.

Ehlers, C. L., and Schuckit, M. A. (1990b). Evaluation of EEG alpha activity in sons of alcoholics. *Neuropsychopharmacology* **4**:199–205.

Ehlers, C. L., Chaplin, R. I., Lumeng, L. and Li, T. K. (1991). Electrophysiological responses to ethanol in P and NP rats. *Alcohol.: Exp. Clin. Res.* **15**:739–744.

Elmasian, R., Neville, H., Woods, D., Shuckit, M. A., and Bloom, F. (1982). Event-related potentials are different in individuals at high risk for developing alcoholism. *Nat. Acad. Sci. Proc.* **79**:7900–7903.

Finn, P. R., and Pihl, R. O. (1987). Men at high risk for alcoholism: The effect of alcohol on cardiovascular response to unavoidable shock. *J. Abnorm. Psychol.* **96**:230–236.

Finn, P. R., and Pihl, R. O. (1988). Risk for alcoholism: A comparison between two different groups of sons of alcoholics on cardiovascular reactivity and sensitivity to alcohol. *Alcohol.: Clin. Exp. Res.* **12**:742–747.

Finn, P. R., Zeitouni, N. C., and Pihl, R. O. (1990). Effects of alcohol on psychophysiological hyperreactivity to nonaversive and aversive stimuli in men at high risk for alcoholism. *J. Abnorm. Psychol.* **99**:79–85.

Gabrielli, W. F., Mednick, S. A., Volavka, J., Pollock, V. E., Schulsinger, F., and Itil, T. M. (1982). Electroencephalograms in children of alcoholic fathers. *Psychophysiology* **19**:494–407.

Garfield, Z. H., and McBrearty, J. F. (1970). Arousal level and stimulus response in alcoholics after drinking. *Q. J. Stud. Alcohol* **31**:832–838.

Goodwin, D. W., Schulsinger, F., Hermansen, L., Guze, S. B., and Winokur, G. (1975). Alcoholism and the hyperactive child syndrome. *J. Nerv. Ment. Dis.* **160**:349–353.

Gorenstein, E. E. (1987). Cognitive-perceptual deficit in an alcoholism spectrum disorder. *J. Stud. Alcohol* **48**:310–318.

Hill, S. Y., Steinhauer, S. R., Zubin, J., and Baugham, F. (1988). Event-related potentials as markers for alcoholism risk in high density families. *Alcohol.: Clin. Exp. Res.* **12**:545–555.

Hillyard, S. A., Picton, T. W., and Regan, D. (1978). Sensation, perception and attention: Analysis using ERP's. In *Event Related Brain Potentials in Man,* E. Callaway, P. Tueting, and S. H. Koslow, eds. New York: Academic Press, pp. 223–321.

Johnson, J. L., and Rolf, J. E. (1990). When children change: Research perspectives on children of alcoholics. In *Alcohol in the Family: Research and Clinical Perspectives,* L. Collins, K. Leonard, and J. Searles, eds. New York: Guilford Press, pp. 162–193.

Kaplan, R. F., Hesselbrock, V. M., O'Connor, S., and Palma, N. (1988). Behavioral and EEG responses to alcohol in nonalcoholic men with a family history of alcoholism. *Prog. Neuropsychopharmacol. Biol. Psychiatr.* **12:**873–885.

Kissin, B., and Hankoff, L. (1959). The acute effects of ethyl alcohol on the Funkenstein mecholyl response in male alcoholics. *Q. J. Stud. Alcohol* **20:**697–703.

Knop, J., Teasdale, T. W., Schulsinger, F., and Goodwin, D. W. (1985). A prospective study of young men at high risk for alcoholism: School behavior and achievement. *J. Stud. Alcohol* **46:**273–278.

Levenson, R. W., Oyana, O. N., and Meek, P. S. (1987). Greater reinforcement from alcohol for those at risk: Parental risk, personality risk and sex. *J. Abnorm. Psychol.* **96:**212–253.

Lukas, S. E., Mendelson, J. H., Benedikt, R. A., and Jones, B. (1986). EEG alpha activity increases during transient episodes of ethanol-induced euphoria. *Pharmacol. Biochem. Behav.* **25:**889–895.

Lumeng, L., Murphy, J. M., McBride, W. J., and Li, T.-K. (1995) Genetic influences on alcohol preferences in animals. In *Alcohol and Alcoholism,* Vol. 1, *The Genetics of Alcoholism,* H. Begleiter and B. Kissin, eds. New York: Oxford University Press, in press.

Luria, A. R., (1980). *Higher Cortical Functions in Man.* Moscow: Moscow University Press.

Miller, W. R., and Brown, J. (1992). Self regulation as a conceptual basis for the prevention and treatment of addictive behaviors. In *Self-Control and the Addictive Behaviors,* N. Heather, W. R. Miller, and J. Greely, eds. New York: Pergamon Press.

Milner, B. (1964). Some effects of frontal labectomy in man. In *The Frontal Grannular Cortex and Behavior,* J. M. Warren and K. Abert, eds. New York: McGraw Hill, pp. 313–324.

Morrison, J., and Stewart, M. (1973). The psychiatric status of the legal families of adopted hyperactive children. *Arch. Gen. Psychiatr.* **130:**791–792.

Morzoratti, S., Lamishaw, B., Lumeng, L., Li, T. K., Bemis, K., and Clemens, J. (1988). Effects of low dose ethanol on the EEG of alcohol preferring and non-preferring rats. *Brain Res. Bull.* **21:**101–104.

Newlin, D. B., and Thomson, J. B., (1990). Alcohol challenge with sons of alcoholics: A critical review and analysis. *Psychol. Bull.* **108:**383–402.

O'Connor, S., Hesselbrock, V., and Tasman, A. (1986). Correlates of increased risk for alcoholism in young men. *Prog. Neuropsychopharmacol. Biol. Psychiatry.* **10:**211–218.

O'Connor, S., Hesselbrock, V., Tasman, A., and DePalma, N. (1987). P3 amplitudes in two distinct tasks are decreased in young men with a history of paternal alcoholism. *Alcohol* **4:**323–330.

Ott, J. (1990). Genetic linkage analysis under uncertain disease definition. In *Barberry Report 33: Genetics and Biology of Alcoholism,* C. R. Cloninger and H. Begleiter, eds. Cold Spring Harbor Laboratory Press, N.Y. pp. 321–331.

Patterson, B. W., H. L., McLean, G. A., Smith, L. T., and Schaeffer K. W. (1987). Alcoholics family history of alcoholism effects on visual and event-related potentials. **4:**265–274.

Peterson, J. B., and Pihl, R. O. (1990). Information processing, neuropsychological function, and the inherited predisposition to alcoholism. *Neuropsychol. Rev.* **1:**3443–369.

Peterson, J. B., Rothfleisch, J., Zelazo, P., and Pihl, R. O. (1990). Acute alcohol intoxication and neuropsychological functioning. *J. Stud. Alcohol* **451:**114–122.

Peterson, J. B., Finn, P., and Pihl, R. O. (1992) Cognitive dysfunction and the inherited predisposition to alcoholism. *J. Stud. Alcohol* **53:**154-160.

Petrides, M., and Milner, B. (1987). Deficits on subject-ordered tasks after the frontal and temporal lobe lesions in man. *Neuropsychologia* **20:**249–262.

Pfefferbaum, A., Rosenbloom, M., and Ford, J. M. (1987). Late event-related potential changes in alcoholics. *Alcohol* **4:**275–281.

Pfefferbaum, A., Ford, J. M. White, P. M. And Mathalon, D. (1991). Event-related potentials in alcoholic men: P3 amplitude reflects family history but not alcohol consumption. *Alcohol* **15**(5):839–850.

Pickens, R. W., Svikis, D. S., McGue, M., Lykken, D. T., Hester, L. L., and Clayton, P. J. (1991). Heterogeneity in the inheritance of alcoholism. *Arch. Gen. Psychiatr.* **48**:19–28.

Pihl, R. O., Peterson, J. B., and Finn, P. R. (1987). Automatic Reactivity and Neuropsychological Deficits in Family Men at High Risk for Alcoholism. Paper presented at the Fourth International Conference on the Treatment of Addictive Behaviors, Bergen, Norway.

Plomin, R. (1983). Developmental behavioral genetics. *Child Dev.* **54**:253–259.

Polich, J., and Bloom, F. E. (1987). P300 from normals and children of alcoholics. *Alcohol* **4**:301–305.

Polich, J., and Bloom, F. E. (1988). Event-related potentials in individuals at high and low risk for developing alcoholism: Failure to replicate. *Alcohol.: Clin. Exp. Res.* **12**:368–373.

Polich, J., and Burns, T. (1987). P300 From identical twins. *Neuropsychologia* **25**(18):299–304.

Polich, J., Haier, R. J., Buchsbaum, M. and Bloom, F. E. (1988). Assessment of young men at risk for alcoholism with P300 from a visual discrimination task. *J. Stud. Alcohol* **49**:186–190.

Polich, J., Pollack, V., and Bloom, F. (1994) Meta-analysis of P300 amplitude from individuals at risk for alcoholism. *Psychol. Bull.* **115**:55-73.

Pollock, V. E. (1992). Meta-analysis of subjective sensitivity to alcohol in sons of alcoholics. *Am. J. Psychiatry.* **149**:1534–1538.

Pollock, V. E., Volavka, J. Goodwin, D. W., Mednick, S. A., Gabrielli, W. F., Knop, J., and Schulsinger, F. (1983). The EEG after alcohol administration in men at risk for alcoholism. *Arch. Gen. Psychiatr.* **40**:857–861.

Pollock, V. E., Volavka, J. Mednick, S. A., Goodwin, D. W., Knop, J., and Schulsinger, F. (1984). A prospective study of alcoholism: Electroencephalographic finding. In *Longitudinal Research in Alcoholism,* D. W. Goodwin, K. Van Dusen, Teilman, and S. A. Mednick, eds. Boston: Kluwer-Nijhoff pp. 125–146.

Porjesz, B., and Begleiter, H. (1985). Human brain electrophysiology and alcoholism. In *Alcohol and the Brain,* R. D. Tarter and D. Van Thiel, eds. New York: Plenum Press, pp. 139–182.

Porjesz, B., Begleiter, H. (1990). Event-related potentials in individuals at risk for alcoholism. *Alcohol* **7**(5):465–469.

Porjesz, B., and Begleiter, H. The effects of alcohol on cognitive event-related potentials in subjects at risk from alcoholism. Presented at Genetics and Alcohol Related Diseases, June 1992, Bordeaux, France.

Porjesz, B., and Begleiter, H. (1993). Neurophysiologic factors associated with alcoholism. In *Alcohol-Induced Brain Damage,* W. Hunt and Nixon, S. J. eds. NIAAA Monograph 22, pp. 89–120.

Porjesz, B., and Begleiter, H. Mismatch negativity and P3a in sons of alcoholic fathers.

Propping, P. (1983). Pharmacogenetics of alcohol's CNS effect: Implications for etiology of alcoholism. *Psychopharm. Biochem. Behav.* **18**:549–553.

Roth, W. T., Tinklenberg, J. R., and Kopell, B. S. (1977). Ethanol and marijuana effects on event-related potentials in a memory retrieval paradigm. *Electroencephalogr. Clin. Neurophysiol.* **42**:381–388.

Rydelius, P. A. (1981). Children of alcoholic fathers: Social adjustment and their health status over twenty years. *Acta Pediatr. Scand.* **286**:1-89.

Schmidt, A. L., and Neville, H. J. (1985). Language processing in men at risk for alcoholism: An event-related potential study. *Alcohol* 2:529–534.

Schuckit, M. A. (1980). Self-rating of alcohol intoxication by young men with and without family histories of alcoholism. *J. Stud. Alcohol* **41:**242–249.

Schuckit, M. A. (1984). Subjective responses to alcohol in sons of alcoholics and control subjects. *Arch. Gen. Psychiatr.* **41:**879–884.

Schuckit, M. A. (1985). Ethanol induced changes in body sway in men at high alcoholism risk. *Arch. Gen. Psychiatr.* **42:**375–379.

Schuckit, M. A. (1992). Advances in understanding the vulnerability to alcoholism. In *Addictive States,* C. P., O'Brien and J. H. Jaffe, eds. pp. 93–108.

Schuckit, M. A., E. O. Gold, and Risch, S. C. (1987). Plasma cortisol levels following ethanol in sons of alcoholics and controls. *Arch. Gen. Psychiatr.* **44:**942–945.

Schuckit, M. A., Gold, E. O., Croot, K., Finn, T., and Polich, J. (1988). P300 latency after ethanol ingestion in sons of alcoholics and controls. *Biol. Psychiatr.* **24:**310–315.

Schuckit, M. A., Duthie, L. A., Mahler, H. I. M., Irwin, M., and Monteiro, M. G. (1991a). Subjective feelings and changes in body sway following diazepam in sons of alcoholics and control subjects. *J. Stud. Alcohol* **52:**601–608.

Schuckit, M. A., Hauger, R. L., Monteiro, M. G., Irwin, M., Duthie, L. A., and H. I. M. Mahler, (1991b). Response of three hormones to diazepam challenge in sons of alcoholics and controls. Alcohol.: *Clin. Exp. Res.* **15:**537–542.

Sher, K. J. (1992). *Children of Alcoholics.* Chicago, IL: University of Chicago Press.

Sher, K. J., and Levenson, R. W. (1982). Risk for alcoholism and individual differences in the stress-response-dampening effect of alcohol. *J. Abnorm. Psychol.* **19:**350–367.

Steinhauer, S. R., Hill, S. Y., and Zubin, J. (1987). Event-related potentials in alcoholics and their first-degree relatives. *Alcohol* 4:307–314.

Steinlein, O., Anokhin, A., Mao, Y., and Schalt, E. (1991). Localization of a Gene for the Human Low-voltage EEG to 20q13.2–20q13.3 and Linkage Heterogeneity. Presented at American Society—Human Genetics, Institute of Human Genetics, University of Heidelberg, Germany.

Tarter, R. E., Alterman, A. I., and Edwards, K. L. (1984a). Alcoholic denial: A biopsychological interpretation. *J. Stud. Alcohol* **45:**214–218.

Tarter, R. E., Hegedus, A., Goldstein, G., Shelly, C., and Alterman, A. (1984b). Adolescent sons of alcoholics: Neuropsychological and personality characteristics. *Alcohol.: Clin. Exp. Res.* 8:216–222

Tarter, R. E., Hegedus, A. M., and Gavaler, J. (1985). Hyperactivity in sons of alcoholics. *J. Stud. Alcohol* **46:**259–261.

Tarter R. E., Alterman, A. I., and Edwards, K. L. (1988). Neurobehavioral theory of alcoholism etiology. In *Theories on Alcoholism,* C. D. Chaudron and D. A. Wilkinson, eds. Ontario: Addiction Research Foundation, pp. 73–102.

Vogel, F. (1970). The genetic basis of the normal human electroencephalogram (EEG). *Humangenetik* **10:**91–114.

Whipple, S. C., Parker, E. S., and Nobel, E. P. (1988). An atypical neurocognitive profile in alcoholic fathers and their sons. *J. Stud. Alcohol* **49:**240–244.

Whipple, S. C., Berman, S. M., and Noble, E. P. (1991). Event-related potentials in alcoholic fathers and their sons. *Alcohol* 8:321–327.

Zucker, R. A., Lisansky-Gomberg, E. S. (1986). Etiology of alcoholism reconsidered: The case for a biopsychosocial process. *Am. Psychol.* **41:**783–793.

12

Behavioral Genetics
and the Etiology of Alcoholism

RALPH E. TARTER, HOWARD B. MOSS
AND MICHAEL M. VANYUKOV

The overarching aim of behavioral genetic research is to explain phenotypic variation in behavior with respect to genotypic and environmental variation in the population. This research strategy provides a framework for understanding the etiology of alcoholism insofar as the alcoholism phenotype can be characterized in quantifiable behavioral terms such as amount, frequency, and pattern of drinking. Furthermore, the expression of behavioral traits has been shown to contribute to the variability of the risk for alcoholism. A significant proportion of the phenotypic variance in these traits can be explained by genotypic variation. Hence, investigating these psychological traits affords the opportunity of understanding how genetic and environmental variability interact so as to determine psychological functioning, which in turn influences the onset and maintenance of alcohol consumption and its consequences.

There are almost 100 permutations of signs and symptoms within DSM-III-R criteria that theoretically could qualify an individual for a diagnosis of alcoholism or, to be taxonomically precise, a "Psychoactive Substance Use Disorder—Alcohol Abuse/Alcohol Dependence" (American Psychiatric Association, 1987). Individuals assigned this diagnostic label thus form a very heterogeneous population. The problems inherent in contemporary nosological systems for the clinical diagnosis of alcoholism have recently been addressed from both conceptual and empirical perspectives (Tarter et al., 1987; Mezzich et al., 1991; Tarter et al., 1992). Aggregating individuals into one broad diagnostic category obscures understanding individual variability with respect to such salient factors as the rate of development of tolerance and physical dependence, initial reasons for drinking, contingencies maintaining regular consumption, psychiatric comorbidity, and psychological predisposition. Thus, at the outset, it is essential to point out that research aimed at elucidating etiology from a behavioral genetic perspective must define alcoholism in ways that are more narrow and strict than current taxonomic systems permit. Recent investigations demonstrating a genetic contribution to specific behavior topologies of drinking represent a major advance in this direction (Heath et al., 1991a, 1991b).

Because of the vast heterogeneity of the population of putative alcoholics, this chapter is confined to an analysis of early onset alcoholism from the viewpoint of developmental behavioral genetics. Those whose alcoholism begins at an early age, variously labeled as having essential (Rudie and McGaughran, 1961), primary (Tarter et al., 1977), or type II (Cloninger et al., 1981) alcoholism, present a rather consistent clinical picture of conjoint alcoholism and antisocial behavior. The behavioral genetic approach, although applicable to understanding alcoholism commencing at any time in the lifespan, is especially informative for early onset alcoholism (Tarter, 1991). This is because the liability (Falconer, 1965) to early onset of alcoholism has a higher heritability than the liability to later onset of alcoholism (Cloninger et al., 1981).

This chapter advances an epigenetic theoretical framework accompanied by an examination of the empirical literature pertinent to the etiology of early onset alcoholism. The advantage of an epigenetic theoretical orientation is that it affords the opportunity to elucidate the outcome condition, alcoholism, within the context of variations in childhood development. As is discussed below, certain behavioral traits with significant heritability contribute to the variation in psychological development. The main task from a developmental perspective therefore is to *determine how environmental factors, operating during childhood and adolescence, interact chronologically with particular phenotypes for emerging behavioral traits to place the youngster onto a trajectory toward alcohol abuse.* Upon surpassing a consensually accepted, albeit arbitrary threshold of severity with respect to consumption pattern and its consequences, drinking behavior is diagnosed as *alcoholism.* This epigenetic perspective is not only useful in elucidating the etiology of early onset alcoholism, but equally importantly, it can guide primary and secondary prevention strategies (Tarter, 1992).

Temperament and Behavioral Epigenesis

Definition of Temperament

Many definitions and characterizations of temperament have been proffered since ancient philosophers first considered the origins of psychological individuality. One definition that captures the flavor of a person's style of psychological functioning was given by Allport (1961):

> the characteristic phenomena of an individual's nature, including his susceptibility to emotional stimulation, his customary strength and speed of response, the quality of his prevailing mood, and all the peculiarities of fluctuation and intensity of mood, these being phenomena regarded as dependent on constitutional makeup, and therefore largely hereditary in origin (p. 34).

This definition encompasses the core features of temperament, including both mood and behavior. In contemporary terms, one could say that individual differences in temperament reflect variability in neurobiological processes that have a strong genetic basis.

Behavior Genetics

A substantial proportion of the phenotypic variation in temperament traits can be explained by genotypic differences in the population. Twin and adoption studies reveal significant genetic influences on the phenotypic variation of temperament (Plomin and Rowe, 1977; Plomin et al., 1977; Goldsmith and Gottesman, 1981; Loehlin et al., 1981, 1985; Plomin, 1983; Plomin and DeFries, 1985; Cyphers et al., 1990; Bouchard et al., 1990). In addition, the genotypic contribution to phenotypic variation in temperament is similar in children and middle-aged adults (Plomin et al., 1988). Besides being anchored in the genetic determination of individual differences in the population, temperament traits are measurable in infants. Hence, they comprise the primary psychological characteristics from which personality and complex behavior develop.

Epigenetic Framework

New behavioral phenotypes, developing from temperament, successively progress toward increasingly higher levels of complexity in response to changing biological and environmental influences. This ontogenetic process, termed *behavioral epigenesis,* is the theoretical underpinning for elucidating the liability to early onset alcoholism. Epigenesis, in which new phenotypes arise from the influence of existing ones, determines phenotypic diversity in the population because of idiosyncratic person–environment interactions. In effect, complex behavior is the outgrowth of primary temperament phenotypes concomitant to continuous and reciprocal interactions with the environment. Hence, an epigenetic framework has the advantage of clarifying the predisposing phenotypic features of alcoholism within a developmental perspective as well as encompassing the different avenues toward this outcome.

Liability to Alcoholism

Divergence in temperament trait expression paves the way for a developmental trajectory that may culminate in nonnormative behavior (e.g., delinquency, anxiety, social withdrawal). The reasons for this are that temperament deviation per se increases the probability of future personality and behavior deviations and may evoke adverse reactions in parents, siblings, and others in the social environment that further disrupt the child's psychological development. For example, a difficult temperament in early childhood may be characterized by slow adaptability, social withdrawal, negative mood, high intensity of emotional reactions and dysrhythmia (Thomas et al., 1968; Thomas and Chess, 1977). This constellation of temperament characteristics is related to a heightened risk for conduct problems by middle childhood (Maziade et al., 1990), delinquency (Windle, 1992), and alcohol and drug use in early adolescence (Lerner and Vicary, 1984; Tarter et al., 1994). On the other hand, adverse interactions with the social environment occurring throughout development typically precede alcohol and drug use. Temperamentally difficult children frequently are a disciplinary problem and have school and peer adjustment disturbances (Thomas et al., 1968; Martin et al., 1983). Poor marital adjustment, even before the child's birth, may influence the subsequent emergence of a difficult temperament (Esterbrooks and Ende, 1988), illustrating the strong impact that a disruptive home environment has on early childhood development. In this regard, it is noteworthy that marriages are commonly dysfunctional and conflict-laden where one or both partners is alcoholic. Further underscoring the importance of the family environment during early childhood development, it has been shown that children are perceived more negatively after a heated discussion between parents (Markman and Jones-Leonard, 1985). Under these circumstances, coercive and aversive child-rearing strategies are more likely to be employed, particularly if the child is already perceived as difficult (Buss, 1981; Lee and Bates, 1985).

With respect to alcoholism, there is evidence that an affectionate temperament among infant offspring of alcoholics, by eliciting positive reactions in parents, protects against maladjustment in adolescence (Werner, 1986). This finding indicates that the risk for alcoholism can be attenuated among high-risk individuals if they have a favorable temperament disposition, which in turn promotes positive interactions with others. On the other hand, it has been found that a difficult affective temperament disposition in male offspring of substance-abusing fathers who also have this disposition is associated with behavior problems in the boys that are well-established precursors of alcoholism (Blackson et al., 1994). In effect, negative interactions with parents, influenced in large part by temperament makeup, appears to predispose to the development of behavior that is associated with a heightened risk of alcoholism. In a laboratory study of the effects of child behavior on adult behavior, it has been observed that child actors who are trained to behave disruptively induce greater alcohol consumption in adults who have a positive family history of alcoholism, even though they are not alcoholic themselves (Pelham, unpublished manuscript). Child-rearing efficacy is clearly compromised by acute and chronic alcohol intoxication in parents. The main conclusions to be drawn from these studies, however, are that ongoing bidirectional interaction between the child and others is important in the etiology of behavior disorder, and ultimately alcoholism, and that the quality of this interaction can either protect or predispose the youngster to this outcome.

In elucidating the basis of adverse person–environment interactions, it is essential to recognize that temperament deviation manifests early in life and predisposes to deviant psychological development. Figure 12-1 depicts the development of alcoholism from a behavior genetic perspective. At birth (age 0) behavior phenotypes, vis-à-vis temperament characteristics, are defined according to the individual's position relative to the population mean within a normal distribution. A deviation in temperament phenotype (d) determines the outset point of the epigenetic trajectory of the liability phenotype. In its relation with the liability to alcoholism, each temperament phenotype (t) can also be conceptualized as a vector (v_t) that biases the infant towards ($+$) or away from ($-$) the adverse outcome. The individual differences in the value and direction of v_t are determined to large degree by genetic factors.

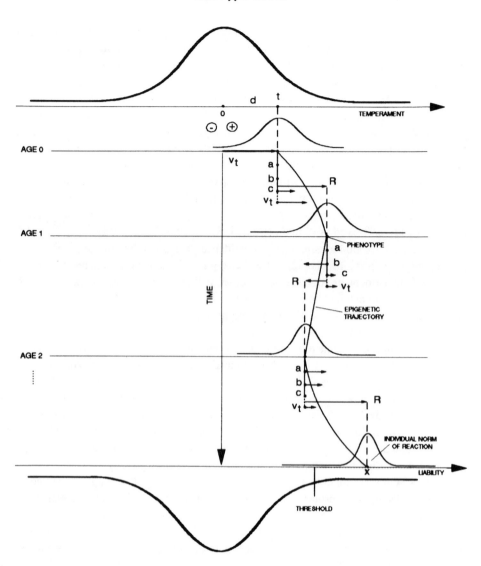

Fig. 12-1 Development of alcoholism. Deviation (d) in temperament (t) comprises a vector (v_t) that in combination with other vectors (**a, b, c, . . .**), biases the person toward or away from a threshold diagnosis of alcoholism. (In the illustration, the liability is shown to shift with age because the constituent vectors fluctuate throughout life.)

    In addition to temperament ($\mathbf{v}_t$), many other vectors (**a, b, c, . . .**, etc.) contribute to the variation in the epigenesis of the liability phenotype to alcoholism. For instance, other vectors besides $\mathbf{v}_t$ include, but are not limited to, parental supervision, religion, culture, gender, and availability of alcohol. Collectively, they determine the probability of an adverse outcome at any time during the life span. Their resultant vector (**R**), being the sum of all the vectors, is amplified or attenuated as the relative contribution of these component vectors ($\mathbf{a}$, $\mathbf{b}$, $\mathbf{c}$,. . . $\mathbf{v_t}$) change with age (Labouvie, Pandina, and Johnson, 1991). Within the epigenetic framework, each value of $\mathbf{R}$ determines the person's phenotype at each following point. Upon surpassing a consensually accepted threshold of severity, the person is deemed to qualify for a diagnosis of alcoholism. In Fig. 12-1, this is represented as the "beyond the threshold" position (X) of the person's phenotype on the axis of the liability.

Figure 12-2 depicts one hypothetical scenario for early age onset of alcohol problems. As can be seen, an inborn deviation in expression of the temperament trait behavioral activity level, via interactions with family, peers, and authority figures, culminates in deviant behavior. This behavior pattern in turn places the person at increased risk for a psychiatric diagnosis of alcohol abuse, defined as the surpassing of

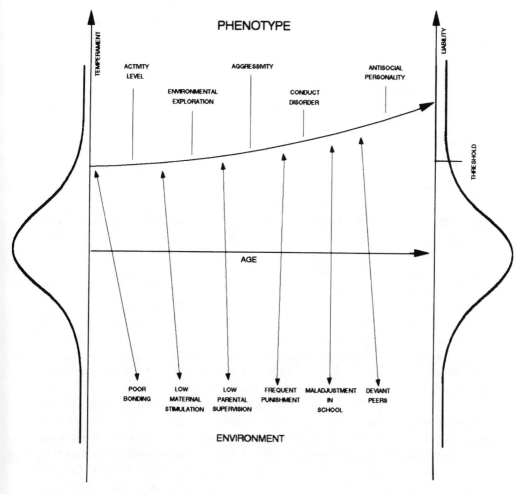

Fig. 12-2 Hypothetical scenario of the development of alcoholism from the epigenetic perspective.

an arbitrary threshold of severity of alcohol use and its physical and psychosocial consequences.

As depicted in Fig. 12-2, children with a temperament phenotype of high behavioral activity level experience more punishment, but less verbal communication from their mothers compared to children with a normative temperament disposition (Webster-Stratton and Eyberg, 1982; Dunn and Plomin, 1986). These negative parent–child interactions early in the youngster's life compromise the opportunity for affectional bonding or secure infant-to-mother attachment. In a study of subhuman primates, it has been shown that the absence of opportunity for attachment between mother and infant is associated with increased levels of alcohol consumption in monkeys by adolescence or young adulthood (Higley et al., 1991).

Furthermore, children who are temperamentally active commonly have tantrums, refuse requests and oppose authority figures; indeed they are often management problems before 4 years of age (Billman and McDevitt, 1980; Stevenson-Hinde and Simpson, 1982). Also, recall that it has been observed that in a conflictual home environment, children with a high behavioral activity level are perceived more negatively after an argument between the parents (Markman and Jones-Leonard, 1985). Being perceived negatively by parents may further promote the development and stabilization of a disruptive behavior disorder in the child. Aggression directed at children takes various forms, including verbal criticism, coercive discipline, and physical maltreatment. Because physical abuse and maltreatment are common in children of alcoholics, it is probable that these adverse interactions with parents augment further their genetically high risk to develop alcoholism. Evidence supporting this conclusion was recently provided by Tarter et al. (1993a), who found that children of substance-abusing fathers received more severe and inconsistent punishment than other children, and that these discipline practices explained a significant proportion of variance on externalizing and internalizing scores of the Child Behavior Checklist. Difficult temperament scores were also higher in the children of substance-abusing fathers. In addition, greater mutual dissatisfaction between mother and offspring is reported where there is a substance-abusing father, and the magnitude of this negative interaction pattern covaries with the severity of child's behavior disturbance (Tarter et al., 1993b). Specifically, the results of this latter study point to the presence of externalizing behaviors in children where unfavorable interactions characterize the parent–offspring relationship.

Children who experience aggression are more likely than other children to perpetrate aggression (Stewart and du Blois, 1981). They also have difficulty sustaining play behavior, engage in a more frenetic pattern of play, are less compliant, and are more oppositional than other children (Halverson and Waldrop, 1976). As shown in Fig. 12-2, a conduct disorder typically ensues as an outcome of an aggressive disposition in childhood. Relating back to the infant's disposition, it is salient to point out that high behavioral activity level commonly presages a conduct disorder. Indeed, viewed from a psychiatric perspective, a conduct disorder is the most frequently diagnosed comorbid condition in children with hyperactivity, ranging from 40% to 70% of cases (August and Stewart, 1982; Szatmari et al., 1989). Moreover, poor bonding between parent and child has been shown to antedate the child's development of impulsivity

(Carey et al., 1977). This behavior propensity is a cardinal feature of hyperactivity, conduct disorder, and alcoholism.

Conduct disorder in youth commonly evolves into an antisocial personality disorder in adulthood. Alcohol abuse is almost universal among individuals who qualify for a diagnosis of antisocial personality disorder. Considered, therefore, in the context of an epigenetic process, early onset of alcoholism is one end point of deviant psychological development. As shown in Fig. 12-2, there are several intermediary behavioral phenotypes for emerging behavior traits (aggressivity, conduct disorder, antisocial personality) linking the temperament phenotype of high behavioral activity level to alcoholism. Each of these intermediary phenotypes has been shown to be associated with an increased risk for alcoholism (McCord and McCord, 1960; Robins, 1966; Kellam et al., 1983; Tarter et al., 1985). These phenotypes, termed *liability promoters,* are composed of the combined effects of genetic and environmental factors determining, at any time in life, the probability of developing alcoholism.

Once the liability threshold is exceeded (that is, consensually accepted diagnostic criteria are satisfied), as shown in the developmental trajectory depicted in Figs. 12-1 and 12-2, the case is demarcated as affected, thereby defining the presence of alcoholism. In this regard, it is interesting to note that findings from the Epidemiologic Catchment Area Study indicate that age of first drink, age of first intoxication, and the apparent presence of an age-dependent risk for the onset of alcoholism peak between 15 and 19 years of age (Burke et al., 1990). Hence, viewed from the epigenetic perspective, individual temperament phenotype, first measurable soon after birth, develops into increasingly complex behavioral dispositions concomitant to reciprocal and continuous interaction between the person and social environment such that the person is placed on a trajectory to an alcoholism outcome. However, it is essential to emphasize that the earliest point in the trajectory to the outcome liability phenotype is defined according to individual differences in temperament expression in the population and not as an abnormal condition. During psychological development, consisting of idiosyncratic interactions with the social environment, behavior is continuously shaped such that it biases the person toward or away from the alcoholism outcome. End-point typological characterizations of early onset alcoholism (e.g., primary, essential, or type 2 alcoholism) thus do not capture the dynamic person–environment interactions occurring during development that are argued herein to be necessary for understanding the etiology of alcoholism.

Specificity in the Ontogenetic Patterning of Behavior

The discussion up to this juncture has addressed the need to understand alcoholism as one outcome of a deviant developmental process. As previously noted, this ontogenetic process consists of the temporal emergence of phenotypes that have their origins in the individual's temperament phenotype. An important question emanating from this discussion, and one that has received virtually no attention by researchers, concerns the *specificity* of person–environment interactions that place the youngster onto a trajectory for alcoholism.

The *organismic specificity hypothesis* asserts that the child's phenotype evokes particular reactions from others in the social environment that resonate back to affect the child's development in specific ways, depending on the child's phenotype (Wachs and Gruen, 1982). In other words, "early experiences differentially influence development because the impact of the environment is mediated by individual differences in the organism" (Gandour, 1989, p. 1093). For example, highly active toddlers who receive a large amount of stimulation from their primary caretaker exhibit less exploratory behavior than highly active children whose caretakers provide little stimulation (Gandour, 1989). Children with low behavioral activity level and high caretaker stimulation also exhibit vigorous exploratory behavior, whereas children with low activity level and low stimulation exhibit comparatively little environmental exploration. In effect, exploratory behavior is determined by the interaction between the characteristics of the caretaker and the child's phenotype. Hence, in understanding the development pathway to an alcoholism outcome, it is necessary to disaggregate both the quality and mechanisms driving person–environment interaction patterns.

The preceding example regarding exploratory behavior is especially relevant for elucidating the developmental course toward alcoholism. Children of alcoholics, compared to children of normal parents, are more likely to have elevated behavioral activity level (for a review, see Tarter, 1991). For a variety of reasons, several of which may be related directly to parental alcoholism, highly active children, as noted previously, receive less supervision and communication from parents than normally active children. Consequently, environmental exploration, consisting of novelty or sensation seeking, is more likely to occur in such children. This motivational propensity has been strongly linked to early age involvement with alcohol and other drugs. Indeed, because alcohol is readily available and consumed in a wide variety of situations, high levels of exploratory behavior or novelty seeking behavior will result in a greater exposure to alcohol beverages and opportunities to drink. The main conclusions to be drawn, however, from the research to date are that (1) complex motivational propensities (viz, novelty or sensation seeking) are amenable to an epigenetic analysis in which temperament phenotype and the social environment interact in particular fashion; and (2) the organismic specificity hypothesis provides a heuristic rubric in which to undersatand and potentially predict behavioral development in the context of a coherent process.

Within the interactional perspective proposed herein, the teleological basis underlying the specific behavior needs to be carefully considered. For example, in Gandour's study reviewed earlier, high exploration of the environment occurs in conjunction with two different types of interactional patterns between child and caretaker. However, it is only in the condition of low caretaker stimulation and high childhood activity level that the behavior may be a vector for subsequent maladjustment and ultimately for alcohol abuse because of its unsupervised and apparent dysregulated quality.

Temperament and Developmental Continuity

The genetic contribution to the phenotypic variability of temperament traits is approximately the same in adulthood as it is in childhood (Plomin et al., 1988). Temperament expression also tends to be relatively stable during development (Hagekull, 1989; Rothbart, 1989). Although the behavioral topography changes, the underlying quality tends to remain unchanged. For example, high emotional reactivity at age 2 (expressed usually as crying or tantrums) has, under normal circumstances, a very different presentation at age 20 (when the person's behavioral functioning is at a higher level of complexity). Hence, whereas the expression of emotional distress changes across the life span, emotionality per se remains stable.

Temperament phenotypes generally maintain *ipsative* and *normative* stability. Insofar as ipsative stability is concerned, the complement of phenotypes temporally retain their relative magnitude of expression within the individual; that is, their ordinal position does not change. Thus, if high emotionality is the most salient temperament phenotype in early childhood, it remains so during development. With regard to normative stability, the phenotype tends to maintain the same position over time in relation to the population mean (Rothbart, 1989). Thus, an individual who deviates in temperament from the population mean by a certain quantity at one time is likely to show the same magnitude of deviation if reexamined at a subsequent occasion.

Temperament phenotypes, although generally stable, are, however, potentially modifiable. As previously discussed, the extent of modifiability is determined by the norm of reaction for the particular trait. Babies characterized by low capacity for sustained attention and negative affectivity shift toward more normative behavior if the mother is spontaneous, expressive, and living in an emotionally secure and cohesive family (Matheny, 1986; Matheny et al., 1987). If the mother has emotional problems, or is in a state of emotional distress, the child's temperament disposition shifts toward disruptiveness (Engfer, 1986). Low support from family and friends exacerbates temperament deviations, particularly with respect to the construct of the "difficult" disposition (Windle, 1992). These latter findings have important implications for understanding the etiology of alcoholism. Specifically, they underscore the need to determine the extent and mechanisms by which the environment shifts the person having certain phenotypes toward behavioral deviancy such that the risk for an alcoholism outcome is increased. Alternatively, the extent to which the person can be protected from alcohol abuse by manipulating the environment in temperamentally vulnerable individuals also remains to be determined.

These matters notwithstanding, it is important to emphasize that even though temperament phenotype variation is influenced strongly by genetic variability and mediated by neurobiological mechanisms, the probability of any particular behavioral reactions is changeable. However, as the child matures, flexibility diminishes because habitual patterns of behavior are firmly established. This crystallization of the behavioral repertoire during development not only makes it increasingly difficult to apply interventions that can deflect the child off a trajectory toward maladjustment (e.g., conduct disorder) but also is associated with progressive narrowing of options with respect to the range of environments in which the youngster can make a socially normative adjustment. In other words, opportunities to adapt to an environment that can reduce the liability to alcoholism become progressively less available. For example, once a conduct disorder is established, usually by late childhood, the opportunity to shift to normative behavior is diminished because the social environment in which the child has best adjusted, or at least made a "good fit," is restricted to nonnormative peers. In effect, stabilization of deviance has occurred and crystallization of the behavior pattern as a beyond-the-threshold phenotype for the liability to alcoholism and antisocial personality has become highly probable.

Temperament and Psychopathology

Deviations in temperament phenotype are associated with an increased risk for maladjustment. Psychopathology and behavior disorder in middle childhood are more common among children with a difficult temperament disposition (Graham et al., 1973; Earls and Jung, 1987). Children with a difficult temperament are at about 2.5 times increased risk of developing psychopathology by adolescence compared to children with normative temperament (Maziade et al., 1990). Indeed, about half the cases of difficult temperament develop into clinical disorders by adolescence (Maziade et al., 1990). Significantly, a difficult temperament has been linked particularly to a predisposition to develop externalizing and oppositional behavior disorders (Maziade et al., 1984); these behavior disturbances frequently occur in conjunction with early onset alcohol and drug use. Importantly, however, this outcome is the culmination of bidirectional interactions between the child and the social environment (Bell, 1968). For example, children with a difficult temperament but having high intelligence and living in normal supportive families can be protected from an adverse outcome (Maziade et al., 1985).

One theoretically important issue concerns whether there is an association between a specific temperament phenotype and type of psychiatric or adjustment disorder. The available evidence indicates that a tightly connected relationship does not exist (Lee and Bates, 1985; Maziade et al., 1990). Difficult temperament, for example, has also been linked to conduct anxiety, and depressive disorders in late childhood and early adolescence (Maziade et al., 1984; Maziade, 1989; Windle, 1992). As is discussed later, these disorders appear to increase the risk for the development of alcoholism. Thus, deviations in temperament expression predispose to psychopathology; however, the specific form and manifestation of psychopathology is determined ultimately by the quality of person–environment interactions.

Another question that has yet to be addressed empirically concerns whether deviation of temperament phenotypes in either a high or low direction from the population mean is associated with an increased risk for alcoholism. For example, high and low sociability, each temperament phenotype for different reasons, could place the child on a developmental trajectory that culminates in alcoholism. In effect, the reasons the socially avoidant person initiates and sustains drinking are likely to be different from the reasons drinking is initiated and maintained by a highly sociable person. Thus, despite the dearth of research, it appears reasonable to conclude that a deviation in temperament trait expression in either a high or low direction covaries in a U-shape relationship with the risk for subsequent psychological disorder, and ultimately, alcoholism.

Finally, it is important to underscore the importance of characterizing temperament as the product of phenotypes reflecting all trait dimensions. The example provided in Fig. 12-2 with respect to behavioral activity level should be viewed in the perspective of outcome being determined by all of the trait dimensions combined and not just this one dimension. An important task for researchers is to identify particular configurations of traits that produce phenotypes that are salient to an alcoholism outcome. For instance, the combination of high motor activity level and high fearfulness produce a phenotype "inhibition to the unfamiliar" (Kagan and Snidman, 1991). Thus, in addition to global characterizations of temperament phenotype combinations such as "difficult," "easy" or "slow to warm up" (Thomas et al., 1968; Thomas and Chess, 1977), it is essential to identify other more specific aggregates of phenotypes that are associated with an increased liability to alcoholism.

Temperament Dimensions Applied to Alcoholism Liability

Combining the scales from the New York Longitudinal Study (Thomas et al., 1968) and Colorado Adoption Project (Plomin and DeFries, 1985), Rowe and Plomin (1977) extracted six temperament dimensions: (1) behavior activity level; (2) attention-span persistence; (3) emotionality; (4) reaction to food; (5) sociability; and (6) soothability. The extent to which deviations on each of these six traits are associated with the risk for alcoholism is considered below. This complement of traits is related herein to the risk for alcoholism because the traits integrate the two most comprehensive research programs on temperament conducted to date involving longitudinal and behavior genetic paradigms.

Behavior Activity Level

Family studies indicate that hyperactivity in childhood aggregates with paternal alcoholism. Morrison and Stewart (1973) and Cantwell (1972) found that hyperactive children are more likely than nonhyperactive children to have a biological, but not adoptive father, who is alcoholic. Goodwin et al. (1975) reported that adopted children who become alcoholic, most of whom were sons of alcoholics, exhibited more childhood hyperactivity symptoms than controls.

Prospective studies also suggest that high behavioral activity level in childhood is associated with an increased risk for subsequent problem alcohol abuse. McCord and McCord (1960) and Jones (1968) observed that alcoholics were often characterized as hyperactive children compared to controls. In a prospective study, Hechtman et al., (1984a, 1984b) found that childhood hyperactivity was an important predictor of subsequent alcoholism. A number of other longitudinal investigations have obtained similar findings; however, the prevalence and method of measurement of alcohol abuse as the outcome variable differed widely among the studies (Borland and Heckman, 1976; Blouin et al., 1978; Gittelman et al., 1985). A recent longitudinal study by Barkley and colleagues (1990) is particularly noteworthy. In a sample fo 123 children, they found twice the prevalence of alcohol abuse at follow-up in hyperactive children (42.5%)

compared to normal (22.7%) controls. Also, they observed a higher prevalence of alcohol abuse in the fathers of hyperactive children (34%) compared to fathers of normal children (14%). Paralleling these findings, Manuzza et al. (1991) reported that 44% of hyperactive children developed a substance abuse disorder compared to 20% of their nonhyperactive siblings. Probably because of small sample size, this difference did not, however, attain statistical significance.

In two studies of college freshmen, Loper et al. (1973) and Kammeier et al. (1973) found that as a group, individuals who subsequently became alcoholic scored higher on the MMPI hypomania scale than nonalcoholics. Also, in a follow-up study of a sample of college students, Vaillant (1983) noted that there was faster behavioral tempo among individuals who became problem drinkers later in life.

Primary alcoholics, namely, individuals who did not begin drinking concomitant to a psychiatric disorder or a life crisis, retrospectively reported 2–5 times more childhood hyperactivity features than secondary alcoholics whose drinking began following another psychiatric disorder (DeObaldia et al, 1983a; Tarter et al., 1977). In the study by DeObaldia et al., 77% of primary alcoholics were classified as being high in childhood hyperactivity symptoms compared to only 27% of secondary alcoholics. In a follow-up study, DeObaldia and Parsons (1983) found that the retrospective reports of childhood hyperactivity using Tarter et al.'s (1977) checklist were highly reliable across two testings and concurred with independent reports by a parent or older sibling. These findings suggest that the results of retrospective research, despite its limitations, yield valid information regarding childhood behavior disposition. In this vein, Alterman et al. (1982), also administering the childhood history checklist developed by Tarter et al. (1977) to document childhood hyperactivity, observed that alcoholics who had a family history of alcoholism retrospectively reported significantly more hyperactivity features than alcoholics in which none of their first-degree relatives were alcoholic. In addition, Gomberg (1982) noted that young early onset alcoholics were twice as frequently described as being hyperactive as children compared to older later onset alcoholics. The former individuals were also more likely to have an alcoholic parent. Contrasting subgroups of alcoholics according to their level of psychosocial maturity using the essential-reactive scale, Tarter (1982) found that early onset ("essential") alcoholics reported significantly more features of childhood hyperactivity than socially competent, later onset ("reactive") alcoholics. Indeed, the score on the childhood history checklist (documenting hyperactivity characteristics) combined with the essential-reactive score explained almost 50% of the variance on the general alcoholism scale of the Alcohol Use Inventory.

Administering the revised Dimensions of Temperament Scale, Tarter et al. (1990a) found that male offspring of alcoholics were rated higher on dimensions of behavioral activity level compared to sons of nonalcoholic controls. In a subsequent study, it was found that adolescent substance abusers scored higher on behavioral activity level than normal controls (Tarter et al., 1990b). Furthermore, activity level covaried with severity of substance use, psychiatric disorder, and psychosocial maladjustment as measured by the Drug Use Screening Inventory (Tarter, 1990). Employing an actigraph to directly quantify motor activity, Moss et al. (1992) observed greater motor activity in

10- to 12-year-old sons of substance abusers compared to sons of normal men during tasks requiring sustained attention and behavioral suppression, but not while the subjects were in a resting condition.

Hyperactive adolescents are more prone than their nonhyperactive peers to excessively consume alcohol (Mendelson et al., 1971). This propensity for alcohol misuse cannot be explained on the basis of either general academic failure or the presence of a learning disability (Blouin et al., 1978). There is, however, indication that alcohol abuse among hyperactive adolescents occurs primarily in conjuction with a conduct disorder (Mendelson et al, 1971; Hoy et al, 1978; Tarter et al, 1985b; Barkley et al., 1990; Windle, 1990). This observation is consistent with the previously discussed concept of an epigenetic patterning of emergent traits—that is, high behavioral activity phenotype—in interaction with the environment culminating in conduct or disorder that in turn predisposes to problematic alcohol use.

Attention-Span Persistence

Tarter el al. (1984) observed that adolescent sons of alcoholics performed less well on certain neuropsychological tests measuring attention capacity compared to sons of nonalcoholic. Schaeffer et al. (1984) found that adult nonalcoholic relatives of alcoholics performed more poorly on the average than nonalcoholics without a family history of alcoholism on a battery of abstracting, problem-solving, and perceptual-motor tests. Most of the tests employed in this latter study required sustained concentration for optimal performance. Elmasian et al. (1982) found a greater time-related deterioration of performance on a reaction time task in nonalcoholic young adults with a family history of alcoholism compared with individuals who did not have a family history of alcoholism.

Event-related potential (ERP) findings additionally implicate the presence of attentional disturbances in persons at high risk for alcoholism. It is important to note, however, that ERP waveforms are poorly understood with respect to their neuroanatomical substrate and their psychological significance. These caveats aside, and despite inconsistency across studies, there is mounting evidence suggesting that the P3 component of the ERP is discriminable with respect to its latency and amplitude between high- and low-risk subjects (Begleiter et al., 1984; Hill et al., 1990). Although these findings are intriguing, it is important to emphasize that deviation in the P3 waveform have been reported for a number of different psychiatric disorders, and with respect to individuals at high risk for alcoholism, that some investigators have found differences according to latency whereas others have found differences on amplitude compared to subjects at low risk for alcoholism. Nonetheless, the neurophysiological results concur with the psychological evidence implicating deficient attentional processes.

In a seminal longitudinal study of conduct-disordered youth, Robins (1966) found that inattention and daydreaming were more common among the children who subsequently developed alcoholism. Goodwin et al. (1975) also found a high prevalence of childhood daydreaming in biological offspring of alcoholics who became alcoholics even though they were reared by adoptive parents. In a large Swedish cohort of young adults reporting for military registration, Rydelius (1983a) found that 35% of high alcohol consumers were rated by an examining psychologist as having difficulties in concentration and low mental endurance in contrast to 5% of nonconsumers. Restlessness was described in 40% of high consumeres compared to 4% of nonconsumers.

Psychiatric and psychometric findings additionally suggest that an attentional disturbance in childhood is a risk factor for the subsequent development of alcoholism. Wood et al. (1983) found that 33% of alcoholics met the criteria for an attention deficit disorder, residual type. This observation is consistent with the results obtained by Tarter et al. (1977), who noted that 44% of primary alcoholics reported having a short attention span as children, and Shekim et al. (1990), who found that 34% of adults with attention deficit disorder qualified for a diagnosis of alcoholism.

Evidence for attentional deficits and impersistence is also obtained from studies employing the MMPI. The elevated psychopathic deviate scale of the MMPI, commonly observed in alcoholic men, points to a behavioral disposition featured by high impulsivity, low goal persistence, and low frustration tolerance. Furthermore, the high score on the MacAndrew Alcoholism Scale of the MMPI describes a rancorous, disorganized, and disinhibited behavioral disposition that is marked by little or no concern for future consequences (MacAndrew, 1981). It has been found that university students who subsequently become alcoholic scored higher on this scale than individuals who did not develop alcoholism (Hoffmann et al., 1974). Furthermore, a high score on the MacAndrew Scale is more characteristic of younger than older alcohol abusers (MacAndrew, 1979). On tests measuring impulse control and persistence, Alterman et al. (1984) found that young alcoholics performed more deficiently than older alcoholics. The studies by MacAndrew (1979) and Alterman et al. (1984) suggest that these behavioral disturbances presaged the onset of alcoholism inasmuch as younger alcoholics were more impaired than older alcoholics. Taken together, the available evidence indicates that behavioral impersistence and attentional limitations are associated with an increased liability to alcoholism. It is also noteworthy that impulsivity, a characteristic commonly found to presage alcoholism, is associated with poor attentional capacity (Mischel, 1983). Among young adults, poor self-control or impulsivity has been found to correlate .79 with drinking behavior (Earleywine et al., 1990).

Soothability

Soothability is operationally defined as the facility to be calmed after experiencing emotional distress. At the physiological level of analysis, soothability can be interpreted to mean an ability to return to homeostasis following emotional arousal.

Rosenberg and Buttsworth (1969) reported that young alcoholics were less able than older alcoholics to attenuate anxiety, suggesting that the incapacity to be calmed either predates drinking onset or emerges very early during the course of the alcoholism. Suggestive evidence indicates that alcoholics, after exposure to stress, are slow to return to physiological homeostasis. Holmberg and Martens (1955) found that alcoholics and nonalcoholics exhibited an increase in heart rate after the administration of a challenge dose of alcohol. However, whereas the nonalcoholic returned to below the prealcoholic baseline level 15–30 minutes after alcohol absorption, the majority of alcoholics sustained the heart rate increment. These findings indicate that they are less efficient in returning to homeostasis after sympathetic arousal. Coopersmith and Woodrow (1967) also found that alcoholics and nonalcoholic do not differ in basal arousal level. Only when stressed did group differences become apparent, at which time they noted that the alcoholic "becomes physiologically and verbally more responsive and is much more likely to deny all stimuli that impinge upon him. Since he does not discriminate between affective and more neutral stimuli, he responds to all stimuli maximally and is thus more likely to be stimulated into greater and presumably more distressing reactivity" (pp. 30–31). Thus, once aroused, alcoholics tend to remain physiologically activated longer than nonalcoholic.

The slowness in returning to physiological homeostasis, that is, the capacity to be calmed after stress, may be an influential factor underlying the decision to continue drinking following first alcohol exposure and perhaps may explain the rapid transition from initial use to habitual problematic ingestion that is commonly found in young alcoholics. In this regard, it is noteworthy that young adults ascertained to be at high risk for alcoholism experience a greater stress-dampening effect from alcohol than other individuals in the population (Sher and Levenson, 1982). Extrapolating these findings to the clinical context, it would appear that alcohol ingestion affords the opportunity to both obtain quick relief from tension and to recover from stress.

Emotionality

Emotionality is defined, at the psychological level of analysis, as the tendency to become easily and intensely distressed (Buss and Plomin, 1975). At the physiological level it can be defined as excessive autonomic reactivity or lability. A high degree of association exists between physiological lability and psychological instability (Eysenck, 1983).

With respect to physiological lability, Kissin and Hankoff (1959) observed that alcohol had a normalizing effect on autonomic functioning in alcoholics. In effect, alcoholics who were initially low in sympathetic reactivity were stimulated by alcohol, whereas those who were high in sympathetic reactivity were sedated after alcohol consumption. Thus, depending on the individual's baseline physiological state, alcohol either increased or decreased autonomic arousal. Other investigators have reported that alcohol increases arousal (Docter and Bernal, 1964; Docter et al., 1966) as well as reduces autonomic reactivity to external stimuli in alcoholics (Coopersmith and Woodrow, 1967; Garfield and McBrearty, 1970). In a comprehensive review of the literature, Pihl et al. (1990) conclude that autonomic hyperreactivity characterizes sons of alcoholics (but not daughters) and that this propensity underlies both neurocognitive and behavioral disturbances that have been observed to precede the onset of alcoholism.

Investigations of psychological functioning also indicate that high emotionality might be associated with an increased risk for alcoholism. On the Eysenck Personality Inventory (EPI), alcoholics have been found to score higher than nonalcoholics on the neuroticism–stability dimension, but not on the introversion–extraversion dimension (for a review, see Barnes, 1983). According to Eysenck (1983), neuroticism is the behavioral manifestation of limbic and autonomic lability. It has been estimated from twin studies that up to 50% of the phenotypic variance on neuroticism is determined by genotype variation in the population (Loehlin and Nichols, 1976; Floderus-Myhred et al., 1980). Sieber and Bentler (1982) studied 750 19-year-old men and retested them when they were 22 years old. They found that high excitability, dominance, and aggressiveness were directly related to subsequent substance misuse. Neuroticism was found to be indirectly related to substance misuse. Tarter (1982) found that essential alcoholics scored significantly higher than reactive alcoholics on the EPI neuroticism scale, but not on the extraversion–introversion scale. Rosenberg and Buttsworth (1969) found that alcoholics under 30 years of age scored higher on the EPI neuroticism scale than alcoholics over 30 years of age, leading the authors to conclude that young alcoholics have abnormally high levels of anxiety that they are unable to regulate. The observation that younger alcoholics, not having a long-standing history of alcohol misuse, exhibited greater neuroticism than older alcoholics (a finding contrary to what one would expect if this feature covaried with duration of alcoholism), suggests that the psychological and inferred physiological lability either predated the onset of problematic drinking or developed soon thereafter.

Indirect evidence for impaired emotional regulation has also been presented by Gomberg (1982), who observed that young alcoholics (30 years of age or younger) had numerous anxiety like behavioral disturbances in childhood. These features included nail biting, shyness, nightmares, phobias, tantrums, tics, stuttering, thumb sucking, and eating problems. Rydelius (1983a) observed that 18-year-old military conscripts who were heavy alcohol consumers (1000 to 4999 g of alcohol/month) were more frequently described as irritable, restless, and tense compared to abstainers. In a second study, using a personality test developed at the Karolinska Institute, Rydelius (1983b) observed that heavy alcohol consumers also scored higher on scales measuring somatic anxiety, psychic anxiety, psychasthenia, irritability, and impulsiveness.

Costello (1981) factor analyzed the Sixteen Personality Factors Questionnaire and found that 74 of 120 alcoholic subjects scored strongly in the direction of high emotional lability. In contrast, only 17 alcoholic subjects scored low on this dimension. Of additional interest was the finding that "shrewdness" and "low superego strength" clustered with high lability, illustrating the possible overlap between antisocial characteristics and emotional lability in alcoholics. The coexistence of heightened anxiety and antisocial behavior was also observed by Rydelius (1983a, 1983b) in his sample of 18-year-old military conscripts.

A number of investigators have observed elevated anxiety levels in alcoholics (for a review, see Barnes, 1983). It is pertinent to note that heightened anxiety is particularly characteristic of young, early onset alcoholics, whether it is measured as a concurrent feature (Rosenberg and Buttsworth, 1969) or inferred from retrospective reports about childhood behavior disturbance (Gomberg, 1982). Male offspring of alcoholics have also been reported to exhibit a high level of emotionality. Lund and Landesman-Dwyer (1979) found that sons of alcoholics were rated as less emotionally controlled than children of nonalcoholic on the Devereaux Adolescent Behavior Rating Scale. Comparing delinquent adolescent sons of alcoholics and nonalcoholic on the MMPI, Tarter et al. (1984), found that the former group scored higher than the nonalcoholics' sons on the neurotic triad (hypochondriasis, depression, hysteria) scales, but on none of the other clinical or validity scales. Aronson and Gilbert (1963) contrasted preadolescent sons of alcoholics to classmates who did not have an alcoholic father. Teachers more frequently endorsed such characteristics as "emotionally immature," "unable to take frustration in stride," "sensitive to criticism," "anger open and direct," "impulsive," and "moody and depressed" in the sons of alcoholics. Sher et al. (1991) and Chasin et al. (1991) have similarly observed greater negative affectivity in offspring of alcoholics.

In a longitudinal study of conduct disordered children, Robins (1966) found a higher prevalence of nail biting in adolescents who subsequently became alcoholics. Block (1971) evaluated the outcomes of children who originally participated in the Berkeley and Oakland California studies of child development. Two types of personality configurations characterized the subjects who developed problem drinking. The first type tended to cry easily, become angry readily, and worry excessively even though they outwardly appeared cheerful, gregarious, and assertive. These individuals were classified as "anomic extroverts." The second group of adolescents was described as extrapunitive, irritable, and hostile. They were classified as "unsettled undercontrollers." Both of these personality profiles are characterized by disturbances in emotional regulation.

Emotional immaturity, low frustration tolerance, and moodiness have also been described in the preadolescent sons of alcoholic fathers (Aronson and Gilbert, 1963). Goodwin et al. (1975) found that the adopted-out sons of alcoholics who themselves became alcoholics were reported to be hot tempered, hypersensitive, and insecure as children more often than controls.

Reaction to Food

This temperament dimension describes the propensity to seek out new and different tasting foods. Studies have not yet been conducted directly linking reaction to food to the liability to alcoholism.

It is interesting to note, however, that individuals with bulimia not only possess an intense drive state with respect to the pursuit and ingestion of food but also that bulimics typically consume foods that are either sweet or starchy, have a high calorie content, and require little chewing. About 30% of bulimics experience cravings for certain foods, and up to 25% have an uncontrollable appetite (Pyle et al., 1981). In addition, following food consumption, negative emotional experiences are common (Mitchell et al., 1985).

Studies directed to clarifying the primary temperament characteristics of individuals who develop an eating disorder have not yet been performed. Considering the aggregation of alcoholism and bulimia, both within the individual (Mitchell et al., 1985) and among family members (Hudson et al., 1983), it is intriguing to advance the hypothesis that a similar diathesis may be present in both disorders. Because of gender differences in social demands and acceptance of deviancy behavior, bulimia is the more likely outcome in females, whereas an antisocial disorder is more likely among males. Significantly, several reports link eating problems in childhood to the risk for alcoholism. However, systematic investigations remain to be conducted that are aimed at clarifying the role of food preference and reaction to food as components of the temperament phenotype predisposing to bulimia and alcoholism.

Sociability

Commenting on the characteristics measured by a high score on the MacAndrew Scale of the MMPI, Finney et al. (1971) stated that alcoholics are "bold, uninhibited, self-confident, sociable people who mix well with others" (p. 1058). Nonalcoholic young adults scoring high on these traits combined with a low score on the Socialization Scale of the California Personality Inventory experience a greater stress-dampening effect following alcohol consumption compared to controls (Sher and Levenson 1982). These findings indicate that alcohol consumption may be particularly reinforcing for individuals who are disinhibited and not normatively socialized. Hence, pharmacologic factors may interact with behavioral disposition to augment the risk for alcoholism. Support for the conclusion that these behavioral propensities predispose alcoholism, is provided by the observation that prealcoholics (Hoffman et al., 1974) as well as offspring of alcoholics also tend to score high on the MacAndrew Scale (MacAndrew, 1979; Saunders and Schuckit, 1981). Paralleling these findings, McCord and McCord (1960) found that the prealcoholic male commonly presented himself as outwardly aggressive and self-confident. Jones (1968) reported that the prealcoholic is typically talkative, spontaneously expressive, and prone to initiating humor in interpersonal situations.

The preceding findings could be interpreted to indicate that the prealcoholic and the person at elevated risk for alcoholism are more sociable than others in the general population. Closer examination of the qualitative aspects of the behavior demonstrates, however, that this is not the case. Rather, what appears to reflect high sociability actually comprises a disinhibited or dysregulated behavioral disposition. Disturbances in behavioral self-regulation have been linked to alcoholism etiology (Gorrenstein and Newman, 1980; Tarter et al., 1985a). Of the follow-up studies that have been conducted to date, all except Vaillant (1983) have reported that antisocial tendencies, to a more or less extent, often predate alcoholism. The absence of such an association in Vaillant's follow-up study may be due to the fact that his sample consisted of graduates from an elite university. Significantly, Robins (1966) reported that sadism and school truancy, as well as theft and other serious offenses, were common among prealcoholics. Prealcoholics were also found to be more sadistic than their peers by McCord and McCord (1960). Weak peer loyalty (Berry, 1967) and a negativistic outlook (Jones, 1968) were also reported to be common among prealcoholics. Studying male offspring who were adopted away from alcoholic parents, Goodwin et al. (1975) found that there was a higher prevalence of school truancy, antisocial behavior, aggressivity, and emotional insecurity compared to controls.

The preceding studies indicate that antisocial propensities characterize many prealcoholics. What appears superficially as sociability is in actuality, however, the expression of a highly active, disinhibited, labile, and impulsive disposition. The finding by Jones (1968) that prealcoholics are often inconsiderate and unaware of the impressions created on others underscores the manipulative and aggressive interpersonal style. In this regard, it is noteworthy that secondary school students scoring high on the MacAndrew Scale are more likely than their peers to have a history of drunkenness, crimes against property, and physical aggressiveness toward others (Rathus et al., 1980). In addition, adolescent problem drinkers are more likely to sustain their drinking behavior if inclined toward deviant behavior, have poor self-control, and are not involved with church or school (Donovan et al., 1983). The observation that teenage heavy alcohol consumers score lower than teenage abstainers on scales measuring socialization, aggression, suspicion, and impulsivity (Rydelius, 1983a, 1983b) further underscores the conclusion that the gregariousness reported to characterize prealcoholics is instead the manifestation of behavioral disinhibition. This disinhibition is expressed behaviorally as impulsivity and aggressivity, as well as in the more florid context of a conduct disorder or antisocial personality.

Summary

To recapitulate, deviations of primary temperament characteristics appear to be associated with an increased risk for alcoholism. Prealcoholics, as well as samples of individuals at high average risk for alcoholism (e.g., offspring of alcoholics), exhibit marked deviations in five of these characteristics: behavioral activity level, attention-span persistence, emotionality, soothability, and sociability. Formal studies of reaction to food have yet to be undertaken. Despite the paucity of research conducted to date, the findings suggest that interindividual differences in the liability to alcoholism can be understood to a large degree within the context of phenotypic variation in temperament traits. Assuming, as the evidence suggests, that the trait dimensions are orthogonal (Rowe and Plomin, 1977), it can be readily seen why each individual in the population is unique with respect to their temperament makeup. In effect, there is an infinite number of phenotypic combinations. Consequently, no specific temperament phenotype can be presumed to predispose to alcoholism. Rather, the magnitude and quality of phenotypic deviation among the complement of temperament dimensions via unique interactions with the environment underlies an idiosyncratic pathway to alcoholism for each person in the population.

Reciprocal Interactions between Behavior Phenotype and Environment

To this point we have examined the basis for the interindividual differences in the liability to alcoholism conceptualized within a life-span epigenetic perspective. Variations in the phenotypic expression of temperament traits provide a heuristic framework for characterizing this variability early in the child's life. Because alcoholism can occur only where alcohol beverages are available in the environment, neither the phenotypic characteristics of the individual alone (e.g., deviations in temperament traits) or the environment (e.g., poverty, parental abuse) are sufficient to determine the adverse outcome. Rather, it is the individually specific quality of interaction between phenotypic and environmental variables that is the condition required to produce this outcome. Figure 12-3 illustrates how variations in the phenotypic expression of temperament traits, through dynamic and reciprocal interaction with manifold environments, propels the child toward either a good or adverse outcome. In this conceptualization, there are both positive and negative forces in the environment operating simultaneously on the person throughout life to determine risk status. Because the type and balance (e.g., stressors relative to buffers) of environmental influences are distinctive for each person, it follows that the pathway to an alcoholism outcome is likewise idiosyncratic. From the standpoint of prevention and treatment, therefore, interventions must be directed to not only modifying the individual's behavior but also to engineering changes in the environment that attenuate the risk for problem alcohol use (Tarter, 1993b). The following discussion examines the key environmental factors that need to be elucidated with respect to how they specifically impact on the individual phenotype to determine the risk for an alcoholism outcome.

The home is the first and perhaps most important environment that interacts with the temperament phenotype to shape future behavior disposition. In this context, the first

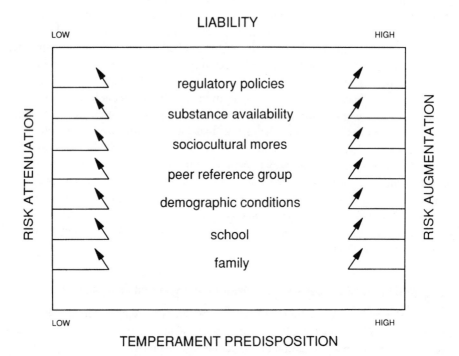

Fig. 12-3 Interaction between predisposition and environmental influences having either enhancing or attenuating effects on the liability to alcoholism.

developmental process is the formation of attachment or emotional bonding between the mother and baby (Ainsworth et al., 1978). It is interesting to note in this regard that rhesus monkeys separated early in life from their mothers and not afforded the opportunity for affectional bonding are more likely than monkeys raised by their mothers to subsequently consume alcohol (Higley et al., 1991).

Children with adverse temperament features whose parents are under stress or have emotional problems are more likely to be the target of criticism (Rutter, 1970). Mothers typically withdraw from temperamentally difficult sons but not difficult daughters (Macoby et al., 1984). Buss (1981) observed that fathers interact positively with sons who have a high behavioral activity level but negatively with highly active daughters. Thomas et al. (1968) found that temperamentally difficult children do not respond to maternal caregiving as readily as children with easy temperaments. These studies amply illustrate that deviations in temperament by neonates and infants jeopardizes the opportunity for parent–child bonding. In the absence of effective parenting skills, aversive control tactics are likely to be employed in managing the behavior of the temperamentally difficult child (Lee and Bates, 1985). Hence, in the context of the epigenetic model described herein, it is not surprising that Crockenberg (1987) noted that infants at 3 months of age are rated as more irritable, noncompliant, and hostile by 2 years of age if mothers exercised a punitive rearing style. In effect, a difficult temperament during infancy, in conjunction with a home environment characterized by parents with poor child-rearing skills, molds the preschooler's behavior such that it is prodromal to a conduct disorder (Bates and Bales, 1988) and subsequently to school failure, commitment to a deviant peer group, and delinquency (Patterson et al., 1989). Alcohol consumption is typical, albeit age-inappropriate, among youths with this type of problem behavior (Donovan et al., 1983; Jessor et al., 1991). In summary, the importance of the quality of interaction between the parents and child in contributing to a conduct disorder outcome cannot be overemphasized; affectionate mothers, for example, can lower the liability to a conduct disorder (McCord, 1986), whereas anxious, commanding, permissive, or neglectful parents promote the development of such a disorder in their children (Loeber and Dishion, 1983).

The preceding studies underscore the prominence of the parent–child interaction pattern in establishing a behavioral disposition in children that predisposes to alcoholism. Additionally, these studies illustrate the critical role of unshared environmental influences, that is, factors that uniquely affect one child and not the other in a sibship. Interestingly, the unshared environment appears to contribute more to variability in the risk of the development of psychopathology than shared environmental influences (Reiss et al., 1991). Moreover, research to date clearly demonstrates the importance of bidirectional effects on the development of behavior problems in children. For example, babies who resist cuddling are more active and restless; they are also less comforted by soothing from the mother (Schaffer and Emerson, 1964). Hence, in attempting to understand the development of successive phenotypes that place the child on a trajectory toward alcoholism, it is essential to clarify how the child's phenotype at any point induces effects on the environment that resonate back to influence subsequent development according to the type of response by others in the environment.

Adjustment to the school environmental is usually the first development challenge for adjustment outside the home. Martin et al. (1983) report that the temperament traits of persistence, distractibility, and behavioral activity level explained 20–30% of the variance on a measure of "constructive self-directed activity" among children in the first grade. Magnitude of expression of these temperament traits also correlates significantly with achievement test scores (Martin, 1989). Children in kindergarten who are held back from the first grade are more likely to be rated by teachers as less persistent and more distractable than children who are promoted (D'Agastino, 1987). Performance on standard achievement tests by fifth graders has also been shown to be related to behavior activity level, persistence, and distractibility (Martin, 1989). Interestingly, good and poor achievers in school are discriminable on the temperament traits of persistence, approach/withdrawal, and distractibility (Martin, 1983). This temperament cluster is also associated with teachers' perceptions of the child's learning potential (Keogh, 1982). These studies illustrate the association between temperament traits and the quality of adjustment in school. Maladjustment therein, in addition to the home, may thus comprise a vector to adaptational failure. Children who are behaviorally maladjusted or are unable to adequately meet age concordant academic challenges are at risk for school dropout and ostracism from peers who do make a satisfactory adjustment. The point to be made is that individual differences in temperament traits influence academic performance and social adjustment in the school environment. Failure to adjust optimally to this environment contributes to the risk for psychopathology and social deviancy that in turn is associated with alcohol abuse.

As the child matures and disengages from parental control, peer influences on behavior become increasingly strong. There is little doubt that the structure of the social environment with respect to the degree of social integration in a network of friends and other community members is important. Peers provide functional support so as to buffer stress, provide advice, and enhance self-esteem. Importantly, the networks—family and peer—interact so as to affect the risk for alcohol-use onset. For example, emotional support from the family can have a protective influence over drug use in adolescents where there is a high level of substance abuse among peers (Wills, 1990). Alternatively, where family influence is limited, the peer group can exercise control over the child's behavior. Thus, beginning at around puberty, as the child asserts increasing autonomy, family and peer networks each influence the youngster's behavior. Not surprisingly, alcohol and drug use is initiated most commonly during this transition phase from parental to peer influence as the latter becomes an increasingly important regulator of behavior.

A substantial literature has developed over the past five decades detailing the relationship between occupational (Plant, 1979), cultural (Heath, 1984), and psychosocial (Sadava, 1987) factors on alcohol consumption behavior. No research has been conducted, however, that examines specific phenotype–environment interactions; rather this line of investigation has been confined to characterizing, as main effects, only the environmental influences. Research in this area is thus required to determine how specific environmental demands, contingencies, and social policies interact with particular temperament phenotypes (as well as other behavioral dispositions) that can promote or protect the person from an alcoholism outcome.

Implications of the Epigenetic Perspective

An epigenetic perspective is clearly helpful in elucidating the factors involved in the variability of the liability to alcoholism. One advantage of such an approach is the opportunity to conduct controlled research using animal models. By systematically manipulating environmental contingencies in paradigms using animals selectively bred to be high or low in a particular trait, it is possible to elucidate gene–environment correlations and interactions with respect to alcohol consumption. For instance, rodents have been selectively bred for behavioral traits (e.g., emotionality, activity level, sociability) that appear to be associated with the liability to alcoholism. Furthermore, recognizing that variation in these behaviors has a polygenic basis, the application of molecular genetic techniques may be valuable for detecting DNA marker loci for these traits. Recombinant inbred strains having specific behavior phenotypes are particularly applicable to investigations directed toward isolating the proportion of genetic variance contributed to by many genes (Plomin, 1990). Quantitative trait loci, reflecting polygenic influences, have been identified in rodents in a test of behavioral activity level in an open field (Plomin et al., 1991). Also the effects of ethanol on behavior in this procedure have been examined (McClearn et al., 1991). These studies are especially intriguing considering the preliminary evidence linking high behavior activity level in humans to increased risk for alcoholism. The general point to be made, however, is that behavior-genetic studies of humans could guide research with animals that can inform about potential DNA markers for the liability to alcoholism.

Animal studies can also provide important information in situations where the behavioral phenotype cannot be experimentally controlled, as in research on humans. For example, parent–offspring interactional style, particularly the supervisory involvement of the parent, might be linked to the risk for an alcohol abuse outcome. One aspect of this relationship that may be especially important and has been examined in a primate model, concerns the influence of parent–offspring bonding. Separation from the mother and being raised by peers (Highley et al., 1991) are associated with a propensity for alcohol consumption among subhuman primates. The extent to which alcohol consumption in adolescence is mediated or moderated by temperament deviation concomitant to deficient affectional bonding soon after birth is not known. Nonetheless, it would appear to be an important topic for study from an epigenetic perspective.

The individual norm of reaction for the liability to alcoholism exists from the moment of conception. However, the phenotypic distribution for this trait remains a statistical abstraction until such time as the variation in the liability can be directly observed; that is, when the presence of affected and nonaffected phenotypes can be identified in the population. Since only phenotypes from the beyond-the-threshold range are currently described, a large portion of the distribution, estimated at approximately 85% from the Epidemiologic Catchment Area study (Helzer and Pryzbeck, 1988), is obscure because all nonaffected phenotypes are collapsed into one category (i.e., not alcoholic). The search for the predictors of the liability, including genetic markers, should therefore be recognized as directed to making the total liability distribution visible rather than as the search for the causes of alcoholism.

Behavioral genetic research in humans and animals could potentially elucidate the neurobiological substrate underlying the variation in expression of temperament. Insofar as individual differences in temperament phenotypes are due to variations in the biological substrate (i.e., neurochemical and neurophysiological processes), it is heuristic to guide the search for neurochemical and physiological mechanisms that might underlie the association between certain temperament phenotypes and risk for alcoholism. Such research may in fact also contribute ultimately to revealing the relevant gene loci inasmuch as biological processes, compared to behavioral traits, are more proximal to primary gene action. Several connecting threads from a number of different lines of research point to the potential value of searching for biobehavioral mechanisms underlying the liability to alcoholism. For example, there is evidence that the concentrations of 5-HIAA, the serotonin metabolite, is lower in cerebrospinal fluid among persons who are violent (Brown and Linnoila, 1990). Aggressivity, as pointed out earlier, may have its origins in certain temperament phenotypes, particularly high behavioral activity level. Significantly, the level of 5-HIAA is correlated with aggressivity in alcoholics (Limson et al., 1991). Furthermore, altered serotonergic functioning has been reported to be associated with aggression among antisocial substance abusers (Moss et al., 1990). Although research has yet to be conducted that links variation in serotonin metabolism to temperament, the available findings are nonetheless suggestive of such an association.

Finally, the epigenetic perspective has practical ramifications. It underscores the need to elucidate how phenotypic characteristics and environmental variables interact during development to direct the person toward or away from an alcoholism outcome. From the standpoint of primary prevention, interventions must begin early in life; that is, long before the developmental trajectory is established. Negative peer status, for example, is well known to comprise an important risk factor for subsequent serious maladjustment (Parker and Asher, 1987), and is also associated concurrently with aggressivity (Olson and Brodfeld, 1991). Both these factors are easily detectable early in the child's life and are related to an increased risk for alcohol abuse. Once such children are identified, methods need to be employed that conjointly change the child's behaviors as well as the others (e.g., parents, peers, siblings) in the social environment. In this manner, the vector responsible for placing the child into the high-risk trajectory (vis-à-vis person–environment interaction pattern) can be both reduced in force and altered with respect to its direction.

Acknowledgements: This was supported by grants DA05605 and AA8746. From the National Institute on Drug Abuse and National Institute on Alcohol Abuse and Alcoholism. Appreciation is expressed to Jessie Chiang for her technical assistance.

References

Ainsworth, M., Blehar, M., Waters, E., and Wall, S. (1978). *Patterns of Attachment.* Hillsdale, NJ: Erlbaum.

Allport, G. (1961). *Pattern and Growth in Personality.* New York: Holt, Reinhart, Winston.

Alterman, A., Petrarulo, E., Tarter, R., and McCowan, G. (1982). Hyperactivity and alcoholism: Familial and behavioral correlates. *Addict. Behav.* **7**:413–421.

Alterman, A., Tarter, R., Petrarulo, E., and Baughman, T. (1984). Evidence for impersistence in young male alcoholics. *Alcohol.: Clin. Exp. Res.* **8**:448–450.

American Psychiatric Association (1987). *Diagnostic and Statistical Manual of Mental Disorders,* 3d ed. Washington, DC.

Aronson, H., and Gilbert, A. (1963). Preadolescent sons of male alcoholics. *Arch. Gen. Psychiatr.* **8**:47–53.

August, G., and Stewart, M. (1982). Is there a syndrome of pure hyperactivity? *Br. J. Psychiatr.* **140**:305–311.

Barkley, R., Fischer, M., Edelbrock, C., and Smallish, L. (1990). The adolescent outcome of hyperactive children diagnosed by research criteria: 1. An 8-year prospective follow-up study. *J. Am. Acad. Child Adolesc. Psychiatr.* **29**:546–557.

Barnes, G. (1983). Clinical and prealcoholic personality characteristics. In *The Pathogenesis of Alcoholism,* B. Kissin and H. Begleiter, eds. New York: Plenum Press, pp. 113–195.

Bates, J., and Bales, K. (1988). The role of attachment in the development of behavior problems. In *Clinical Implications of Attachment,* J. Belsky and T. Nezworski, eds. Hillsdale, NJ: Erlbaum, pp. 253–295.

Begleiter, H., Porjesz, B., and Kissin, B. (1984). Event-related brain potentials in children at risk for alcoholism. *Science* **225**:1493–1495.

Bell, R. (1968). A reinterpretation of the direction of effects in studies of socialization. *Psychol. Rev.* **75**:81–95.

Berry, J. (1967). Antecedents of Schizophrenia, Impulsive Character, and Alcoholism in Males. Ph.D. dissertation, Columbia University.

Billman, J., and McDevitt, S. (1980). Convergence of parent and observer ratings of temperament with observations of peer interaction in nursery school. *Child Dev.* **51**:395–400.

Blackson, T., Tarter, R., Martin, C., and Moss, H. (1994) Temperament mediates the effects of family history of substance abuse on externalizing and internalizing child behavior. *Am. J. Addict.* **3**:58-66.

Block, J. (1971). *Lives Through Time* Berkeley, CA: Bancroft.

Blouin, A., Bornstein, R., and Trites, R. (1978). Teenage alcohol use among hyperactive children: A four-year follow-up study. *J. Pediatr. Psychiatr.* **3**:188–194.

Borland, B., and Heckman, H. (1976). Hyperactive boys and their brothers: A 25-year follow-up study. *Arch. Gen. Psychiatr.* **33**:669–675.

Bouchard, T., Lykken, D., McGue, M., Segal, N., and Tellegen, A. (1990). Sources of human psychological differences: The Minnesota Study of Twins Reared Apart. *Science* **250**:223–228.

Brown, G., and Linnoila, M. (1990). CSF Serotonin metabolite (5-HIAA) studies in depression, impulsivity, and violence. *J. Clin. Psychiatr.* **52**(suppl.):31–41.

Burke, K., Burke, J., Regier, D., and Rae, D. (1990). Age at onset of selected mental disorders in five community populations. *Arch. Gen. Psychiatr.* **47**:511–518.

Buss, D. (1981). Predicting parent-child interactions from children's activity level. *Dev. Psychol.* **17**:59–65.

Buss, A., and Plomin, R. (1975). *A Temperament Theory of Personality Development.* New York: Wiley.

Cantwell, D. (1972). Psychiatric illness in families of hyperactive children. *Arch. Gen. Psychiatr.* **27**:414–417.

Carey, W., Fox, M., and McDevitt, C. (1977). Temperament as a factor in early school adjustment. *Pediatrics* **60**:621–624.

Chassin, L., Rogush, F., and Barrera, M. (1991). Substance use and symptomatology among adolescent children of alcoholics. *J. Abnorm. Psychol.* **100**:449–463.

Cloninger, C., Bohman, M., and Sigvardsson, S. (1981). Inheritance of alcohol abuse: Cross fostering analyses of adopted men. *Arch. Gen. Psychiatr.* **38**:861–868.

Coopermith, S., and Woodrow, K. (1967). Basal conductance levels of normals and alcoholics. *Q. J. Stud. Alcohol* **28**:27–32.

Costello, R. (1981). Alcoholism and the "alcoholic personality." In *Evaluation of the Alcoholic. Implications for Research, Theory and Treatment.* R. Meyer, B. Glueck, J. O'Brien, T. Babor, J. Jaffe, and J. Stabenau, eds. Washington, DC, NIAAA Monograph No. 5 (DHHS publ. no. (ADM) 81-1033), pp. 69–83.

Crockenberg, S. (1987). Predictors and correlations of anger toward and punitive control of toddlers by adolescent mothers. *Child Dev.* **58**:964–975.

Cyphers, L., Phillips, K., Fulker, D., and Mrazek, D. (1990). Twin temperament during the transition from infancy to early childhood. *J. Am. Acad. Child Adolesc. Psychiatr.* **29**:392–397.

D'Agostino, J. (1987). Children's Characteristics Related to Promotion and Nonpromotion in Kindergarten. Unpublished doctoral dissertation. University of Southern California, Los Angeles, CA.

DeObaldia, R., and Parsons, O. (1983). Reliability studies on the primary-secondary alcoholism classification questionnaire and the HK/MBD childhood symptoms checklist. *J. Clin. Psychol.* **40**:1257–1257.

DeObaldia, R., Parsons, O., and Yohman, R. (1983). Minimal brain dysfunction symptoms claimed by primary and secondary alcoholics: Relation to cognitive functioning. *Int. J. Neurosci.* **20**:173–181.

Docter, R., and Bernal, M. (1964). Immediate and prolonged psychophysiological effects of sustained alcohol intake in alcoholics. *Q. J. Stud. Alcohol* **25**:438–450.

Docter, R., Naitoh, P., and Smith, J. (1966). Electroencephalographic changes and vigilance behavior during experimentally induced intoxication with alcoholic subjects. *Psychosom. Med.* **28**:605–615.

Donovan, J., Jessor, R., and Jessor, L. (1983). Problem drinking in adolescence and young adulthood. A follow-up study. *J. Stud. Alcohol* **44**:109–137.

Dunn, J., and Plomin, R. (1986). Determinants of maternal behavior towards 3-year-old siblings. *Br. J. Dev. Psychol.* **4**:127–137.

Earleywine, M., Finn, P., and Martin, C. (1990). Personality risk and alcohol consumption: A latent variable analysis. *Addict. Behav.* **15**:183–187.

Earls, F., and Jung, K. (1987). Temperament and home environment characteristics in the early development of child psychopathology. *J. Am. Acad. Child Psychiatr.* **26**:491–498.

Elmasian, R., Neville, H., Woods, D., Schuckit, M., and Bloom, F. (1982). Event-related brain potentials are different in individuals at high and low risk for developing alcoholism. *Proc. Nat. Acad. Sci.* **79**:7900–7903.

Engfer, A. (1986). Antecedents of perceived behavior problems in infancy. In *Temperament Discussed,* G. Kohnstamm, ed., New York: Wiley, pp. 165–180.

Esterbrooks, A., and Ende, R. (1988). Marital and parent-child relationships. The role of affect in the family system. In *Relationships Within Families: Mutual Influences,* R. Hinde and J. Stevensen-Hinde, eds. New York: Oxford University Press, pp. 104–141.

Eysenck, H. (1983). Neurotic conditions. In *The Child at Psychiatric Risk,* R. Tarter, ed. New York: Oxford, pp. 245–285.

Falconer, D. (1965). The inheritance of liability to certain diseases estimated from the incidence among relatives. *Ann. Hum. Genet.* **29**:51–86.

Finney, J., Smith, D., Skeeters, D., and Auvenchine, C. (1971). MMPI alcoholism scales: Factor structure and content analysis. *Q. J. Stud. Alcohol* **32**:1055–1060.

Floderus-Myhred, B., Pederson, M., and Rasmuson, J. (1980). Assessment for heritability for personality based on a short form of the Eysenck Personality Inventory. A study of 12,898 twin pairs. *Behav. Genet.* **10**:153–162.

Gandour, M. (1989). Activity level as a dimension of temperament in toddlers: Its relevance for the organismic specificity hypothesis. *Child Dev.* **60**:1092–1098.

Garfield, Z., and McBrearty, J. (1970). Arousal level and stimulus response in alcoholics after drinking. *Q. J. Stud. Alcohol* **31**:832–838.

Gittelman, R., Manuzza, S., Shenker, R., and Bonagura, N. (1985). Hyperactive boys almost grown up. *Arch. Gen. Psychiatr.* **42**:937–947.

Goldsmith, H., and Gottesman, I. (1981). Origins of variation in behavioral style. A longitudinal study of temperament in young twins. *Child Dev.* **52**:91–103.

Gomberg, E. (1982). The young male alcoholic: A pilot study. *J. Stud. Alcohol* **43**:683–701.

Goodwin, D., Schulsinger, F., Hermansen, L., Guze, S., and Winokur, G. (1975). Alcoholism and the hyperactive child syndrome. *J. Nerv. Ment. Dis.* **160**:349–353.

Gorrenstein, E., and Newman, J. (1980). Disinhibitory psychopathology: A new perspective and model for research. *Psychol. Rev.* **87**:301–315.

Graham, R., Rutter, M., and George, S. (1973). Temperamental characteristics as predictors of behavior disorder in children. *Am. J. Orthopsychiatr.* **43**:328–339.

Hagekull, B. (1989). Longitudinal stability of temperament within a behavioral style framework. In *Temperament in Children,* G. Kohnstamm, J. Bates, and M. Rothbart, eds. New York: Wiley, pp. 283–297.

Halverson, C., and Waldrop, M. (1976). Relations between preschool activity and aspects of intellectual and social behavior at age 7;n1/;d2. *Dev. Psychol.* **12**:107–112.

Heath, D. (1984). Cross-cultural studies of alcoholism. In *Recent Developments in Alcoholism,* M. Galanter, ed. New York: Plenum, pp. 405–415.

Heath, A., Meyer, J., Eaves, L., and Martin, N. (1991a). The inheritance of alcohol consumption patterns in a general population twin sample: I. Multidimensional scaling of quantity/frequency data. *J. Stud. Alcohol* **52**:345–352.

Heath, A., Meyer, J., Jardine, R., and Martin, N. (1991b). The inheritance of alcohol consumption in a general population twin study: II. Determinants of consumption frequency and quantity consumed. *J. Stud. Alcohol* **52**:425–433.

Hechtman, L., Weiss, G., and Perlman, T. (1984b). Hyperactives as young adults: Past and current substance abuse and antisocial behavior. *Am. J. Orthopsychiatr.* **54**:415–425.

Hechtman, L., Weiss, G., Perlman, R., and Amsel, R. (1984a). Hyperactives as young adults: Initial predictors of outcome. *J. Am. Acad. Child Psychiatr.* **23**:250–260.

Helzer, J., and Pryzbeck, T. (1988). The co-occurrence of alcoholism with other psychiatric disorders in the general population and its impact on treatment. *J. Stud. Alcohol* **49**:219–224.

Higley, J., Hasert, M., Suomi, S., and Linnoila, M. (1991). Nonhuman primate model of alcohol abuse: Effects of early experience, personality, and stress on alcohol consumption. *Proc. Natl. Acad. Sci.* **88**:7261–7265.

Hill, S., Steinhauer, S., Park, J., and Zubin, J. (1990). Event-related potential characteristics in children of alcoholics from high density families. *Alcohol.: Clin. Exp. Res.* **14**:6–16.

Hoffman, H., Loper, R., and Kammeier, M. (1974). Identifying future alcoholics with MMPI alcoholism scales. *Q. J. Stud. Alcohol* **35**:490–498.

Holmberg, G., and Martens, S. (1955). Electroencephalographic changes in man correlated with blood alcohol concentration and some other conditions following standardized ingestion of alcohol. *Q. J. Stud. Alcohol* **16**:411–424.

Hoy, E., Weiss, G., Minde, K., and Cohen, H. (1978). The hyperactive child at adolescence: Cognitive, emotional and social functioning. *J. Abnorm. Child Psychol.* **6**:311–324.

Hudson, J. I., Pope, H. J., Jonas, J. M., and Yurgelun-Todd, D. (1983). Family history study of anorexia nervosa and bulimia. *Br. J. Psychiatr.* **142**:133–138.

Jessor, R., Donovan, J., and Costa, F. (1991). *Beyond Adolescence. Problem Behavior and Young Adult Development.* New York: Cambridge University Press.

Jones, M. (1968). Personality correlates and antecedents of drinking patterns in adult males. *J. Consult. Clin. Psychology* **32**:2–12.

Kagan, J., and Snidman, N. (1991). Infant predictors of inhibited and uninhibited profiles. *Psychol. Sci.* **2**:40–44.

Kammeier, M., Hoffman, H., and Loper, R. (1973). Personality characteristics of alcoholics as college freshmen at time of treatment. *Q. J. Stud. Alcohol* **34**:390–399.

Kellam, S., Brown, H., Rubin, B., and Ensminger, M. (1983). Paths leading to teenage psychiatric symptoms and substance use: Developmental epidemiological studies in Woodlawn. In *Child Psychopathology and Development,* S. Guze, F. Earls, and J. Barrett, eds. New York: Raven Press, pp. 17–47.

Keogh, B. (1982). Children's temperament and teachers' decisions. In *Temperamental Differences in Infants and Young Children,* R. Porter and G. Collins, eds. London: CIBA Foundation Symposium 89, Pitman, pp. 269–279.

Kissin, B., and Hankoff, L. (1959). The acute effects of ethyl alcohol on the Funkenstein mecholyl response in male alcoholics. *Q. J. Stud. Alcohol* **20**:696–703.

Labouvie, E., Pandina, R., and Johnson, V. (1991). Developmental trajectories of substance use in adolescence: Difference and predictors. *Int. J. Behav. Dev.* **14**:305–328.

Lee, C., and Bates, J. (1985). Mother-child interaction at age two years and perceived difficult temperament. *Child Dev.* **56**:1314–1326.

Lerner, J., and Vicary, J. (1984). Difficult temperament and drug use: Analysis from the New York Longitudinal Study. *J. Drug Educ.* **14**:1–8.

Limson, R., Goldman, D., Roy, A., Lamparski, D., Ravitz, B., Adinoff, B., and Linnoila, M. (1991). Personality and cerebrospinal fluid monoamine metabolites in alcoholics and controls. *Arch. Gen. Psychiatr.* **48**:437–441.

Loeber, R., and Dishion, T. (1983). Early predictors of male delinquency: A review. *Psychol. Bull.* **94**:68–99.

Loehlin, J., and Nichols, R. (1976). *Heredity, Environment and Personality.* Austin, TX: University of Texas Press.

Loehlin, J., Horn, J., and Willerman, L. (1981). Personality resemblance in adoptive families. *Behav. Genet.* **11**:309–330.

Loehlin, J., Willerman, L., and Horn, J. (1985). Personality resemblances in adoptive families where the children are late adolescent or adult. *J. Pers. Soc. Psychol.* **48**:376–392.

Loper, R., Kammeier, M., and Hoffman, H. (1973). MMPI characteristics of college freshman males who later became alcoholics. *J. Abnorm. Psychol.* **82**:159–162.

Lund, C., and Landesman-Dwyer, S. (1979). Pre-delinquent and disturbed adolescents: The role of parental alcoholism. In *Currents in Alcoholism: Biomedical Issues and Clinical Effects of Alcoholism,* M. Galanter, ed. New York: Grune & Stratton, pp. 339–345.

MacAndrew, C. (1979). On the possibility of the psychometric detection of persons who are prone to the abuse of alcohol and other substances. *Addict. Behav.* **4**:11–20.

MacAndrew, C. (1981). What the MAC Scale tells us about men alcoholics: An interpretive review. *J. Stud. Alcohol* **42**:604–625.

McClearn, G., Plomin, R., Gora-Maslak, G., and Crabbe, (1991). The gene chase in behavioral science. *Psychol. Sci.* **2**:222–229.

McCord, J. (1986). Instigation and insulation: How families affect antisocial aggression. In *Development of Antisocial and Prosocial Behavior: Research Theories and Issues,* D. Olweus, J. Block, and M. Radke-Yarrow, eds. San Diego: Academic Press, pp. 343–358.

McCord, W., and McCord, J. (1960). *Origins of Alcoholism.* Stanford, CA: Stanford University. Mendelson, W., Johnson, N., and Stewart, M. (1971). Hyperactive children as teenagers: A follow-up study. *J. Nerv. Ment. Dis.* **153**:273–279.

Macoby, E., Snow, M., and Jacklin, C. (1984). Children's disposition and mother child interaction at 12 and 18 months. A short-term longitudinal study. *Dev. Psychol.* **20**:259–272.

Mannuzza, S., Gittelman, R., and Addalli, K. (1991). Young adult mental status of hyperactive boys and their brothers: A prospective follow-up study. *J. Am. Acad. Child Adolesc. Psychiatr.* **30**:743–751.

Markman, H., and Jones-Leonard, D. (1985). Marital discord and children at risk: Implications for research and prevention. In *Identification of the Child at Risk. An International Perspective,* W. Frankenburg and R. Ende, eds. New York: Plenum, pp. 59–77.

Martin, R. (1983). Temperament: A review of research with implications for the school psychologist. *Sch. Psychol. Rev.* **12**:266–273.

Martin, R. (1989). Activity level, distractibility, and persistence: Critical characteristics in early schooling. In *Temperament in Childhood,* G. Kohnstamm, J. Bates, and M. Rothbart, eds. New York: Wiley, pp. 451–461.

Martin, R., Nagle, R., and Paget, K. (1983). Relationship between temperament and classroom behavior, teacher attitudes, and academic achievement. *J. Clin. Psychol.* **39**:1013–1020.

Matheny, A. (1986). Stability and change of infant temperament: Contributions from the infant, mother and family environment. In *Temperaments Discussed,* G. Kohnstamm, ed. Kisse, The Netherlands: Swetz & Zeitlinger, pp. 49–58.

Matheny, A., Wilson, R., and Thoben, A. (1987). Home and mother: Relations with infant temperament. *Dev. Psychol.* **23**:323–331.

Maziade, M. (1989b). Should adverse temperament matter to the clinician? An empirically based answer. In *Temperament in Childhood,* G. Kohnstamm, J. Bates, and M. Rothbart, eds. New York: Wiley, pp. 421–435.

Maziade, M., Caperaa, P., LaPlante, B., Boudreault, M., Thiverge, J., Cote, R., and Boutin, P. (1985). Value of difficult temperament among 7-year-olds in the general population for predicting psychiatric diagnosis at age 12. *Am. J. Psychiatr.* **142**:943–946.

Maziade, M., Caron, C., Cote, R., Boutin, P., and Thiverge, J. (1990). Extreme temperament and diagnosis: A study in a psychiatric sample of consecutive children. *Arch. Gen. Psychiatr.* **47**:477–484.

Maziade, M., Cote, R., Boudreault, M., Caperaa, P., and Thiverge, J. (1984). The NYLS model of temperament: Gender differences and demographic correlates in a French speaking population. *J. Am. Acad. Child Psychiatr.* **23**:582–587.

Mezzich, A., Arria, A., Tarter, R., Moss, H., and Van Thiel, D. (1991). Psychiatric comorbidity in alcoholism: Important of ascertainment source. *Alcohol.: Clin. Exp. Res.* **5**:893–898.

Mischel, W. (1983). Delay of gratification as a process and as a person variable in development.

In *Human Development: An Interactional Perspective,* D. Magnusson and V. Allen, eds. New York: Academic Press, pp. 149–165.

Mitchell, J. E., Hatsukami, D., Eckert, E. D., and Pyle, R. L. (1985). Characteristics of 275 patients with bulimia. *Am. J. Psychiatr.* **142**:482–485.

Morrison, J., and Stewart, M. (1973). The psychiatric status of the legal families of adopted hyperactive children. *Arch. Gen. Psychiatr.* **28**:888–891.

Moss, H., Blackson, T., Martin, C., Vanyukov, M., and Tarter, R. (1992). Heightened motor activity level in male offspring of substance abusing parents: Association with temperament and behavior disposition. *Biol. Psychiat.* **32**:1135–1147.

Moss, H., Yao, J., and Panzak, G. (1991). Serotonergic responsivity and behavioral dimensions in antisocial personality disorder with substance abuse. *Biol. Psychiatr.* **28**:325–338.

Olson, S., and Brodfeld, P. (1991). Assessment of peer rejection and externalizing behavior problems in preschool boys: A short-term longitudinal study. *J. Abnorm. Psychol.* **19**:493–503.

Parker, J., and Asher, S. (1987). Peer relations and later personal adjustment. Are low-accepted children at risk? *Psychol. Bull.* **102**:357–389.

Patterson, G., DeBaryshe, B., and Ramsey, E. (1989). A developmental perspective on antisocial behavior. *Am. Psychol.* **44**:329–335.

Pelham, W., Lang, A., Atkeson, B., Murphy, D., Gnagy, E., Greiner, A., Vodde-Hamilton, M., and Greenslade, K. Stress Induced Alcohol Consumption in Parents Interacting with Confederate Children: Effects of Child Behavior, Offspring Psychopathology, and Family History of Alcohol Problems. Unpublished manuscript.

Pihl, R., Peterson, J., and Finn, P. (1990). Inherited predisposition to alcoholism: Characteristics of sons of male alcoholics. *J. Abnorm. Psychol.* **99**:291–301.

Plant, M. (1979). Occupation, drinking patterns, and alcohol related problems: Conclusion from a follow-up study. *Br. J. Addict.* **74**:267–273.

Plomin, R. (1983). Developmental behavioral genetics. *Child Dev.* **54**:253–259.

Plomin, R. (1990). The role of inheritance in behavior. *Science* **248**:183–188.

Plomin, R., and DeFries, J. (1985). *Origins of Individual Differences in Infancy. The Colorado Adoption Project.* New York: Academic Press.

Plomin, R., and Rowe, D. (1977). A twin study of temperament in young children. *J. Psychol.* **97**:107–115.

Plomin, R., DeFries, J., and Loehlin, J. (1977). Genotype-environment interaction and correlation in the analysis of human behavior. *Psychol. Bull.* **84**:309–322.

Plomin, R., Petersen, N., McClearn, G., Nesselroade, J., and Bergman, C. (1988). EAS temperament during the last half of the life span: Twins reared apart and twins reared together. *Psychol. Aging* **3**:43–50.

Plomin, R., McClearn, G., Gora, Maslak, G., and Neiderhiser, J. (1991). Use of recombinant inbred strains to detect quantitative trait loci associated with behavior. Behav. Genet. **21**:99–116.

Pyle, R. L., Mitchell, J. E., and Eckert, E. D. (1981). Bulimia: A report of 34 cases. *J. Clin. Psychiatr.* **42**:60–64.

Rathus, S., Fox, J., and Ortins, J. (1980). The MacAndrew Scale as a measure of substance abuse and delinquency among adolescents. *J. Clin. Psychol.* **36**:579–583.

Reiss, D., Plomin, R., and Hetherington, M. (1991). Genetics and psychiatry: An unheralded window on the environment. *Am. J. Psychiatr.* **148**:283–291.

Robins, L. (1966). *Deviant Children Grown Up. A Sociological and Psychiatric Study of Sociopathic Personality.* Baltimore: Williams and Wilkins.

Rosenberg, C., and Buttsworth, F. (1969). Anxiety in alcoholics. *Q. J. Stud. Alcohol* **30:**729–732.

Rothbart, M. (1989). Temperament and development. In *Temperament in Childhood,* G. Kohnstamm, J. Bates, and M. Rothbart, eds. New York: Wiley, pp. 187–247.

Rowe, D., and Plomin, R. (1977). Temperament in early childhood. *J Pers. Assess.* **41:**150–156.

Rudie, R., and McGaughran, L. (1961). Differences in developmental experiences, defensiveness and personality organization between two classes of problem drinkers. *J. Abnorm. Soc. Psychol.* **62:**659–655.

Rutter, M. (1970). Psychological development: Predictions from infancy. *J. Child Psychol. Psychiat.* **15:**49–62.

Rydelius, P. (1983a). Alcohol-abusing teenage boys: Testing a hypothesis on alcohol abuse and personality factors using a personality inventory. *Acta Psychiatr. Scand.* **68:**381–385.

Rydelius, P. (1983b). Alcohol-abusing teenage boys: Testing a hypothesis on the relationship between alcohol abuse and social background factors, criminality and personality in teenage boys. *Acta Psychiatr. Scand.* **68:**368–380.

Sadava, S. (1987). Interactional theory. In *Psychological Theories of Drinking and Alcoholism,* H. Blane and K. Leonard, eds. New York: Guilford, pp. 90–130.

Saunders, G., and Schuckit, M. (1981). MMPI scores in young men with alcoholic relatives and controls. *J. Nerv. Ment. Dis.* **169:**456–458.

Schaeffer, K., Parsons, O., and Yohman, J. (1984). Neuropsychological differences between male familial alcoholics and nonalcoholics. *Alcohol.: Clin. Exp. Res.* **8:**347–351.

Schaffer, H., and Emerson, P. (1964). Patterns of response to physical contact in early human development. *J. Child Psychol. Psychiatr.* **5:**1–13.

Shekim, W., Asarnow, R., Hess, E., Zaucha, K., and Wheeler, N. (1990). A clinical and demographic profile of a sample of adults with attention deficit hyperactivity disorder, residual state. *Compr. Psychiatr.* **31:**416–425.

Sher, K., and Levenson, R. (1982). Risk for alcoholism and individual differences in the stress-response-dampening effect of alcohol. *J. Abnorm. Psychol.* **19:**350–367.

Sher, K., Walitzer, D., and Wood, P. (1991). Characteristics of children of alcoholics: Putative risk factors, substance use and abuse, and psychopathology. *J. Abnorm. Psychol.* **10:**427–448.

Sieber, M., and Bentler, P. (1982). Kausalamodelle zur personlichkeit und dem spateren konsum legaler und illegaler drogen. *Schweizrisch Zeitschrift fur Psychologie und Ibre Anwendugen.* **41:**1–5.

Stevenson-Hinde, J., and Simpson, A. (1982). Temperament and relationships. In *Temperamental Differences in Infants and Young Children,* R. Porter and G. Collins, eds. London: CIBA Foundation Symposium 89, Pittman, pp. 51–61.

Stewart, M., and duBlois, C. (1981). Wife abuse among families attending a child psychiatry clinic. *J. Am. Acad. Child Psychiatr.* **20:**845–862.

Szatmari, P., Boyle, M., and Offord, D. (1989). ADDH and conduct disorder: Degree of diagnostic overlap and differences among correlates. *J. Am. Acad. Child Adolesc. Psychiatr.* **28:**865–872.

Tarter, R. (1982). Psychosocial history, minimal brain dysfunction and differential drinking patterns of male alcoholics. *J. Clin. Psychol.* **38:**867–873.

Tarter, R. (1990). Evaluation and treatment of adolescent substance abuse: A decision tree method. *Am. J. Drug Alcohol Abuse* **16:**1–46.

Tarter, R. (1991). Developmental behavior-genetic perspective of alcoholism etiology. In *Recent Developments in Alcoholism,* M. Galanter, ed. New York: Plenum, pp. 71–85.

Tarter, R. (1992). Prevention of drug abuse. Theory and application. *Am. J. Addict.* **1:**2–20.

Tarter, R., McBride, H., Buonpane, N., and Schneider, D. (1977). Differentiation of alcoholics: Childhood history of minimal brain dysfunction, family history, and drinking pattern. *Arch. Gen. Psychol.* **34:**761–768.

Tarter, R., Hegedus, A., Goldstein, G., Shelly, C., and Alterman, A. (1984). Adolescent sons of alcoholics: Neuropsychological and personality characteristics. *Alcohol.: Clin. Exp. Res.* **8:**216–222.

Tarter, R., Alterman, A., and Edwards, K. (1985a). Vulnerability to alcoholism in men. A behavior-genetic perspective. *J. Stud. Alcohol* **46:**329–356.

Tarter, R., Hegedus, A., and Gavaler, J. (1985b). Hyperactivity in sons of alcoholics. *J. Stud. Alcohol* **46:**259–261.

Tarter, R., Arria, A., Moss, H., Edwards, N., and Van Thiel, D. (1987). DSM-III criteria for alcohol abuse. Association with alcohol consumption behavior. *Alcohol.: Clin. Exp. Res.* **11:**541–543.

Tarter, R., Kabene, M., Escallier, E., Laird, S., and Jacob, T. (1990a). Temperament deviation and risk for alcoholism. *Alcohol.: Clin. Exp. Res.* **14:**380–382.

Tarter, R., Laird, S., Kabene, M., Bukstein, O., and Kaminer, Y. (1990b). Drug abuse severity in adolescents is associated with magnitude of deviation in temperament traits. *Br. J. Addict.* **85:**1501–1504.

Tarter, R., Moss, H., Arria, A., Mezzich, A., and Vanyukov, M. (1992). Psychiatric diagnosis of alcoholism: Critique and reformulation. *Alcohol.: Clin. Exp. Res.* **16:**106–116.

Tarter, R., Blackson, T., Martin, C., Loeber, R., and Moss, H. (1993a). Characteristics and correlates of child discipline practices in substance abuse and normal families. *Am. J. Addict.* **2:**18–25.

Tarter, R., Blackson, T., Martin, C., Seilhamer, R., Pelham, W., and Loeber, R. (1993b). Mutual dissatisfaction between mother and son in substance abuse and normal families. *Am. J. Addict.* **2:**1–10.

Tarter, R., Kirisci, L., Hegedus, A., Mezzich, A., and Vanyukov, M. (1994). Heterogeneity of adolescent alcoholism. *Ann. NY Acad. Sci.* **708:** 172–180.

Thomas, A., and Chess, S. (1977). *Temperament and Development.* New York: Brunner/Mazel.

Thomas, A., Chess, S., and Birch, H. (1968). *Temperament and Behavioral Disorders in Childhood.* New York: New York University Press.

Vaillant, G. (1983). Natural history of male alcoholism. V: Is alcoholism the cart or the horse to sociopathy. *Br. J. Addict.* **78:**317–326.

Wachs, T., and Gruen, G. (1982). *Early Experience and Human Development.* New York: Plenum.

Webster-Stratton, C., and Eyberg, S. (1982). Child temperament: Relationship with child behavior problems and parent-child interactions. *J. Clin. Child Psychiatr.* **11:**123–129.

Werner, E. (1986). Resilient offspring of alcoholics: A longitudinal study from birth to age 18. *J. Stud. Alcohol* **47:**34–40.

Wills, T. (1990). Multiple networks and substance use. *J. Soc. Clin. Psychol.* **9:**78–90.

Windle, M. (1990). HK/MBD questionnaire: Factor structure and discriminant validity with an adolescent sample. *Alcohol.: Clin. Exp. Res.* **14:**232–237.

Windle, M. (1992). Temperament and social support in adolescence: Interrelations with depressive symptoms and delinquent behaviors. *J. Youth Adolesc.* **21:**1–21.

Wood, D., Wender, P., and Reimherr, F. (1983). The prevalence of attention deficit disorder, residual type, or minimal brain dysfunction in a population of male alcoholic patients. *Am. J. Psychiatr.* **140:**95–98.

13

Strategies for the Search for Genetic Influences on Alcohol-related Phenotypes

GERALD E. MCCLEARN
AND ROBERT PLOMIN

The field of alcohol research provides an interesting case study of change in scientific attitude toward nature and nurture. From a pervasive and scarcely challenged view a few decades ago, that alcoholism was caused exclusively by environment, there has been a shift toward general acceptance of a significant etiological role of heredity, and in some forums even an air of expectancy that the identification of the gene for alcoholism is simply a matter of time.

There are reasons for judging this expectation to be, at best, overly optimistic. The purpose of this chapter is to discuss some of the considerations underlying this cautionary note, and to provide a framework for reasonable expectations about the gene chase in alcoholism and other alcohol-related attributes.

Mendelian Phenomena, Continuous Distributions and the Two Cultures of Genetics

Before Mendel's discoveries, the biology of inheritance was a confusing jumble of descriptions of specific relationships among relatives, differing from one attribute to another and from one species to another. Mendel's genius lay in concentrating on attributes that conformed to certain simple rules. The explication of these rules, and the hypothesizing of underlying paired elements to account for the way the rules worked, provided the foundation for modern genetics. Mendel's success, and that of the many dedicated pioneers who extended the field in the early years of the century, is largely attributable to the fact that they studied the rules of inheritance where they were most clearly and simply manifested. It has been a spectacular success story of looking where the light is best, and the Mendelian light shone brightest on categorical, dichotomous variables.

Not nearly so well illuminated were those variables that are continuously distributed. Indeed, for quite a while there was serious doubt that the Mendelian rules applied at all to situations other than those in which one class of the dichotomy is a clearly abnormal condition. When dealing with the normal range of variation of body height, for example, there is no gap separating one group from another. The Galtonian biometrical approach to this kind of situation sought to describe the regularities of inheritance by calculating the degree of resemblance of relatives. The theoretical reconciliation of Mendelian categories and Galtonian continuities, particularly the contribution of Fisher (1918), has been often told (e.g., Plomin et al., 1990). Briefly, the resolution postulated the existence of many different genes, each behaving according to Mendelian rules, and each having a small effect on the same characteristic. This model rationalized the correlations among relatives that had been empirically found by the biometricians, and laid the groundwork for the elaboration of quantitative genetic theory.

In spite of this theoretical merger, however, the tools, the methods of inquiry, and the analytic logic have continued to differ greatly depending upon whether the characteristic under investigation (the *phenotype*) is continuously or discontinuously distributed.

Categorical Phenotypes

In the early Mendelian research, elementary all-and-only causal logic appeared to be adequate: all cases of membership in one category (e.g., the abnormal category) were due to a particular genotype, and only individuals with that genotype were in that category. That is to say, the particular genotype was both necessary and sufficient to generate the abnormal phenotype. Soon it became apparent, however, that the effect of genotype at any particular single locus might be influenced, perhaps greatly influenced, by its environmental and genetic context. The term, *epistasis,* is used to describe genetic context-dependence, and examples abound. A pertinent example is that of the diabetes locus in the mouse. Coleman and Hummel (1975) studied the diabetic condition associated with homozygous *db/db* status in two inbred strains, C57BL/6J and C57BL/KsJ, and in various crosses of these strains. On the genetic background of the former, the condition is relatively mild and is associated with hypertrophy of the islets of Langerhans of the pancreas. On the latter genetic background, the diabetes is severe, and is associated with islet *atrophy.* Results in the F1 and backcross generations permitted the conclusion that there was more than one modifying locus, and that there was average dominance of these plural loci in the direction of those of the C57BL/6J parent. Thus, in this case, a classic single-gene influence is seen to be insufficient for determining the phenotypic expression. Indeed, a correct characterization would seem to be that the *diabetes* locus is an identified locus, obviously an important one, but only one, in a polygenic system that influences the diabetic condition, with its companion loci not as yet identified.

The work of Coleman and Hummel provides yet another heuristic illustration. In addition to the *diabetes* locus, which is on mouse chromosome 4, there is another locus, *obese,* on chromosome 6, that, when homozygous for the recessive *ob* allele can result in a diabetic condition. In fact, the phenotypes of *ob/ob* and *db/db* mice are highly similar when on the same inbred background, either C57BL/6J or C57BL/KsJ. Thus, just as the *db/db* genotype is not sufficient to determine the diabetic condition, it is also not necessary. A similar outcome can be the result of a different locus on a different chromosome, and an "either-or" rather than "all-and-only" causation must be considered. Further supportive evidence for an either-or view comes from the recent discovery of two genes, *Idd-3* and *Idd-4,* that independently confer susceptibility to type 1 (insulin-dependent) diabetes; both genes lie outside the major histocompatibility complex known to be associated with type 1 diabetes, and both show human homologues (Todd et al., 1991).

Another type of gene interaction engages "both-and" causation, in which a particular genotype is required at two or more loci in order to generate a particular phenotype. Simple illustrations are provided by mouse coat color. The smooth, uniform lightbrown appearance of DBA/2 mice, for example, is dependent upon the animal being homozygous for particular recessive alleles at three loci: *dilute, brown,* and *agouti* (hence the name of the strain). Formally, this situation, in which the proper allelic configurations at several loci can be regarded as severally necessary and jointly sufficient (Hull, 1974), can be described as conjunctive plurality of causes and can be reduced to simple causation (Bunge, 1979). From the point of view of the geneticist oriented to segregation or linkage analyses, however, this reduction is inappropriate, for the (formally) unitary cause is distributed over several chromosomes, and each of its components is dancing to its own stochastic tune in meiotic segregation. Furthermore, it is only an approximation to regard this three-locus configuration as jointly sufficient for the DBA coat color. The animal must be *not* homozygous for the recessive allele at the *albino* locus, else it will be white; it must also not have the genotypes that will give rise to hairlessness (*hairless, rhino,* etc.), or it will not have a coat at all.

Some early Mendelian analyses were complicated by the fact that some animals or plants that, according to theory, must have a particular genotype did not display the appropriate phenotype. This phenomenon was described as *incomplete penetrance.* Another term that was found necessary in the Mendelian literature was *variable expressivity,* which described situations in which organisms with the same genotype at a particular locus had widely differing manifestations of the phenotype. Cases of incomplete penetrance and variable expressivity, which are matters of great importance in segregation and linkage analysis, must be due either to genetic or environmental contexts, and further illustrate that, though a particular locus may be a ringleader, it is not an oligarch in determining a phenotypic outcome.

Continuous Phenotypes

The starting point for the quantitative genetic analysis of continuously distributed phenotypes is a model of an indefinitely large number of loci, each having an equal, small

effect on the phenotype under examination. Very sophisticated theoretical developments have built upon this foundation (see Falconer, 1989). These developments
underlie the analysis of twins, adoptees, and family members in human alcohol
research, and the use of inbred strains, selectively bred lines, and other animal model
approaches in alcohol studies. The key idea in this type of analysis is to assess contributions to variance in the phenotype of interest. Two principal domains of influence
are considered—genetic and environmental—and each is in turn divisible into sub-
components. In the genetic domain, for example, additive and nonadditive components
are often sought. The latter is sometimes divisible into dominance and epistatic effects.
The environment is divisible in a variety of ways, depending upon the nature of the
study. A particularly interesting subdivision in human research, for example, is into
those environmental effects that are shared by relatives and those that are not shared
(Plomin and Daniels, 1987). Central ideas in this type of analysis include that of heritability (proportion of phenotypic variance due to genetic differences among individuals in the population), its converse, environmentality, and genetic and environmental
contributions to phenotypic correlations among phenotypes.

In this basic model, the genetic loci are anonymous. The causal model most suited to
this type of situation is that of multiple causal elements with partially interchangable,
summing (or multiplying) effects.

Effect Size and Research Strategies

The major locus research strategy is enormously attractive. If a single gene can be
found, there are prospects of discovering its chromosomal location, its base sequences,
and its primary polypeptide product. Such information is of major importance for diagnosis, genetic counseling, and the design of rational therapies.

The prospects are different if a prototypic polygenic situation exists. The virtue of
an estimate of quantitative genetic parameters is that it is a bottom-line estimate
(Plomin, 1990), summing all of the transmissable genetic effects whether they be of
regulatory or structural genes. Heritability estimates do not provide an immediate route
to exploration of mediating mechanisms—the molecular biology, biochemistry, and
physiology—of the genetic influence. However, the examination of genetic correlations between the phenotype of interest and putative mechanisms can serve to narrow
the search by eliminating those mechanistic elements with no genetic overlap with the
phenotype.

The environmental components estimable from quantitative analyses may also be of
great value in pointing toward specific domains of environmental influence from which
preventive or ameliorative interventions might be devised. Clearly, the research
agenda are different if the evidence suggests a single locus than when a pack of anonymous loci are implicated.

It has long been appreciated (e.g., Falconer, 1981) that there are logical alternatives
other than giant genes or tiny genes. Actual biological situations may involve loci with
intermediate effect sizes. Robertson (1984), for example, suggested a negative expo-
nential distribution of effect size, with those of largest effect being rarest and those of
tiny effect most numerous. It is therefore possible to think of a continuum of genetic

architecture, ranging from the prototypic polygenic situation of very many genes of miniscule effect, through configurations in which a few loci account for an appreciable part of the variance, with many others contributing to fine tuning, to those circumstances in which a single locus accounts for sufficient variance to be detectable on most any background of contextual genes or environments. Present methods are best suited for the first and last cases. Until very recently, the discovery and characterization of loci in the middle ground between major loci and polygenes has been arduous. Developments in molecular genetics have led to a recent spate of research on those genes of intermediate impact, described as quantitative trait loci (QTL) (McClearn et al., 1991; Plomin et al., 1991). Striking advances have been made in detecting QTL in a variety of plant species (e.g., Allard, 1988; Paterson et al., 1988), and the general picture that emerges is that very substantial portions of the variance of the quantitative traits examined are attributable to variation at QTL whose effect size is too small for them to have been caught in the wide mesh of the major locus net. Many of them conform well to the image of the puny polygene; some of them, however, do individually account for 5% to 50% of the variance. It may well be that Robertson's (1984) speculation has wide validity.

The QTL approach is currently being extended to animal research (Weir et al., 1988), and one example deals specifically with alcohol-related phenotypes (McClearn et al., 1991). The analysis assesses degree of association between specific marker loci and scores on continuously distributed alcohol-related variables across recombinant inbred (RI) strains of mice. These RI strains were derived by inbreeding from a single F2 between two progenitor inbred strains (Bailey, 1971; Taylor, 1989). The RIs thus represent reshuffling of the genetic differences between the progenitors. For many loci, of course, the progenitors may be in like allelic state, but these loci cannot be assessed by the technique. At many other loci, however, the progenitors will differ. A huge body of information has been generated about the allelic state of the various RIs at many loci and the linkage relationships among these loci (Taylor, 1989). For each locus at which the progenitor strains differ, each RI is homozygous for either the allele of the one or of the other progenitor. If the genotype of one progenitor is scored 0 and the other 1, it becomes a straightforward matter to calculate a biserial correlation coefficient between the quantitative variable of interest and the "progenitor-strain-likeness" at each of the available loci (McClearn et al., 1991; McClearn, 1991; Plomin et al., 1991).

The sampling unit in the analysis is obviously the RI *strain,* so the statistical power is limited by the number of RI strains within a series derived from a common F2. Fortunately, the RI series with one of the largest number of RI strains is the B $\times$ D series derived from C57BL/6 and DBA/2 mice. These strains have proved to be dramatically different in a wide variety of alcohol-related variables. Thus, although any RI series will assess only those loci at which the progenitors differ, a substantial portion of all the mouse genes that are capable of influencing these alcohol traits are probably represented in this series.

Crabbe et al. (1983) reported the results of assessment of the B $\times$ D series on alcohol acceptance, low-dose activation, and withdrawal severity, among other variables. The initial analysis sought major loci, and reported success in respect to ethanol acceptance and possibly in withdrawal severity. The association analysis (McClearn et al., 1991) identified numerous QTL for all of the phenotypes distributed across the mouse chromosomes, as shown in Fig. 13-1.

Some of the QTL have effects sufficiently large to warrant the effort of more precise localization, sequencing, cloning, and so on. For smaller effect sizes, this approach would be inefficient. A new research avenue is immediately opened by the QTL information, however. Genotype-based selection, assigning mates on the basis of markers close to the QTL, offers the prospect of manipulating the genetic system on a locus by locus basis. Lines of animals generated in this way should provide a new order of power to the already well-demonstrated research potential of lines generated by phenotypic selective breeding.

Genetics and Complex Systems

When the Mendelian rules were well described, and when their general applicability had been appreciated, but before the mode of action of genes was guessed at, it was possible to think of genetic causal influence in simplistic terms:

Genotype→Phenotype

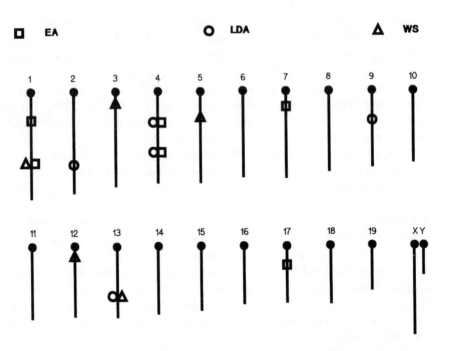

Fig. 13-1 Genome hotspots for alcohol-related processes: chromosomal zones containing one or more significant association with ethanol acceptance, low-dose activation, or withdrawal severity.

Indeed, it was difficult to do otherwise. The nature of the connecting arrow—how the cellular elements, called genes, could bring about differences in whole organism characteristics—was a central biological mystery.

When it was shown that genes could affect enzymes, and when the suspicion grew that this was a general process (the "one gene-one enzyme hypothesis" of the 1950s), it became possible to entertain biochemical notions of how genes influence phenotypes. The paradigm-shifting success of molecular genetics and molecular biology has provided us today with an enormous body of knowledge with respect to the mechanism of gene action. It is clear that the pathway from the gene to a phenotype at any distance downstream from the primary gene product is anything but simple.

Genetic influence can appropriately be regarded as an input to a multiplex system, with the phenotypic outcome being a function of the operation of that system. In this section, we review some consequences of this elementary proposition for expectations concerning the nature of genetic influence on complex phenotypes in general, and those of alcohol use and abuse specifically.

Causal Chains

Serial reactions are a general feature of biochemical systems, with the product of one reaction becoming the substrate for a subsequent reaction. Assuming the serial reactions each to be enzyme-mediated, such a chain exemplifies one type of polygeny, with one gene (at least) for each reaction in the chain.

Kacser and Burns (1979) emphasize that because of biochemical feedback regulation, an allele's influence in such a chain can depend very much on other alleles in the chain: "An enzyme is only 'important' by virtue of its relation to a specific set of fellow enzymes." (p. 1154) They propose a sensitivity coefficient to replace simpler notions of controlling or noncontrolling enzymes and of pacemakers or rate-limiters. For our present purposes, the important lesson is that the effect of an allelic substitution at a given single locus is not a fixed value, but is dependent upon the genetic context.

In other words, we have departed from the neat Newtonian simple causal realm and entered that of circular causality (Sattler, 1986) in which cause and effect are blurred. In a serial reaction system with feedback, which genes are to be given the credit for a particular value of metabolite at any point or of the flux through the entire system? Ward (1990) has given an extended discussion of situations of this type and has proposed an analytic approach to polygenic systems in which the variance of flux plays a central role.

Networks

The conceptual complexities of unbranched chains are increased enormously when branching (which appears to be commonplace) is considered. From a genetic perspective, branching can be regarded as underlying two major phenomena—pleiotropy and polygeny. Through branching, a single locus can have an effect on several phenotypes downstream from the branching point. Such pleiotropy, which is often treated as a special topic, must be a near-ubiquitous phenomenon when phenotypes more than a few steps from the primary gene product are considered.

Through the merging of branches, different loci can have an impact on a common phenotype. Thus, the polygenic system influencing a complex phenotype includes all the genes concerned with sequential steps in all the different branches that ultimately merge to common effect. In summary, the path from genes to complex phenotypes must be a reticulum or network, and the phenomena observed in phenotypes of this sort must be reflections of the way in which networks operate.

The rules of network operation are a far cry from the rules of one- or few-step linear, unidirectional causality. An enormous intellectual effort has recently been devoted to the understanding of these rules and to applying them to specific scientific problems. The literature describing this effort is very extensive and any citations in the present context can only be hints, representing some of the material the present authors have encountered and found applicable to the topic at hand. Particularly accessible are the works by Simon (1969), Yates et al. (1972), Prigogine (1976), Miller (1978), Jantsch (1980), Salthe (1985), and Ford (1987). Specific relevance of the systems approach to genetics has been eloquently presented by, among others, Waddington (1977), Murphy and Trojak (1986), Bonner (1988), Mayr (1988), and Murphy and Berger (1988). From the thought-provoking principles in these works, we cite below a few we believe to be of special relevance for the thesis of this paper.

Nonuniformity of Networks. Although the network or system may be very complex, with many things related to many other things, everything is not equally related to everything else. Some elements of the matrix may have relatively more and stronger relationships and others may have relatively fewer or weaker relationships with other elements in the system. A familiar example is the notion of a final common pathway, wherein a number of causal routes converge onto a particular structure or function that then determines the outcome under investigation. It is quite possible that a number of polygenic systems operate in this way. It is also important to consider that there might be many nodes, not just a final common one, in a system, and that these may vary greatly both in the number and strength of their inputs and outputs. Note that, in the current frame of reference, "a large number of inputs" is another way of saying "a polygenic system," and that "a large number of outputs" describes a rich pleiotropic effect, relatable, perhaps, to Simon's (1969, p. 89) concept of "span of control." These intermediate common nodes are called "soft spots" by Waddington (1977), who, in a statement reminiscent of Kacser and Burns, cautions that ". . . the sensitivity of a particular link is not a fixed characteristic of it, but depends on the state of the rest of the network." (p. 91)

If the scientific purpose requires phenotypic description at a system level far downstream from the genes, investigators must be prepared to encounter multiple determinants. If the scientific purpose requires that single (or very few) determinants be evaluated, then it may often be necessary to select as target phenotype one of the more proximal elements in the determinant system rather than the ultimate downstream phenotype of primary interest. Soft spots would seem to be highly strategic targets for studies of mechanism in polygenic systems. If the total network is so complex as to defy complete description, a description of the major soft spots may provide sufficient information at least for useful approximations.

Regulation. Another characteristic of networks is that they are regulated. At time scales ranging from the momentary to the life span, variation in the values of elements (or nodes) of the system are met by processes from within the system that tend to restore them to some set point or defended value or range of values. These processes, described as homeostatic, homeorhetic (Waddington, 1957), or rheostatic (Mrosovsky, 1990), depending upon whether a more-or-less constant value is defended or some reactive or developmental change in set point is involved, may differ greatly from individual to individual. The attributes of the control system, such as response delay, speed of response, degree of damping, and magnitude of steady-state error, may be more relevant phenotypes than the momentary values of some variable (Murphy and Berger, 1988) such as are often featured in genetic analyses. With the parastatic (Murphy and Berger, 1988) compensation possible when there exist alternate routes from different genes or gene sets to a common node, an unambiguous attribution of effects of any particular locus will obviously be difficult.

Hierarchy and Subsystems. A multinodal, regulated system will often contain discernible subsystems. Because of the near-ubiquity of hierarchical organization in living systems, it is probably a useful default hypothesis that there are hierarchical aspects to the network that we suggest contains the mechanisms of alcohol abuse and alcoholism. Although the elements of a particular hierarchical subsystem will be more closely related to each other than to elements of other subsystems, there will be some communication (i.e., some relationships) across subsystems. This cross talk may be fairly extensive or the total system may be nearly decomposable, with considerable independence of the subsystems (Simon, 1969). Bonner (1988) has related hierarchical systems to the concept of "gene nets," by which term is meant "a grouping of a network of gene actions and their products into discrete units. . . ." (p. 174) In this seminal work, implications of gene nets are explored largely from developmental and evolutionary perspectives. For present purposes, we note the following proposed properties of gene nets: developmental processes in multicellular organisms require the insulation of gene nets from each other; this independence must not be total, but must permit some signals between them; there is a size limitation to a gene net; as complexity increases there will therefore be a tendency for an increase in the number of gene nets; the organization of a multiplicity of gene nets is likely to be hierarchical.

The picture that emerges from these theoretical considerations is of a hierarchical or partially hierarchical reticulum of structures and processes interposed between gene sets and complex phenotypes in which the values of specific elements may be changing from moment to moment in a regulated manner, and changing over the developmental course of the organism in a programmed manner. We have here emphasized the genetic role, but it is essential to understand that the contribution of environmental sources to this reticulum could be as great or greater than the genetic influence.

Heterogeneity. From the genetic point of view, etiologic heterogeneity can be due to the existence of multiple single-locus effects with the same or highly similar phenotypic outcomes, or from differing combinations of more-or-less interchangeable polygenes. If we examine the very first steps in the contribution of a particular locus to the system, with, say, the primary gene product as the phenotype of interest, we can expect to find a major locus effect. As we shift our phenotypic focus further downstream we encounter the nodes and soft spots, which, for different levels of analysis, can be phenotypes in their own right. These nodes, or the most upstream of the hierarchical subsystems, will likely show the effects of multiple-locus input, but some loci may have alleles whose effects are noncompensatable within that subsystem, giving rise to occasional manifestation of single-gene effects. Further downstream, when the phenotypic definition must encompass all of the features of the upstream subsystems, one is dealing with a heterogeneous collection with etiologies being more or less distinct depending, among other things, upon the degree of decomposability of the system. If the system is very complex, the prospects of finding a single-gene locus to account for an overwhelming part of the variance of a thus broadly defined phenotype is small indeed.

It is instructive to consider the domain of mental retardation as an illustration of the applicability of some of these theoretical notions. In the 1930s, it was still possible for investigators to enquire about the role of heredity in the encompassing category of feeblemindedness. Results were far from satisfactory. From our present-day vantage point we can see why. Feeblemindedness is a heterogeneous collection of numerous different single-locus conditions, such as phenylketonuria and Tay-Sachs disease; chromosomal anomalies, such as Down's syndrome, Klinefelter's syndrome, and fragile-X syndrome; polygenic segregants who simply by luck of the meiotic draw received "minus" alleles at a large number of loci relevant to cognitive functioning; and the consequences of environmental insults, such as malnutrition, maternal drug use, perinatal hypoxia, and premature birth. From today's vantage point, we could warn those early investigators of the folly of seeking *the* gene for feeblemindedness. The answer was to be found in the study of differential etiology, initiated, more or less by accident, by Følling et al. (1945) in the case of phenylketonuria.

The strategic posture we assume in dealing with alcohol abuse and alcoholism must be capable of accommodating the possibility of heterogeneity and complexity of an order similar to this exemplar case of mental retardation.

Networks and Alcohol

There is general agreement that alcoholism and alcohol abuse are complex issues. If the network considerations discussed are applicable, then we should not be surprised if it is demonstrated that they are likewise of highly heterogeneous etiology. There may be many genetic loci at which particular allelic configurations lead to an identifiable alcohol abuse problem regardless of environmental influence; there may be chromosomal anomalies with similar result; there may be a continuum of susceptibility to alcoholism on which one's location is established by many loci of interchangable effect and also by environmental influences; there may be cases of alcoholism basically due to environmental influences so powerful that all genotypes are susceptible. If this scenario is even approximately veridical, there is an inescapable conclusion that an urgent research priority is the study of differential taxonomy of alcohol problems.

One approach to differential taxonomy is to examine configurations of components of the complex phenotype at about the same hierarchic level in the system. If upstream elements of the system are included (the nodes and soft spots), then the differential taxonomy search becomes also an exercise in differential etiology. A major problem in instituting such a search is the identification of putative system elements to be measured. Many candidates can be derived from the decades of alcohol research by various disciplines. From pharmacology, for example, we might nominate indices of uptake, distribution, disposition, sensitivity, tolerance, dependence liability, and neurochemical parameters. From psychology, nominees would include notions of stress management, locus of control, personality, peer group pressure, and so on. A strong argument could be made that, at the present stage of understanding of the nosology of alcohol problems, genetic research will be most efficiently applied to studies of these intermediate phenotypes.

Implications for Human Research

The message from the first part of this chapter is that human alcohol use and abuse are paradigm cases of complex systems for which an hypothesis of etiologic heterogeneity seems almost required. At the simplest level, some cases of alcohol abuse may be entirely environmental in origin, and others entirely genetic. A single gene may be the necessary and sufficient cause of alcoholism for some individuals, and for others, different single genes may be at fault. More likely than this all-and-only logic of single genes is the both-and logic in which several genes are necessary and jointly sufficient causes—but a different set of genes for different individuals. Even more likely is the scenario suggested by the either-or logic of multiple causes in which different combinations of serial and parallel polygeny as well as environmental influences are responsible. A crucial implication for genetic research is that strategies are needed to identify small effects of QTL, individual genes in a multiple-gene system.

Identifying Quantitative Trait Loci

For the outbred human species, although the limitations of the traditional linkage approach are becoming recognized, no alternative approach has yet emerged with the cumulative and integrative power of the recombinant inbred strain QTL association methodology. The key element in such an approach will be the ability to detect a continuum of effect size, especially the low end of the continuum where most of the genetic effects in a complex system are expected to reside.

Biochemical Markers. One approach is to examine biochemical markers in alcoholics and nonalcoholics. For example, differences between alcoholics and controls have been reported for monoamine oxidase activity, adenylate cyclase activity, and several other biochemical markers (Devor and Cloninger, 1989). However, this is not a genetic approach—biochemical differences between alcoholic and control individuals could be induced by the use of alcohol or by other environmental factors. Genetic approaches have employed gene markers such as blood types, HLA antigens, and ADH and ALDH isozymes. For example, HLA antigens have been reported to differ for alcoholics and controls (e.g., Corsico et al., 1988).

DNA Markers. Genetic markers are no longer limited to the few markers available from blood because polymorphisms can be found in DNA itself rather than in DNA products. Many thousands of these DNA markers are now available and thousands more will soon emerge as part of the human genome effort. The availability of so many DNA markers makes it reasonable to consider an allelic association strategy that attempts to find differences in allelic frequencies associated with differences in alcohol use and abuse. Because unrelated individuals can be studied, large samples can be used to provide the statistical power to detect small QTL effects. In contrast to linkage analysis in which a DNA marker can easily mark a tenth of a chromosome, a DNA marker in allelic association studies in a population of outbred organisms only marks a few hundred thousand base pairs. For this reason, a systematic search for QTL associations could be conducted only if thousands of closely spaced markers were available. However, the human gene map is currently less than one-tenth the needed density, and cost-effective screening of thousands of markers for each individual in large samples will not be practical until new techniques are developed.

Candidate Genes. As an interim strategy, markers in or near genes with possible impact on alcohol-related processes—including neurally relevant genes such as receptors for the central monoamines—can be used as quasi-candidate genes in what has been called a measured genotype approach (Sing and Boerwinkle, 1987). Of the nearly 2000 cloned genes, more than 150 encode proteins of functional relevance in the nervous system (Kidd et al., 1989). Moreover, new techniques are accelerating the pace of discovery of the more than 20,000 genes uniquely expressed in the brain. For example, cDNA brain libraries have recently been used to sequence parts of more than 200 newly discovered genes expressed in the brain but not in other organs, yielding unique gene identifiers called *expressed sequence tag sites* (Adams et al., 1991). Brain cDNA libraries have also been used effectively in rats to isolate clones that correspond to mRNA molecules expressed only in the brain, which will make it possible to determine whether their expression is affected by alcohol (Milner et al., 1987).

QTL Association. A QTL association approach compares allelic frequencies for groups of individuals. For example, it has been reported that one allele of the D_2 dopamine receptor was present in 69% of 35 alcoholics but in only 20% of 35 control individuals (Blum et al., 1990). Two other polymorphic DNA markers, alcohol dehydrogenase and transferrin, showed no association with alcoholism. Considering the likelihood of genetic heterogeneity for alcoholism, such a strong association is surprising, and requires replication. It may prove important that in this study the alcoholics were apparently severely affected—most had experienced repeated treatment failures and had died from medical complications of alcoholism. A weakness of the study was its retrospective, postmortem diagnosis of alcoholism, relying on medical and autopsy records, interviews with relatives, and alcohol consumption data. Blum et al. (1991) replicated their findings in a study of 52 severe alcoholics, 44 moderate alcoholics, and 43 nonalcoholics. Higher frequencies of the A1 allele were found for severe alcoholics (63%) than for moderate alcoholics (34%) or nonalcoholics (21%). Additional research from the same group investigated binding affinity and the number of binding sites for the D_2 dopamine receptor in the caudate nucleus. They found that the number of binding sites declined linearly for the A2A2, A1A2, and A1A1 genotypes, suggesting a mechanism for the action of the A1 allele in alcoholism (Noble et al., 1991). Association with the A1 allele has also been reported by another group (Parsian et al., 1991). However, failures to replicate have been reported as well (Bolos et al., 1990; Gelernter, 1991). It has been argued that these latter studies did not include severe alcoholics and their control groups did not exclude alcohol abuse (Noble and Blum, 1991). Nonetheless, until additional replications are reported with larger samples, the controversy will continue (Goldman et al., 1991; Conneally, 1991).

The application of molecular genetic techniques to complex systems such as alcohol use and abuse represents an exciting direction for genetic research. For example, identification of a replicable association or linkage for a particular subtype of alcoholism provides the strongest possible evidence for genetic influence and for genetic heterogeneity, leading the way toward identification of individuals at risk, preventive interventions, and isolation and cloning of the QTL in order to understand and perhaps alter its function. More quantitative genetic research is needed, however, to set the stage for molecular genetic analyses. As indicated earlier, quantitative genetic research writes the bottom line for genetic and environmental credits and debits summed across individuals in a population, no matter how complicated the genetic and environmental systems are for each individual. Quantitative genetic research is needed most urgently to address the most fundamental quantitative genetic question. How important is genetic influence for alcoholism? If there is genetic influence, quantitative genetic research can be helpful in going beyond this basic nature–nurture question to address issues such as etiologic heterogeneity, the developmental course of genetic and environmental influence, and etiologic links between the normal and abnormal. These topics are discussed briefly in the following sections.

How Important Is Genetic Influence for Alcoholism?

Regardless of whether the genetic systems underlying alcoholism follow the logic of all-and-only, both-and, or either-or, their genetic effect will be detected by quantitative genetic methods such as twin and adoption studies. That is, even if genetic effects are highly polygenic and interactive (epistatic), the identical genotypes of identical twins require that members of each twin pair be concordant for alcoholism if genetic factors alone are responsible for alcoholism. To the extent that identical twins are less than perfectly concordant for alcoholism, nongenetic factors must be important, at least for some individuals in the population. If nongenetic factors are important in addition to genetic factors, genetic influence can be detected by comparing the resemblance of identical and fraternal twins. Adoption studies that compare first-degree relatives adopted apart can detect additive but not nonadditive genetic influence. In addition to twin and adoption studies, family studies can be used to detect familial resemblance, although they cannot in themselves disentangle genetic effects from the possibility of environmental transmission. These quantitative genetic methods are described in detail elsewhere (e.g., Plomin et al., 1990).

Family Studies. Most areas of human behavioral genetic research, especially cognitive abilities, have met with considerable resistance when genetic influence is found. In contrast, acceptance of genetic influence on alcohol use and abuse has outstripped the data (Murray et al., 1983; Peele, 1986; Lester, 1988; Searles, 1988, 1990; Hodgkinson et al., 1991). Family studies of alcoholism consistently show familial resemblance for alcoholism. On average across dozens of studies, children of alcoholics show a fivefold greater risk of becoming alcoholic than children of nonalcoholic parents (Cotton, 1979). Recent reviews point out that the consistency of this finding is surprising given that definitions of alcoholism have varied widely and only 4 of 40 published family studies have used standardized diagnostic interviews and control groups (Merikangas, 1989; Hodgkinson et al., 1991). It should be emphasized that familial resemblance could be due to shared family environment rather than shared heredity; twin and adoption studies are needed to make this distinction.

Twin Studies. There are few twin studies of alcoholism and no clear picture can as yet be drawn from them. For example, evidence of only modest genetic influence emerged from a recent twin study of 81 monozygotic (MZ) and 86 dizygotic (DZ) twin pairs in which at least one member of each pair received a DSM-III diagnosis of alcohol abuse and/or dependence (Pickens et al., 1991). Concordance rates were 76% and 61% for male MZ and DZ twins, respectively; for females, concordances were 36% and 25%, respectively. An overlapping larger study using questionnaires rather than in-person interviews found similar results (McGue et al., 1992), which led the authors to make this observation:

> Perhaps the most remarkable finding in the present study is the modest magnitude of the genetic influence on alcohol problems. This might seem to run counter to current opinion in the alcohol research field, but other behavioral genetic studies also indicate a modest or weak genetic effect.

In an earlier twin study of diagnosed alcohol dependence (Gurling et al., 1981, 1984), twin concordances were much lower but nonetheless suggested little genetic influence for males (33% concordance for 15 MZ pairs, 25% for 28 DZ pairs) and no genetic influence for females (8% for 13 MZ pairs, 13% for 8 DZ pairs). A study of male twins found concordances of 26% for MZ twins and 12% for DZ twins for alcoholism as diagnosed from medical records of the Department of Veterans Affairs

(Hrubec and Omenn, 1981). Only one twin study suggests strong evidence of genetic influence. Using a combination of records from county Temperance Boards and personal interviews, a sample of 172 Swedish male twin pairs yielded concordances of 71% for MZ twins and 32% for DZ twins for alcohol abuse (Kaij, 1960).

Adoption Studies. It has been suggested that twin studies of alcoholism might be problematic because the drinking habits of one twin can affect those of the cotwin (Hodgkinson et al., 1991). For this reason, studies of individuals adopted away from genetically related alcoholics are particularly valuable in triangulating on an answer to the question of genetic influence on alcoholism. The first adoption study of alcoholism found no excess of alcohol-related problems in adopted-away offspring of heavy drinkers (Roe, 1944), although this study has been criticized for its small sample (27 children adopted away from an alcoholic biological parent), its limited information concerning parental alcoholism, and the questionable comparability of its control group of 22 adopted children with nonalcoholic biological parents (Goodwin et al., 1973). Three other adoption studies suggest genetic influence on alcoholism, but only when selected subsamples were considered. Moreover, the criteria used to select subsamples that show genetic influence are inconsistent across studies. In a Danish study, 18% of 55 adopted-away male offspring of alcoholics were diagnosed as alcoholic as compared to 5% of 78 control offspring of nonalcoholics (Goodwin et al., 1973). Moreover, male offspring of alcoholics only showed an increased risk for alcoholism per se, not for heavy drinking or problem drinking. Female offspring showed no increased risk for alcoholism (Goodwin et al., 1977).

A Swedish adoption study suggested genetic influence for male offspring of moderate (but not mild or severe) alcohol abusers, as derived from the number of registrations with a county Temperance Board and whether the Temperance Board recommended treatment (Cloninger et al., 1981). In the same study, female offspring of alcoholics showed increased risk, but only when fathers' alcoholism was mild and not associated with criminality (Bohman et al., 1981). A recent critique of this study raises issues that cloud the interpretation of these results (Searles, 1990). Finally, in a small U.S. adoption study, problem drinking increased the risk of DSM-III diagnoses of Alcohol Abuse and/or Dependence for both male and female offspring (Cadoret et al., 1985, 1987; Cadoret, 1990). However, this study has also been criticized, for example, for having very limited information on the biological parents and overly broad diagnostic criteria (Searles, 1990).

An unusual adoption design involved 150 half-siblings of 61 alcoholic patients (Schuckit et al., 1972). Of the 150 half-siblings, 28 (18.7%) were considered to be alcoholic, a risk estimate that raises questions because it exceeds that of full siblings. Of these alcoholic half-siblings, 65% had an alcoholic biological parent as compared to only 20% of the nonalcoholic half-siblings. Living with an alcoholic biological parent did not increase the risk for alcoholism; indeed, a recent reanalysis of this study shows that half-siblings who grew up with an alcoholic parent were significantly *less* likely to be alcoholic (Cook and Goethe, 1990).

This brief review suggests that although some behavioral genetic research is consistent with the hypothesis of genetic influence, the case for genetic influence has not yet been made convincingly. As discussed in the following section, more quantitative genetic research is needed, not only to demonstrate genetic influence on diagnosed alcoholism, but also to trace the genetic nexus of relationships among alcohol use, abuse, alcoholism, and alcohol-related processes such as sensitivity, tolerance, and dependence.

Genetic Heterogeneity and Comorbidity

One example of the potential for extending research beyond the basic nature–nurture question is the use of multivariate genetic analysis to address genetic heterogeneity. Attempts to study heterogeneity in alcoholism are often phenotypic, that is, distinguishing subtypes of alcoholism on the basis of symptoms, such as the DSM-III distinction between alcohol abuse and alcohol dependence (i.e., evidence for tolerance or withdrawal). In psychiatric research, three characteristics are most often used in attempts to distinguish subtypes: severity, age of onset, and family history (Plomin and Rende, 1991), and these are also central to research on the heterogeneity of alcoholism. Phenotypic subtyping can also be based on so-called endophenotypes, including electrophysiological markers (Begleiter and Porjesz, 1988), physiological markers, and biochemical markers (e.g., Schuckit, 1987, 1988; Tarter et al., 1990).

Differential Heritability. The usefulness of hypothesized subtypes needs to be assessed by studies of differential prognosis, differences in response to treatment, and differential etiology, which includes genetic heterogeneity. In alcohol research, genetic heterogeneity has been considered primarily in terms of differential heritability. A recent twin study, for example, suggests that the more severe DSM-III diagnosis of alcoholism with physical dependence is more heritable than alcoholism without physical dependence (Pickens et al., 1991). The early twin study by Kaij (1960) also indicated that heritability increases with severity. The adoption study by Cloninger et al. (1981), however, reported greater genetic risk for moderate alcoholism than for mild or severe alcoholism. Nonetheless, from this latter study, two types of alcoholism were proposed that differ in severity and heritability. Heritability was postulated to be greatest for early onset, severely affected males with concomitant drug and conduct disorder problems, called the *male-limited* type of alcoholism, as compared to a milder form of alcoholism called *milieu-limited* (Cloninger, 1987). However, a recent critique suggests that these two subtypes of alcoholism "should be considered, at best, preliminary and, at worst, unfounded." (Searles, 1990, p. 21)

Genetic Correlations. Although differential heritability is one kind of evidence for genetic heterogeneity, it is a weak approach to the issue because two subtypes that show the same degree of genetic influence could be affected by entirely different sets of genes. Alternatively, two subtypes can yield different heritabilities even though the same set of genes affect both, that is, one subtype might simply be more affected by the environment than the other. The key concept in multivariate genetic analysis is the genetic correlation, which is an index of the extent to which genetic effects on one phenotype are correlated with genetic effects on another. The genetic correlation is independent of the heritabilities of the two phenotypes. That is, the genetic correlation for two moderately heritable traits can be high, suggesting that the two traits are genetically the same trait, or the genetic correlation can be low, implying that the two traits are genetically distinct. Eventually, specific QTL examples of genetic heterogeneity will come from molecular genetics, that is, a QTL will be found that is associated with one type of alcoholism but not another.

Multivariate genetic analysis represents the multivariate extension of traditional univariate quantitative genetic strategies. Its focus is on the covariance between traits rather than the variance of each trait considered separately. Any quantitative genetic strategy that can be used to decompose the variance of a trait into genetic and environmental components can also be used to decompose the covariance between two traits (see Plomin et al., 1990). Rather than comparing MZ and DZ resemblance for a single trait X, the basis for multivariate genetic analysis is cross-twin resemblance for one twin on trait X and the cotwin on trait Y. The phenotypic correlation between X and Y is assumed to be mediated genetically to the extent that MZ cross-twin resemblance exceeds DZ cross-twin resemblance. This genetic contribution to the phenotypic correlation can be shown to be the genetic correlation weighted by a function of the heritabilities of the two traits (Plomin and DeFries, 1979). Thus, even if the genetic correlation is high, the genetic contribution to the phenotypic correlation will be low if the heritability of one or both of the traits is low. A second type of question addressed by multivariate genetic analysis focuses on the genetic correlation itself. The genetic correlation indexes the extent to which genetic effects on one trait overlap with genetic effects on the other trait, independent of the heritabilities of the two traits. This question is the essential question of genetic heterogeneity and comorbidity.

Consider the DSM-III categories alcohol abuse and alcohol dependence. These proposed subtypes of alcoholism are correlated phenotypically in the sense that more than half of the individuals who meet diagnostic criteria for alcohol abuse also meet criteria for dependence. If the MZ cross-concordance between abuse and dependence is no greater than DZ cross-concordance, this suggests that genetic factors are not responsible for the phenotypic association between abuse and dependence. If both abuse and dependence are heritable, this implies genetic heterogeneity in the sense that genes that affect abuse are independent of genes that affect dependence.

Genetic Comorbidity. Genetic heterogeneity focuses on splitting alcoholism into etiologically distinct components. An equally important question concerns lumping rather than splitting, and multivariate genetic analysis is just as relevant here. This is the issue of genetic comorbidity: Are genetic effects on certain types of alcoholism shared with other types of psychopathology? Two prime candidates are antisocial personality and depression. For example, if the genetic correlation between alcoholism and antisocial personality is high, it suggests that the diagnosis of alcoholism needs to be broadened to include antisocial personality. Family and adoption studies, however, suggest that transmission of alcoholism, antisocial personality, and depression are independent (Cloninger and Reich, 1983; Merikangas et al., 1985).

Soft Spots. Our preference in multivariate genetic analysis is to follow the lead of mouse researchers by focusing on alcohol-related processes such as preference, behavioral and central nervous system (CNS) sensitivity, acute and chronic tolerance, and psychological and physical dependence rather than symptoms of alcoholism (e.g., Stabenau, 1986; Tabakoff and Hoffman, 1987). We recognize that the issue is one of levels of analysis—each of these processes is itself an exceedingly complex system and could be broken down further into component processes. Levels of analysis are not right or wrong; the issue is their utility for a particular purpose. For the purpose of charting the genetic soft spots underlying alcohol abuse, it is our hunch that componential responses of the whole organism, such as sensitivity and tolerance, may have greater utility than more molecular levels of analysis, such as membrane sensitivity or more molar phenotypes, such as symptoms of alcoholism.

Do Genetic Effects Change During Development?

Development adds to the complexity of the systems of alcohol use and abuse, and here too quantitative genetics can make important contributions. Genes contribute to change as well as to continuity during development, and quantitative genetics provides approaches to the analysis of change and continuity that have not yet been considered in the context of alcohol use and abuse. Genetic research on the development of alcoholism has been limited to two types of findings. As mentioned in the previous section, there is interest in the possibility that, at least in males, alcoholism in early adulthood could be more heritable than alcoholism that first appears later in development (Pickens et al., 1991). Although it makes sense that early onset alcoholism is more severe and thus perhaps more heritable, it is interesting that developmental genetic studies in other areas generally converge on the counterintuitive conclusion that, when heritability changes during development, it increases rather than decreases (Plomin, 1986a). This is counterintuitive because it is often assumed that environmental influences accumulate during development. Moreover, it is often wrongly assumed that genetic effects are unchanging, that genes that affect a disorder or dimension operate at full throttle from the moment of conception. This assumption motivates the second type of developmentally relevant research on alcoholism. Studies of at risk children whose parents are alcoholic assume that these children differ from controls (Schuckit, 1987). It is possible, however, that genes that affect alcoholism do not have any discernible effect until they operate in the developmental context of a mature adult.

Although alcohol abuse and dependence are often implicitly assumed to be permanent disorders, it is clear that they change during development. For example, many young alcohol abusers do not abuse alcohol in adulthood; patterns of alcohol use and abuse also change later in development. It also seems likely that alcohol-related processes such as sensitivity and tolerance change during the life course. In addition to investigating age changes in heritability for such alcohol-related processes, quantitative genetic techniques developed during the past decade can address the issue of the genetic contribution to age-to-age change (Plomin and DeFries, 1981). The simplest way to think about this issue is to consider a genetic analysis of a change score, asking whether genetic factors contribute to change from age to age (Plomin and Nesselroade, 1990). More generally, the concepts and analysis of age-to-age change are similar to the multivariate genetic approach described in the previous section (Plomin, 1986b). Instead of analyzing the covariance between two traits as in multivariate genetic analysis, longitudinal genetic analysis focuses on the covariance between a dimension or disorder assessed longitudinally. The genetic correlation in longitudinal genetic analysis indicates the extent to which genetic effects at one age are correlated with genetic effects at another age; the extent to which the genetic correlation is less than unity indicates that genetic factors contribute to developmental change.

We are aware of no longitudinal behavioral genetic studies in the alcohol domain that can take advantage of these new quantitative genetic techniques to analyze the etiology of change as well as continuity. For this reason, we must add longitudinal studies to the list of needed quantitative genetic research.

Is Alcohol Abuse Influenced by the Same Genetic Factors as Alcohol Use?

The line between normal and abnormal has been of long-standing interest in the study of disorders. To what extent does alcohol abuse represent the extreme end of a spectrum of continuous variation of alcohol use? More specifically, to what extent are genetic factors that affect alcohol abuse only quantitatively, not qualitatively, different from those that cause normal variability in alcohol use? The answers to these questions could have far-reaching implications for diagnosis, prevention, and intervention of alcohol abuse.

A new quantitative technique provides an as-yet unexploited approach to the old problem of the relationship between normal and abnormal that is well suited to the analysis of alcohol use and abuse. If quantitative data are obtained on probands, probands' relatives, and the population, it is possible to assess the extent to which the genetic and environmental etiologies of alcohol abuse differ from the etiologies of alcohol use. The approach has been called *DF analysis* in reference to DeFries and Fulker, who developed it (DeFries and Fulker, 1985, 1988; DeFries et al., 1987).

The DF approach introduces group statistics that address the etiology of the average difference between probands and the population for scores on a quantitative measure. For a quantitative measure relevant to a disorder, diagnosed probands will score toward the extreme of the distribution. The mean of the siblings of the probands will regress to the unselected population mean to the extent that familial factors are unimportant in the etiology of the disorder. The extent to which the probands' siblings do not regress back to the population mean indicates the extent to which familial factors are responsible for the mean difference between probands and the population. This estimate is called *group* familiality to distinguish it from the usual *individual* familiality that is based on familial correlations for individuals in the entire distribution. Group heritability can be assessed, for example, by comparing group familiality for MZ and DZ twins. It should be noted that group heritability is different from asking whether heritability differs for the extreme of a dimension versus the rest of the distribution. This latter question addresses individual differences at the extreme of a dimension, whereas group heritability assesses the etiology of the average difference between probands and the population.

The essential point of the DF analysis is that group heritability can differ from individual heritability. If they differ, this means that the etiology of deviant scores differs from the etiology of individual differences in the population. In other words, the disorder is etiologically distinct from the dimension. Consider mental retardation and the dimension of IQ scores as an example (see Plomin, 1991, for details). The average IQ of siblings of mildly retarded probands (i.e., IQs between 50 and 69 with an average IQ of 65) does not regress back to the population average—their average IQ is 85 (Nichols, 1984). Group familiality for these data has been calculated as 0.43 (i.e., 85–100/65–100), which is similar to the usual individual familiality found for IQ scores. This finding is consistent with the hypothesis that mild mental retardation represents the low end of the IQ distribution. In contrast, siblings of severely retarded probands (i.e., IQs less than 50 with an average IQ of 40) yield an average IQ that is normal (103 in the study by Nichols, 1984). This suggests near-zero group familiality for severe retardation (103–100/40–100) and indicates that the etiology of severe retardation differs from the etiology of the rest of the IQ distribution.

Recognizing the need to take into account a continuous distribution of genetic and environmental liability underlying dichotomous disorders, geneticists typically convert concordances for family members into so-called liability correlations (Falconer, 1965; Smith, 1974). Liability correlations are merely tetrachoric correlations that are routinely computed for data in which continuous, normally distributed data have been reduced artificially to two categories (such as true–false responses). The problem with the liability correlation is that it assesses a discontinuous disorder but assumes a continuous liability. A point often overlooked in the use of the liability correlation is that it does not refer to the disorder as diagnosed but rather to a hypothetical construct of continuous liability to the disorder. Nonetheless, the liability correlation is conceptually similar to group familiality (Plomin, 1991). The critical difference is that the liability correlation assumes an underlying continuous distribution based on dichotomous data, whereas group familiality is based on an empirical assessment of continuous data for probands and their relatives. Nonetheless, if the rather severe assumptions that underlie the computation of the liability correlation from dichotomous data are correct, the liability correlation will be similar to group familiality computed empirically from quantitative measures (Plomin, 1991).

Greater power and conceptual clarity will come from assessing rather than assuming disorder-relevant continua. For some disorders, such as mental retardation, this is easy to do because the disorder is diagnosed in relation to a continuous measure, IQ. The DF analysis has primarily been applied to reading disability, which has been diagnosed as the extreme of a continuous distribution of discriminant function scores. For other disorders, dimensional parallels are less obvious. What disorder-relevant dimensions can be employed in the case of alcoholism? Any of the processes discussed in the previous section would be appropriate for analyses of this type, such as alcohol consumed, behavioral and CNS sensitivity, acute and chronic tolerance, and psychological and physical dependence.

Conclusions

As the complexity of alcohol use and abuse is recognized, the need for a solid foundation of quantitative genetic research will be increasingly felt, especially as the field
contemplates the use of molecular genetic tools. There is an almost embarrassing need
for more quantitative genetic research to pin down an answer to the most elementary
question that can be asked. How important is genetic influence for alcohol abuse?
Although some behavioral genetic research is consistent with the hypothesis of genetic
influence, the case has not yet been made convincingly. After discussing this
nature–nurture issue, we considered three applications of quantitative genetics that go
beyond it. First, multivariate genetic analysis can be used to address the question of
genetic heterogeneity and comorbidity in terms of etiology rather than symptomatology. Second, longitudinal quantitative genetic studies can take advantage of techniques
to assess genetic contributions to age-to-age change as well as continuity of alcohol-
related processes. Third, quantitative genetic techniques can be used to ask whether
genetic effects on alcohol abuse are merely the quantitative extreme of genetic effects
on dimensions of alcohol use.

Simple causal systems are much easier to deal with than complex ones. If the object
of study is a complex system, however, research strategies based explicitly or implicitly on assumptions of simplicity will produce limited visions of reality. Without advo-
cating that all alcohol researchers henceforth adopt a "self-organization science" orientation (Scott, 1991), with attendant multivariate, interdisciplinary, developmental and
nonlinear features, we do believe that the field would benefit from encouraging this
type of research. It should provide new hypotheses and new integrative frameworks for
all scholars working in this particular area.

Acknowledgments: The authors' current research on alcohol-related problems is supported by a
gift from Mr. John Hanley and a grant (AA08125) from the National Institute on Alcohol Abuse
and Alcoholism.

References

Adams, M. D., Kelley, J. M., Gocayne, J. D., Dubnick, M., Polymeropoulos, M. H., Xiao, H.,
    Merril, C. R., Wu, A., Olde, B., Moreno, R. F., Kerlavage, A. R., McCombie, W. R., and
    Venter, J. C. (1991). Complementary DNA sequencing: Expressed sequence tags and
    human genome project. *Science* **252**:1651–1656.
Allard, R. W. (1988). Genetic changes associated with the evolution of adaptedness in cultivated
    plants and their wild progenitors. *J. Hered.* **79**:225–238.
Bailey, D. W. (1971). Recombinant-inbred strains, an aid to finding identity, linkage, and func-
    tion of histocompatibility and other genes. *Transplantation* **11**:324–327.
Begleiter, H., and Porjesz, B. (1988). Neurophysiological dysfunction in alcoholism. In *Alco-
    holism: Origins and Outcome,* R. M. Rose and J. Barrett, eds. pp. 157–172.
Blum, K., Noble, E. P., Sheridan, P. J., Montgomery, A., Ritchie, T., Jagadeeswaran, P.,
    Nogami, H., Briggs, A. H., and Cohn, J. B. (1990). Allelic association of human
    dopamine D_2 receptor gene in alcoholism. *JAMA* **263**:2055–2060.
Blum, K., Noble, E. P., Sheridan, P. J., Finnley, O., Montgomery, A., Ritchie, T., Ozkaragoz, T.,

Fitch, R. J., Sadlak, F., Sheffiend, D., Dahlmann, T., Harbardier, S., and Nogami, H. (1991). Association of the A1 allele of the D_2 dopamine receptor gene with severe alcoholism. *Alcohol.* **8**:409–416.

Bohman, M., Sigvardsson, S., and Cloninger, C. R. (1981). Maternal inheritance of alcohol abuse. *Arch. Gen. Psychiatr.* **38**:965–969.

Bolos, A. M., Dean, M., Lucas-Derse, S., Ramsburg, M., Brown, G. L., and Goldman, D. (1990). Population and pedigree studies reveal a lack of association between the dopamine D_2 receptor gene and alcoholism. *JAMA* **264**:3156–3160.

Bonner, J. T. (1988). *The Evolution of Complexity.* Princeton: Princeton University Press.

Bunge, M. (1979). *Causality and Modern Science,* 3d rev. ed. New York: Dover.

Cadoret, R. J. (1990). Genetics of alcoholism. In *Alcohol and the Family: Research and Clinical Perspectives,* R. L. Collins, K. E. Leonard, and J. S. Searles, eds., New York: Guilford Press, pp. 39–78.

Cadoret, R., J., O'Gorman, T., Toughton, E., and Heywood, E. (1985). Alcoholism and antisocial personality: Interrelationships, genetic and environmental factors. *Arch. Gen. Psychiatr.* **42**:161–167.

Cadoret, R. J., Troughton, E., and O'Gorman, T. W. (1987). Genetic and environmental factors in alcohol abuse and antisocial personality. *J. Stud. Alcohol* **48**:1–8.

Cloninger, C. R. (1987). Neurogenetic adaptive mechanisms in alcoholism. *Science* **236**:410–416.

Cloninger, C. R., and Reich, T. (1983). Genetic heterogeneity in alcoholism and sociopathy. In *Genetics of Neurological and Psychiatric Disorders,* S. S. Kety, L. P. Rowland, R. L. Sidman, and S. W. Matthysse, eds. New York: Raven Pres, pp. 145–166.

Cloninger, C. R., Bohman, M., and Sigvardsson, S. (1981). Inheritance of alcohol abuse: Cross-fostering analysis of adopted men. *Arch. Gen. Psychiatr.* **38**:861–868.

Coleman, D. L., and Hummel, K. P. (1975). Influence of genetic background on the expression of mutations at the diabetes locus in the mouse. II. Studies on background modifiers. *Israeli J. Med. Sci.* **11**:708–713.

Conneally, P. M. (1991). Association between the d_2 dopamine receptor gene and alcoholism: A continuing controversy. *Arch. Gen. Psychiatr.* **48**:664–666.

Cook, W. L., and Goethe, J. W. (1990). The effect of being reared with an alcoholic half-sibling: A classic study reanalyzed. *Fam. Process* **29**:87–93.

Corsico, R., Pessino, O. L., Morales, V., and Jmelninsky, A. (1988). Association of HLA antigens with alcoholic disease. *J. Stud. Alcohol* **49**:546–550.

Cotton, N. S. (1979). The familial incidence of alcoholism: A review. *J. Stud. Alcohol* **40**:89–116.

Crabbe, J. C., Kosobud, A., Young, E. R., and Janowsky, A. J. (1983). Polygenic and single-gene determination of responses to ethanol in BXD/Ty recombinant inbred mouse strains. *Neurobehav. Toxicol. Teratol.* **5**:181–187.

DeFries, J. C., and Fulker, D. W. (1985). Multiple regression analysis of twin data. *Behav. Genet.* **15**:467–473.

DeFries, J. C., and Fulker, D. W. (1988). Multiple regression analysis of twin data: Etiology of deviant scores versus individual differences. *Acta Genet. Medi. Gemellol.* **37**:205–216.

DeFries, J. C., Fulker, D. W., and LaBuda, M. C. (1987). Evidence for a genetic aetiology in reading disability in twins. *Nature* **329**:537–539.

Devor, E. J., and Cloninger, C. R. (1989). Genetics of alcoholism. *Ann. Rev. Genet.* **23**:19–36.

Falconer, D. S. (1965). The inheritance of liability to diseases, estimated from the incidence among relatives. *Ann. Hum. Genet.* **29**:61–76.

Falconer, D. S. (1981). *Introduction to Quantitative Genetics,* 2d ed. London: Longman.

Falconer, D. S. (1989). *Introduction to Quantitative Genetics,* 3d ed. New York: Wiley.

Fisher, R. A. (1918). The correlation between relatives on the supposition of Mendelian inheritance. *Trans. Roy. Soc. Edinburgh* **52**:399–433.

Følling, A., Mohr, O. L., and Ruud, L. (1945). *Oligophrenia phenylpyrouvica,* a recessive syndrome in man. *Nor. Vidensk./Akad. I Oslo. Mat.-Nat.vidensk. Kl.* **13**:1–44.

Ford, D. H. (1987). *Humans as Self-constructing Living Systems.* Hillsdale, NJ: Lawrence Erlbaum.

Gelernter, J. (1991). The Association of DRD2 with Alcoholism. Paper presented at the Eleventh International Workshop on Human Gene Mapping (HGM-11), London, August 21.

Goldman, D., Brown, G. L., Bolos, A. M., Lucas-Derse, S., and Dean, M. (1991). The dopamine D_2 receptor gene and alcoholism. *JAMA* **265**:2668.

Goodwin, D. W., Schulsinger, F., Hermansen, L., Guze, S. B., and Winokur, G. (1973). Alcohol problems in adoptees raised apart from alcoholic biological parents. *Arch. Gen. Psychiatr.* **28**:238–243.

Goodwin, D. W., Schulsinger, F., Knop, J., Mednick, S., and Guze, S. B. (1977). Alcoholism and depression in adopted-out daughters of alcoholics. *Arch. Gen. Psychiatr.* **34**:751–755.

Gurling, H. M. D., Murray, R. M., and Clifford, C. A. (1981). Investigations into the genetics of alcohol dependence and into its effects on brain function. In *Twin Research 3: Part C. Epidemiological and Clinical Studies,* L. Gedda, P. Parisi, and W. E. Nance, eds. New York: Alan R. Liss, pp. 77–87.

Gurling, H. M. D., Oppenheim, B. E., and Murray, R. M. (1984). Depression, criminality and psychopathology associated with alcoholism: Evidence from a twin study. *Acta Genet. Med. Gemellol.* **33**:333–339.

Hodgkinson, S., Mullan, M., and Murray, R. M. (1991). The genetics of vulnerability to alcoholism. In *The New Genetics of Mental Illness,* P. McGuffin and R. Murray, eds. Oxford: Butterworth-Heinemann, pp. 182–197.

Hrubec, Z., and Omenn, G. S. (1981). Evidence of genetic predisposition to alcoholic cirrhosis and psychosis: Twin concordance for alcoholism and its biological endpoints by zygosity among male veterans. *Alcohol.: Clin. Exp. Res.* **5**:207–215.

Hull, D. L. (1974). *Philosophy of Biological Science.* Englewood Cliffs, NJ: Prentice-Hall.

Jantsch, E. (1980). *The Self-organizing Universe.* Oxford: Pergamon Press.

Kacser, H., and Burns, J. A. (1979). Molecular democracy: Who shares the controls? *Biochem. Soc. Trans.* **7**:1149–1160.

Kaij, L. (1960). *Alcoholism in Twins.* Stockholm: Almqvist and Wiksell.

Kidd, K. K., Bowcock, A. M., Schmidtke, J., Track, R. K., Ricciuti, F., Hutchings, G., Bale, A., Pearson, P., and Willard, H. F. (1989). Report of the DNA committee and catalogs of cloned and mapped genes and DNA polymorphisms. *Cytogenet. Cell Genet.* **51**:622–947.

Lester, D. (1988). Genetic theory: An assessment of the heritability of alcoholism. In *Theories on Alcoholism,* C. D. Chaudron and D. A. Wilkinson, eds. Toronto: Addiction Research Foundation, pp. 1–28.

McClearn, G. E. (1991). Tools of pharmacogenetics. In *The Genetic Basis of Alcohol and Drug Action,* J. C. Crabbe and R. A. Harris, eds. New York: Plenum Press.

McClearn, G. E., Plomin, R., Gora-Maslak, G., and Crabbe, J. C. (1991). The gene chase in behavioral science. *Psychol. Sci.* **2**:222–229.

McGue, M., Pickens, R. W., and Svikis, D. S. (1992). Sex and age effects on the inheritance of alcohol problems: A twin study. *J. Abnorm. Psychol.* **101**:3–17.

Mayr, E. (1988). *Toward a New Philosophy of Biology.* Cambridge: Harvard University Press.

Merikangas, K. R. (1989). Genetics of alcoholism: A review of human studies. In I. Wetterberg, ed. *Genetics of Neuropsychiatric Diseases,* London: Macmillan, pp. 269–271.

Merikangas, K. R., Leckman, J. F., Prusoff, B. A., Pauls, D. L., and Weissman, M. M. (1985). Familial transmission of depression and alcoholism. *Arch. Gen. Psychiatr.* **42**:367–372.

Miller, J. G. (1978). *Living Systems.* New York: McGraw-Hill.

Milner, R. J., Randolph, L., Bahr, D., Cappello, M., Lenoir, D., Miller, F. D., and Bloom, F. E. (1987). Molecular biological approaches to the brain and their application to the study of alcoholism. In *Genetics and Alcoholism,* H. W. Goedde and D. P. Agarwal, eds. New York: Alan R. Liss, pp. 291–302.

Mrosovsky, N. (1990). *Rheostasis.* New York: Oxford University Press.

Murphy, E. A., and Berger, K. R. (1988). An approach to the genetics of physiological homeostasis. In *Proceedings, Second International Conference on Quantitative Genetics,* B. S. Weir, E. E. Eisen, M. M. Goodman, and G. Namkoong, eds. Sunderland, MA: Sinauer Associates.

Murphy, E. A., and Trojak, J. L. (1986). The genetics of quantifiable homeostasis: I. The general issues. *Am. J. Med. Genet.* **24**:159–169.

Murray, R. M., Clifford, C. A., and Gurling, H. M. D. (1983). Twin and adoption studies: How good is the evidence for a genetic role? In *Recent Developments in Alcoholism,* Vol. 1, E. Galanter, ed. New York: Plenum, pp. 25–48.

Nichols, P. L. (1984). Familial mental retardation. *Behav. Genet.* **14**:161–170.

Noble, E. P., and Blum, K. (1991). The dopamine D_2 receptor gene and alcoholism. *JAMA* **265**:2667.

Noble, E. P., Blum, K., Ritchie, T., Montgomery, A., and Sheridan, P. J. (1991). Allelic association of the D_2 dopamine receptor gene with receptor-binding characteristics in alcoholism. *Arch. Gen. Psychiatr.* **48**:648–654.

Parsian, A., Todd, R. D., Devor, E. J., O'Malley, K. L., Suarez, B. K., Reich, T., and Cloninger, C. R. (1991). Alcoholism and alleles of the human D_2 dopamine receptor locus. *Arch. Gen. Psychiatr.* **48**:655–663.

Paterson, A. H., Lander, E. S., Hewitt, J. D., Peterson, S., Lincoln, S. E., and Tanksley, S. D. (1988). Resolution of quantitative traits into Mendelian factors by using a complete linkage map of restriction fragment length polymorphisms. *Nature* **335**:721–726.

Peele, S. (1986). The implications and limitations of genetic models of alcoholism and other addictions. *J. Stud. Alcohol* **47**:63–73.

Pickens, R. W., Svikis, D. S., McGue, M., Lykken, D. T., Heston, L. L., and Clayton, P. J. (1991). Heterogeneity in the inheritance of alcoholism. *Arch. Gen. Psychiatr.* **48**:19–28.

Plomin, R. (1986a). *Development, Genetics, and Psychology.* Hillsdale, NJ: Lawrence Erlbaum.

Plomin, R. (1986b). Multivariate analysis and developmental behavioral genetics: Developmental change as well as continuity. *Behav. Genet.* **16**:25–43.

Plomin, R. (1990). The role of inheritance in behavior. *Science* **248**:183–188.

Plomin, R. (1991). Genetic risk and psychosocial disorders: Links between the normal and abnormal. In *Biological Risk Factors for Psychosocial Disorders,* M. Rutter and P. Casaer, eds. Cambridge, UK: Cambridge University Press, pp. 101–138.

Plomin, R., and Daniels, D. (1987). Why are children in the same family so different from each other? *Behav. Brain Sci.* **10**:1–16.

Plomin, R., and DeFries, J. C. (1979). Multivariate behavioral genetic analysis of twin data on scholastic abilities. *Behav. Genet.* **9**:505–517.

Plomin, R., and DeFries, J. C. (1981). Multivariate behavioral genetics and development: Twin studies. In *Progress in Clinical and Biological Research, Twin Research 3: Part B. Intelligence, Personality, and Development,* Vol. 69B, L. Gedda, P. Parisi, and W. E. Nance, eds. New York: Alan R. Liss, pp. 25–33.

Plomin, R., and Nesselroade, J. R. (1990). Behavioral genetics and personality change. *J. Pers.* **58:**191–220.

Plomin, R., and Rende, R. (1991). Human behavioral genetics. *Ann. Rev. Psychol.* **42:**161–190.

Plomin, R., DeFries, J. C., and McClearn, G. E. (1990). *Behavioral Genetics: A Primer,* 2d ed. New York: W. H. Freeman.

Plomin, R., McClearn, G. E., Gora-Maslak, G., and Neiderhiser, J. M. (1991). Use of recombinant inbred strains to detect quantitative trait loci associated with behavior. *Behav. Genet.* **21:**99–116.

Prigogine, I. (1976). Order through fluctuation: Self-organization and social system. In *Evolution and Consciousness,* E. Jantsch and C. H. Waddington, eds. Reading, MA: Addison-Wesley, pp. 99–123.

Robertson, A. (1984). The relevance of molecular biology to animal improvements. In *Genetics: New Frontiers,* V. L. Chopra, B. C. Joshi, R. P. Sharma, and H. C. Bansal, eds. New York: Oxford and IBH Publishing.

Roe, A. (1944). The adult adjustment of children of alcoholic parents raised in foster homes. *Q. J. Stud. Alcohol.* **5:**378–393.

Salthe, S. N. (1985). *Evolving Hierarchical Systems.* New York: Columbia University Press.

Sattler, R. (1986). *Biophilosophy.* Berlin: Springer-Verlag.

Schuckit, M. A. (1987). Biological vulnerability to alcoholism. *J. Consult. Clin. Psychol.* **55:**301–309.

Schuckit, M. A. (1988). A search for biological markers in alcoholism: Application to psychiatric research. In *Alcoholism: Origins and Outcomes,* R. M. Rose and J. Barrett, eds. New York: Raven Press, pp. 143–154.

Schuckit, M. A., Goodwin, D. W., and Winokur, G. (1972). A study of alcoholism in half siblings. *Am. J. Psychiatr.* **128:**1132–1135.

Scott, G. P. (1991). Introduction: Self-organization science and the interdisciplinary tower of Babel syndrome. In *Time, Rhythms, and Chaos in the New Dialogue with Nature,* G. P. Scott, ed. Ames, IA: Iowa State University Press, pp. 3–21.

Searles, J. S. (1988). The role of genetics in the pathogenesis of alcoholism. *J. Abnorm. Psychol.* **97:**153–167.

Searles, J. S. (1990). The contribution of genetic factors to the development of alcoholism: A critical review. In *Alcohol and the Family: Research and Clinical Perspectives,* R. L. Collins, K. E. Leonard, and J. S. Searles, eds. New York: Guilford Press, pp. 3–38.

Simon, H. A. (1969). *The Sciences of the Artificial.* Cambridge, MA: MIT Press.

Sing, C. F., and Boerwinkle, E. A. (1987). Genetic architecture of inter-individual variability in apolipoprotein, lipoprotein and lipid phenotypes. In *Molecular Approaches to Human Polygenic Disease,* G. Bock and G. M. Collins, eds. Chichester, UK: Wiley, pp. 99–122.

Smith, C. (1974). Concordance in twins: Methods and interpretation. *Am. J. Hum. Genet.* **26:**454–466.

Stabenau, J. R. (1986). Genetic factors and human reactions to alcohol. In *Perspectives in Behavior Genetics,* J. L. Fuller and E. C. Simmel, eds. Hillsdale, NJ: Lawrence Erlbaum. pp. 201–266.

Tabakoff, B., and Hoffman, P. L. (1987). Ethanol tolerance and dependence. In *Genetics and Alcoholism,* H. W. Goedde and D. P. Agarwal, eds. New York: Alan R. Liss, pp. 253–269.

Tarter, R. E., Moss, H., and Laird, S. B. (1990). Biological markers for vulnerability to alco-
    holism. In *Alcohol and the Family: Research and Clinical Perspectives,* R. L. Collins, K.
    E. Leonard, and J. S. Searles, eds. New York: Guilford Press, pp. 79–106.

Taylor, B. A. (1989). Recombinant inbred strains. In *Genetic Variance and Strains of the Labo-
    ratory Mouse,* 2d ed., M. F. Lyon and A. G. Searle, eds. Oxford: Oxford University
    Press, pp. 773–789.

Todd, J. A., Aitman, T. J., Cornall, R. J., Ghosh, S., Hall, J. R. S., Hearne, C. M. N., Knight, A.
    M., Love, J. M., McAleer, M. A., Prins, J.-B., Rodrigues, N., Lathrop, M., Pressey, A.,
    DeLarato, N. J., Peterson, L. B., and Wicker, L. S. (1991). Genetic analysis of autoim-
    mune type 1 diabetes mellitus in mice. *Nature* **351:**542–547.

Waddington, C. H. (1957). *The Strategy of the Genes.* New York: MacMillan.

Waddington, C. H. (1977). *Tools for Thought.* New York: Basic Books.

Ward, P. J. (1990). The inheritance of metabolic flux: Expressions for the within-sibship mean
    and variance given the parental genotypes. *Genet. Soc. Am.* **125:**655–667.

Weir, B. S., Eisen, E. J., Goodman, M. M., and Namkoong, G. (1988). *Proceedings, Second
    International Conference on Quantitative Genetics.* Sunderland, MA: Sinauer Associ-
    ates.

Yates, F. E., Marsh, D. J., and Iberall, A. S. (1972). Integration of the whole organism—a foun-
    dation for a theoretical biology. In *Challenging Biological Problems: Directions Toward
    Their Solution,* J. A. Behnke, ed. Oxford: Oxford University Press, pp. 110–132.

14

Linkage Analysis in the Study of the Genetics of Alcoholism

ALEXANDER F. WILSON AND
ROBERT C. ELSTON

If genetic components are involved in the etiology of alcoholism, it will be necessary to determine where these components reside in the human genome. Given that the human haploid genome contains about 3 billion base pairs and that a gene may span as few as 1000 bases, the mapping of a gene for alcoholism to a specific region in the genome resembles the proverbial search for a needle in a haystack. Linkage analysis is a statistical method of determining the location of genes that underlie a disease or trait phenotype relative to marker loci with known chromosomal locations. Linkage analysis can be used to determine, to within a few million base pairs, the approximate physical location of genetic components that may be involved in the etiology of alcoholism.

Terminology and Background

Linkage analysis is based on the physical characteristics and properties of reproductive cells as they undergo meiosis. Humans have 23 pairs of chromosomes, 22 pairs of autosomal chromosomes (numbered from 1 to 22) and 1 pair of sex chromosomes (denoted X and Y), in the nucleus of each spermatogonium and oögonium. Members of the same pair of autosomal chromosomes are called *homologous* chromosomes. The chromosomes are composed of both protein and deoxyribonucleic acid (DNA), and DNA consists of an alternating deoxyribose sugar-phosphate backbone with a nitrogenous base attached to each sugar. There are four different bases in DNA: adenine, guanine, thymine, and cytosine. The proteins that are responsible for our biochemical and physical makeup (e.g., ABO and Rh blood types, eye color, the structural proteins, and specific activity of enzymes) are determined by the sequence of these bases in specific chromosomal regions. These sequences are called *genes*, and it is estimated that there are between 50,000 and 200,000 genes in the human genome. The physical location of each gene along the chromosome is referred to as its *locus*. At a given locus there are two copies of each gene—one on each member of the homologous chromosome pair. Different forms of a gene (i.e., different sequences of bases that occur at the same genetic locus) are called *alleles*. Individuals inherit one allele from their father (the paternal allele) and one from their mother (the maternal allele). Similarly, individuals contribute one of their own alleles randomly to each of their offspring. The pair of alleles at a genetic locus is referred to as the *genotype* at that locus, while a measurable characteristic is referred to as the *phenotype*.

Mendel's Laws

In 1865, Gregor Mendel postulated the principle of unit inheritance, and the laws of random segregation and independent assortment (Mendel, 1866). Mendel's discrete units of inheritance (which he called *factors*) are now recognized as genes. Mendel's law of segregation, which states that alleles at a given genetic locus segregate randomly into separate gametes, has its biological basis in the process of meiosis. During the first meiotic division, the members of each pair of homologous chromosomes segregate into separate gametes—separating the alleles at a given locus. Mendel's law of independent assortment, which states that alleles at a given genetic locus assort independently with respect to alleles at other genetic loci, is based on the random orientation of the homologous chromosomes during this same division. The orientation and separation of one member of a chromosome pair is independent of that of the members of other chromosome pairs. Thus, the 23 pairs of chromosomes can theoretically form at least 8,388,608 (2^{23}) different gametes, each with one member of each of the 23 pairs.

If two genes have their loci on different chromosomes, the alleles at these two loci will assort independently of one another during meiosis according to Mendel's second law. Because there are thousands of genes and only 23 chromosomes, however, a large number of genes reside on each chromosome. If the physical basis of independent assortment were due solely to the orientation and separation of the homologous chromosomes, the alleles at all of the loci on a particular chromosome would be transmitted together to the same gamete—seriously violating Mendel's second law. Although Mendel's second law is, in fact, violated, the nonindependent assortment is limited to loci that are physically close to one another on the same chromosome.

Crossover and Recombination

Each chromosome contains two identical strands of DNA known as *chromatids*. During the process of meiosis, segments of the chromatids of homologous chromosomes are often exchanged. The point of exchange of chromosomal material is termed a *crossover*. Figure 14-1 illustrates five heterozygous loci on a pair of homologous chromosomes, and the occurrence of two crossovers during the first meiotic division. The

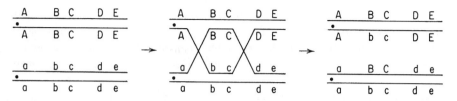

Fig. 14-1 The formation of two crossovers between the chromatids of homologous chromosomes during meiosis. The centromere is represented as ●, alleles at 5 loci are indicated.

loci are *A, B, C, D,* and *E,* with two alleles at each locus represented by upper- and lowercase letters, and the crossovers occur between loci *A* and *B,* and *C* and *D.* When a crossover occurs, alleles on a given chromatid are exchanged for the corresponding alleles on a chromatid of the homologous chromosome. This exchange may alter the allelic composition of two of the four chromatids, resulting in a *recombination.* During the second meiotic division, the chromatids of each homologous chromosome separate and are passed to different gametes. A recombination between two loci is observed in the genotype of an offspring and results from the rearrangement of genotypes that occurred during the process of meiosis. In Fig. 14-1, these crossovers result in recombinations occurring between pairs of loci *AB, AC, BD, BE, CD,* and *CE* on two of the four chromatids. It is important to note that only an odd number of crossovers between two loci can result in an observable recombination. Thus, there is no recombination between the pairs of loci *AD, AE, BC,* and *DE* on these chromatids even though two crossovers have occurred. An offspring whose genotype indicates that a recombination has occurred between two loci is referred to as a *recombinant;* if no recombination between two loci is observed in an offspring, then that offspring is referred to as a *nonrecombinant.*

If two genetic loci on the same chromosome are so far apart that the probability of an odd number of crossovers between them is equal to the probability of an even number of crossovers, then the number of recombinants and nonrecombinants among the offspring will occur with equal frequency; the alleles at each locus will appear to segregate independently with respect to the alleles at the other locus. However, if two loci are physically close enough together on the same chromosome so that the probability of a recombination between them is less than one-half, then the alleles at these two loci will not assort independently; they will tend to be transmitted to the gametes together, and such loci are said to be linked. *Linkage* is the nonindependent assortment of alleles at a given locus with respect to alleles at another locus. Genetic loci that physically reside on the same chromosome are said to be *syntenic,* and although all linked loci are syntenic, all syntenic loci are not necessarily linked.

The *recombination fraction,* a measure of the genetic distance between two loci, can be obtained from the number of recombinants observed among the genotypes of the offspring. The recombination fraction is expressed as

$$\theta = \frac{\text{Number of recombinants}}{\text{Number of recombinants} + \text{number of nonrecombinants}}$$

The minimum value of the recombination fraction is 0 and occurs when no recombinants occur among the genotypes of the offspring. The maximum recombination fraction is often taken to be one-half, representing independent assortment, although in a small sample all the offspring could be recombinants, resulting in a recombination fraction of 1.

Figure 14-2 illustrates a double backcross mating and the expected proportions of genotypes in the offspring. In this illustration there are two loci, *A* with alleles A and a, and *B* with alleles B and b. We denote the father's genotype AB/ab and the mother's genotype ab/ab (the solidus is used to separate the genotypes of homologous chromosomes). The mother's gametes are all identical (ab) in this example. In Fig. 14-2(a), the two loci are physically very close to each other on the same chromosome and their alleles always assort together. If none of the observed genotypes of the offspring are the recombinant type (Ab/ab or aB/ab), but are all the nonrecombinant type (AB/ab or ab/ab), the recombination fraction is estimated to be 0.

In Fig. 14-2(b) the two loci are further apart on the same chromosome. If for example 10% of the offspring are recombinants (Ab/ab or aB/ab), then the recombination fraction is estimated as 0.1. If the loci are on different chromosomes, the alleles at locus *A* would assort independently with respect to alleles at locus *B*. The father's gametes (AB, Ab, aB, ab) would be expected to be observed in equal proportions of recombinant (Ab, aB) and nonrecombinant (AB, ab) types among the genotypes of the offspring. Since on average 50% of the offspring would be expected to be recombinants, the recombination fraction would then be one-half.

Association

When a specific allele is correlated with a particular trait in the general population, there is said to be an *association* between the trait and that allele. If a high correlation

	Father's genotype AB/ab	Mother's genotype: ab/ab	Possible genotypes of the offspring and their expected proportions	
a)	AB • AB	ab • ab	AB/ab	50% (non-recombinants)
			Ab/ab	0% (recombinants)
	ab • ab	ab • ab	aB/ab	0% (recombinants)
			ab/ab	50% (non-recombinants)
b)	A B • A ✕ B a ✕ b • a b	a b • a b • a b	AB/ab	45% (non-recombinants)
			Ab/ab	5% (recombinants)
			aB/ab	5% (recombinants)
			ab/ab	45% (non-recombinants)

Fig. 14-2 Results of a double backcross mating. (a) The *A* and *B* loci are so tightly linked that no recombination occurs. (b) The *A* and *B* loci are far enough apart for 10% recombination to occur.

exists between the presence of a specific allele and a trait phenotype, this suggests that the allele is either tightly linked and in disequilibrium with an allele responsible for the expression of that phenotype, or that the marker allele itself has a pleiotropic effect on the trait. This latter case can also be formally considered as an effect of linkage—it corresponds to the case of linkage in which there is a recombination fraction of zero and complete allelic disequilibrium. An association between a trait and a marker may also occur as a result of chance sampling variation; of an epistatic effect on the viability of two loci, one hitchhiking with the trait locus and the other hitchhiking with the marker locus; or as a result of stratification in the sample, such as may occur if the sample is ethnically heterogeneous. It is important to note, however, that linkage between a trait and a specific locus does not typically result in an association between specific phenotypes and genotypes at the population level. The hallmark of linkage is that it results in an intrafamilial association between the trait and marker, even though there may be no overall population association. Tight linkage is necessary to produce an association across the whole population.

The detection of an association between a trait and a specific allele is the basis of the candidate gene approach. This approach can use two samples of independent individuals, with and without the trait, who are genotyped for a polymorphism at the candidate gene or at a locus tightly linked to it.

A number of early studies focused on associations between alcoholism and polymorphic blood group markers. Billington (1956) and Nordmo (1959) reported a significantly greater proportion of individuals with ABO blood type A in groups of individuals with portal cirrhosis or alcoholism, when compared to groups of nonalcoholics. Subsequent studies did not confirm this finding (Camps and Dodd, 1967; Reid et al., 1968; Camps et al., 1969; Swinson and Madden, 1973), although several of these studies suggested that there were significantly more nonsecretors of the ABO A, B, and H antigens than secretors of these antigens in alcoholic groups, particularly in individuals with blood type A (Camps and Dodd, 1967; Camps et al., 1969; Swinson and Madden, 1973).

Recently, evidence has been reported for an association between alcoholism and the A1 allele of the dopamine D2 receptor (Blum et al., 1990; Parsian et al., 1991; Noble et al., 1991), although one study has failed to confirm this association (Bolos et al., 1990). A family analysis using an odds-ratio method showed no evidence of linkage between alcoholism and the dopamine D2 receptor locus (Parsian et al. 1991). Other recent reports of associations include the association of a structural mutation in aldehyde dehydrogenase and flushing in Orientals (Agarwal et al., 1981; Bosron et al., 1983; Yoshida et al., 1984), and associations between various HLA alleles and alcoholism (Anderson et al., 1988; Monteiro et al., 1988; Corsico et al., 1988). Loci that have been postulated as candidate loci involved in the expression of alcoholism include catechol-o-methyltransferase, monoamine oxidase, dopamine-β-hydroxylase, catalase, cytochrome P450, alcohol dehydrogenase, aldehyde dehydrogenase, norepinephrine, serotonin, imipramine binding sites, and other dopamine and serotonin receptors (Radouco-Thomas et al., 1984; el-Guebaly, 1986; Goldman, 1988).

Clinical and Genetic Heterogeneity in Alcoholism

The assumption is often made in linkage analysis that the trait under study is a distinct single entity at both the clinical and genetic levels and that the variability at the genetic level is at least partly responsible for variation at the phenotypic level. Although the assumptions of clinical and genetic homogeneity may be appropriate for rare autosomal disorders such as Huntington disease, the invocation of these assumptions is problematic with respect to syndromes like alcoholism where the mode of inheritance is not well defined. The term *clinical heterogeneity* refers to differences at the phenotypic level. The presence of clinical heterogeneity is often taken as an indication of genetic differences, but this is not necessarily the case; a single genotype may be responsible for a wide spectrum of different observable clinical phenotypes, a situation termed *variable expressivity. Genetic heterogeneity,* on the other hand, exists if the same phenotype can be produced by different underlying genetic mechanisms.

With respect to clinical and genetic heterogeneity, Cloninger et al. (1981) and Gilligan et al. (1987) have proposed that there are two different forms of alcoholism: type 1, or milieu-limited alcoholism, and type 2, or male-limited alcoholism. Type 1 alcoholism occurs in both males and females and is characterized by adult onset of alcohol abuse and the absence of antisocial or criminal behavior; type 2 is mostly present in males and is characterized by an earlier age of onset of alcohol abuse and associated criminal behavior. Gilligan et al. (1987) suggested different underlying genetic mechanisms for these two forms of alcoholism: the pattern of inheritance in type 2 alcoholism was attributed to the effect of a single major locus together with a multifactorial-polygenic background, while the inheritance of type 1 alcoholism was attributed solely to a multifactorial-polygenic effect.

With respect to clinical heterogeneity, considerable controversy exists as to whether alcoholism is a distinct entity or is part of a broader syndrome. Cadoret and Winokur (1974) reported that 39% of alcoholic patients in their study also had primary or secondary major depression. Weissman and Myers (1980) reported that 68% of patients with alcoholism also met RCD criteria for major or minor depressive disorder. A case-control study by Merikangas et al. (1985) found that first-degree relatives of probands with both depression and alcoholism had increased rates of alcoholism, depression, and antisocial personality when compared to relatives of controls. However, first-degree relatives of probands with depression without alcoholism had increased rates of depression, anxiety disorders, and antisocial personality, but rates of alcoholism were not significantly different between the two groups. Cloninger et al. (1979) also reported the independence of alcoholism and depression. Winokur et al. (1971), Winokur et al. (1975), and Tanna et al. (1976) have suggested that alcoholism may be part of a broader syndrome encompassing depression, alcoholism, and antisocial personality, i.e., depression spectrum disease (DSD), for which the presence of alcoholism may be taken as a familial marker.

Genetic Markers

Polymorphic Markers

The normal variation, or polymorphism, that is found in the phenotypes of well-characterized marker loci is used in linkage analysis to map other traits to the human genome. The cosegregation of a trait and a marker locus suggests that there is a genetic locus physically near the location of the marker locus that is responsible, at least in part, for the expression of the trait.

There are currently thousands of genetic polymorphisms distributed throughout the human genome that can be used as markers. A partial list of polymorphic markers that have been used in linkage studies of alcoholism is given in Table 14-1 (Wilson et al., 1991a; Dumont-Damien and Duyme, 1991). These marker loci include red cell antigens, enzymes, structural proteins, specific sequences of DNA, and candidate loci (loci thought to be involved in the metabolic pathway of the trait). Until a decade ago, the variation in most marker loci was observed at the protein level. Variability in red cell antigens was observed as differences in antigen–antibody reactions; and variation in enzymes and structural proteins was typically observed as differences in electrophoretic mobility. Over the last decade, the use of restriction enzyme methods has improved the resolution from the protein level to the DNA level itself, although the differences are still observed as differences in electrophoretic mobility. DNA markers currently include restriction fragment length polymorphisms (RFLPs) and short tandem repeat polymorphisms (STRPs). RFLPs are polymorphisms based on variation in single nucleotides of DNA. Each restriction enzyme recognizes a specific DNA base sequence, often 4–6 base pairs long, and cuts the DNA at that site. If a single base is altered in the recognition sequence, the restriction enzyme will not cut at that site, resulting in a single large DNA fragment instead of two smaller fragments (Botstein et al., 1980). STRPs are based on variation in the number of repeats of a few bases (often the dinucleotides CA and GT). These markers can be typed using the polymerase chain reaction (PCR) to amplify the appropriate DNA sequence, followed by electrophoresis to determine how many repeats it contains (Litt and Luty, 1989; Weber and May, 1989). Both RFLPs and STRPs are widely distributed throughout the genome.

Heterozygosity and Polymorphic Information Content

Linkage analysis can only be performed in families that exhibit variation at both the trait and marker loci. A family in which all the individuals have the same genotype for the trait and/or the marker locus provides no information about the number of recombinations, and thus no information about linkage. Therefore, one of the most important characteristics of a marker locus is the extent to which it is polymorphic. A marker can be defined to be polymorphic when its most frequent allele occurs with a frequency of not more than 0.99. Genetic markers that have many alleles in the population are the most useful in linkage studies.

The degree of polymorphism of a marker locus can be measured in several ways.

Table 14-1 Polymorphic Markers Used in Linkage Studies of Alcoholism

Red cell antigens	
Rhesus blood group	(RH, 1p36-p34)
Duffy blood group	(FY, 1q21-22)
MNS blood group	(MNS, 4q28-q31)
ABO blood group	(ABO, 9q34)
Kidd blood group	(JK, 18q11-q12)
Lewis blood group	(LE, 19p13)
P blood group	(P1, 22q11-qter)
Kell blood group	(KEL, unassigned)
Enzymes	
6-phosphogluconate dehydrogenase	(PGD, 1p36)
Phosphoglucomutase	(PGM1, 1p22)
Acid phosphatase	(ACP1, 2p25)
Glyoxylase I	(GLO1, 6p21)
Glutamic pyruvic transaminase	(GPT, 8q24)
Adenylate kinase-1	(AK1, 9q34)
Esterase D	(ESD, 13q14)
Adenosine deaminase	(ADA, 20q13)
Structural proteins/immunoglobulins	
Immunoglobulin κ	(IGK, 2p12)
Transferrin	(TF, 3q21)
Group specific component	(GC, 4q12)
Properdin factor B	(BF, 6p21)
Orosomucoid	(ORM, 9q34)
Hemoglobin beta	(HBB, 11p15)
Proline rich protein	(PR, 12p13)
Immunoglobulin γ heavy chain	(IGHG, 14q32)
Haptoglobin	(HP, 16q22)
Third component of complement	(C3, 19p13)
Candidate loci	
Alcohol dehydrogenase	(ADH3, 4q22)
Carboxypeptidase	(CPA, 7q22)
Dopamine D2 receptor	(DRD2, 11q23)
Phenylalanine hydroxylase	(PAH, 12q24)
DNA markers	
Esterase D	(ESD, 13q14)

Heterozygosity is the probability that an individual will be heterozygous at a given locus and is determined as the sum of the frequencies of all the heterozygous genotypes at that locus. The *polymorphic information content* (PIC) of a marker locus is the sum of the frequencies of each mating type multiplied by the probability that an offspring of that mating type will be informative for linkage, on the assumption that one parent is heterozygous at the trait locus (Botstein et al., 1980). In general, markers with a large number of alleles have higher heterozygosities and PICs than markers with only a few alleles, and markers with equally frequent alleles have higher heterozygosities and PICs than similar markers with some very frequent and some very infrequent alleles.

Philosophical Approaches to Linkage Analysis

In addition to mapping, genetic linkage analysis can be used to identify single-locus effects. The demonstration of genetic linkage between a known polymorphic marker locus and a trait phenotype suggests that the trait has a genetic component involved in its underlying etiology. A subtle distinction thus exists between two different ways that linkage analysis can be used to investigate the genetic etiology of complex traits (i.e., traits thought to have a genetic component, but for which the etiology of that component is as yet unknown). These have been called the phenometric and the genometric approaches (Elston and Wilson, 1990).

Phenometric Approach

In the phenometric approach, the phenotype of a trait is assumed to be well-defined and usually represents a distinct clinical entity (such as Huntington disease). Segregation analysis is first used to describe the mode of inheritance of the genetic component and to determine relevant parameter estimates. These estimates are then used in a linkage analysis to find the physical location(s) in the genome that may be relevant to that trait. This is the traditional sequence followed in genetic segregation and linkage studies and it is most effective when the phenotype is actually determined in large part by segregation at a single Mendelian locus. Phenometric analysis seeks to determine the genotypes underlying well-defined phenotypic traits. It can be a less effective approach, however, when the phenotype is not well defined or when the underlying genetic component of the trait is responsible for a relatively small portion of the phenotypic variation, as may occur if the phenotype is a quantitative trait.

Genometric Approach

The genometric approach assumes that alleles at a putative single locus are involved in the etiology of a clinical or biological entity and that the different genotypes at that locus have a measurable effect on the phenotype. The genotypes of the putative locus are assumed to be known through their Mendelian segregation, which can be measured precisely if data are available at tightly linked marker loci. With this knowledge, an attempt is made to determine the kinds of phenotypic variation, if any, for which the various genotypes are responsible. Genometric analysis seeks to measure the phenotypic actions and interactions of specific genotypes. Use is made of this fact in the stepwise oligogenic method for segregation and linkage analysis (Wilson et al., 1990) and in a multivariate approach suggested by Amos et al. (1990). In the most extreme form of this approach, the marker locus and the putative locus are identical, leading to the measured genotype method of Boerwinkle et al. (1986) and the marker association method of George and Elston (1987).

In addition to the identification of single loci with major effects, the genometric approach may allow the identification of single loci with relatively minor effects, the identification of oligogenic loci that affect single traits, and the identification of single loci that have pleiotropic effects (i.e., that affect several phenotypic traits) (Wilson et al. 1991b).

Candidate Gene Approach

Linkage analyses have also been done using a candidate gene approach. Morton (1990) notes that a linkage test in complex disease is well motivated under either of two conditions: if a prior segregation analysis has given evidence for a major locus, or if there is a candidate locus that may influence liability. The latter motivation is inherently different from the former. The notion of a candidate locus—for example, a locus in a biochemical pathway thought to influence the phenotype, without such an effect having been actually demonstrated—is actually a restricted application of the genometric approach.

The candidate gene approach focuses on loci in a metabolic pathway thought to have an effect on the expression of the trait. The most efficient study design to investigate candidate loci is a case-control study. This design is used to determine if the allelic frequencies at any of the candidate loci are different between two groups that differ with respect to the disease trait of interest. If a difference can be demonstrated, then this implies an association between that candidate locus and the trait (see the section titled "Association"). In the absence of confounding factors, an association implies that the candidate locus is involved in the expression of the trait. This approach is particularly appropriate if the metabolic pathways underlying a particular trait are well characterized. If none of the proposed candidate loci is involved in the etiology of a trait, typically no association will be found even though one or more of these candidate loci may be linked to an unknown locus that is involved in the etiology of that trait. For this reason candidate loci are often used as markers in linkage studies, based on family data. In this way it is possible to detect an effect due either to the candidate locus itself, or to another locus that is linked to the candidate locus. An association study will detect the effect of linkage to a candidate gene only if the linkage is so tight that there is allelic disequilibrium.

Statistical Methods

Two major types of statistical analysis have been used in linkage studies of alcoholism: lod-score and sib-pair methods.

Lod-Score Method

As noted in the section on crossover and recombination, the most direct method used to estimate the recombination fraction is to count the number of recombinants (k) and express it as a fraction of the total number of offspring (n) so that the recombination fraction is $\theta = k/n$. In order to determine this fraction, the genotypes of both parents must be known; typically one parent is heterozygous at both loci and the other parent is homozygous at both loci, i.e., a double backcross mating. Unfortunately, these restrictions limit the size of the sample that can be obtained for linkage analysis. A less restrictive procedure using an inverse-probability ratio (a likelihood ratio) was proposed by Haldane and Smith (1947). This method can be used to accept or reject a hypothesis of independent assortment as well as to obtain an estimate of the recombination fraction. Given trait and marker data in a family or set of families, this test compares the likelihood of a hypothesis of linkage between a putative genetic locus underlying the trait and a marker locus (a specific recombination fraction $\leq 1/2$), against that of the hypothesis of independent assortment of alleles at these two loci (a recombination fraction of 1/2). Smith (1953) proposed taking the log of this ratio

$$z = \log \frac{\text{Likelihood (data given recombination fraction } \theta)}{\text{Likelihood (data given independent assortment, } \theta = \frac{1}{2})}$$

The term *lods* was derived from the backward *log odds* ratio (Barnard 1949).

The formulation of the likelihood for a set of data can be illustrated quite simply. Consider a double-backcross mating where the father has the two-locus genotype AB/ab and the mother has genotype ab/ab. Four possible genotypes, AB/ab, Ab/ab, aB/ab, and ab/ab can occur among the genotypes of the offspring. These are derived from the maternal gamete (ab) and the paternal gametes AB and ab (nonrecombinant types) and Ab and aB (recombinant types). If the probability of recombination between the two loci is denoted θ, then the likelihood for exactly one recombinant (Ab/ab, for example) among the genotypes of four offspring is $4(\theta^1)(1 - \theta)^3$, i.e., the probability of observing exactly one recombinant and three nonrecombinants in any one of the four orders in which these two types can occur. The log likelihood ratio would then be

$$z = \log \frac{4(\theta^1)(1 - \theta)^3}{4(\frac{1}{2}^1)(1 - \frac{1}{2})^3}$$

or $\log \{\theta(1 - \theta)^3/(\frac{1}{2})^4\}$. By setting the derivative of the log likelihood ratio equal to 0 and solving for θ, we find that the recombination fraction that maximizes θ is 0.25, which is identical to the result obtained using the direct counting method ($\theta = 1/4$). Unlike the counting method, however, the general method of maximizing the likelihood can be used to estimate the recombination fraction in a wide variety of situations. Thus the method based on the likelihood ratio can be used for all types of family data.

Morton (1955) applied Wald's (1947) sequential probability ratio test to combine results from a series of samples. Morton recommended summing lod or Z-scores calculated at a series of specific recombination fractions (0.0, 0.1, 0.2, 0.3, 0.4) over families and provided tables of these scores for various mating types of the parents and numbers of recombinants and nonrecombinants among the genotypes of the offspring. The value of the recombination fraction that makes this sum largest is taken to be an estimate of the recombination fraction between the genetic locus underlying the trait and the marker locus. Traditionally, when this lod score (calculated over the range 0 to 1/2) exceeds 3 (a backward odds ratio of 1000:1), the null hypothesis of independent assortment is rejected and linkage is inferred. If this log ratio is less then -2, then the null hypothesis of independent assortment is not rejected and linkage between the trait and marker locus is considered to be excluded. A total lod score between -2 and 3 is taken as evidence that more families are needed to make a decision between linkage and exclusion of linkage. The critical limits of 3 and -2 are widely used but somewhat arbitrary; a maximum lod score of 3 corresponds in a large sample to a significance level of less than 0.0005. Results from a lod-score analysis are typically presented either in tabular or graphical form.

Lod-score methods have been extended to quantitative traits and larger simple families (Elston and Stewart, 1971; Ott, 1974), and to complex families (Lange and Elston, 1975; Cannings et al., 1978). Other modifications include allowing for variable age of onset (Hodge et al., 1979) and for genetic heterogeneity (Smith, 1961; Ott, 1983). Lod-score linkage analysis is discussed in detail in Ott (1985, 1991). It is important to note that lod-score methods require that specific assumptions be made concerning the genetic model underlying the trait and values of the parameters that describe the mode of inheritance, such as gene frequency and penetrance parameters. Although these assumptions can be legitimately made for some disorders, the invocation of these assumptions may not be appropriate for disorders such as alcoholism, where the nature of the genetic component is not yet completely understood.

Sib-Pair Methods

The term *sib-pair method* is often used to denote a type of analysis, typically performed on pairs of siblings, that is not based directly on a model likelihood. Although the most powerful of these sib-pair linkage methods requires approximately twice the sample size of lod-score methods when there is single locus inheritance (Demenais and Amos, 1989), sib-pair methods do not require any assumptions about the mode of inheritance for a particular trait, nor any knowledge of the parameters specifying the mode of inheritance or age of onset distribution for that trait. They are model-free in the sense that they are not based on any particular genetic model, although some kind of statistical model must be assumed in order to perform a test of linkage. This test is usually based on a *t*- or chi-square statistic that is known to have robust properties in large samples.

Sib-pair linkage methods can be classified into those based on the identity-by-state relationships of the sib pairs at the marker locus, such as the Penrose method (1953), and those based on the sib-pair's identity-by-descent relationships, such as the method of Haseman and Elston (1972). The Haseman and Elston sib-pair method uses information from both the sibs' and their parents' marker phenotypes to estimate, using Bayesian methods, the proportion of allelic genes each sib-pair shares identical by descent (IBD) at the marker locus. Different types of relatives share different proportions of genes IBD. For example, identical twins share 100% of their genes IBD at each locus, parents and their offspring share 50%, and unrelated individuals share 0%. Siblings share, on average, 50% of their genes IBD at each locus, but the actual proportion can be 0, 50, or 100% for a specific sib pair at a given locus. In the case of sibships of size two or larger, it has been shown that in large samples a valid test results if all possible sib pairs are included in the analysis as though they were independent (Blackwelder and Elston, 1982; Amos et al., 1989). These model-free methods are not limited to sib pairs, but can also be applied to other relative pairs who share a variable proportion of their genes IBD at any particular locus (e.g., grandparent–grandchild pairs, cousin pairs, avuncular pairs, and half-sibling pairs).

For quantitative traits, the squared sib-pair trait difference is regressed on the estimated proportion of genes each sib pair shares IBD at a marker locus. If a particular polymorphic marker is tightly linked to a locus responsible for at least some of the phenotypic variation of a trait, the alleles at the marker and trait locus should segregate together. Sibs with an estimated proportion of genes IBD that is high (more likely to be concordant for the marker alleles) should also have a high probability of having the same alleles at the linked trait locus, and so the difference between the sibs' phenotypes should be relatively small. Conversely, if the estimated proportion of genes IBD for the marker locus is low (more likely to be discordant), the probability of having the same alleles at the linked locus should similarly be low and the difference between the sibs' phenotypes should be relatively large. Thus, as the estimated proportion of genes IBD for the marker locus increases from 0 to 1, the difference between the sibs' trait phenotypes should on average decrease, if a locus tightly linked to the marker is responsible for part of the trait variation (i.e., the slope of the regression line should be negative). On the other hand, if the marker locus is not linked to a locus responsible for some of the phenotypic variation of the trait, the difference between the phenotypes of the sibs would not be expected to change with the proportion of genes IBD at the marker locus (i.e., the slope of the regression line would be expected to be 0).

Most of the information from the sib-pair method is derived from pairs of sibs with estimated proportions of genes IBD near 0 or 1. The distribution of these estimates depends in part on the number and frequency of the alleles at the marker locus. The number of sib pairs with estimated proportions of genes IBD near 0 or 1 can be small, especially if the marker is not very polymorphic. However, this does not appear to affect the validity of this test (Wilson and Elston, 1993).

For a dichotomous trait, the Haseman–Elston test reduces to testing whether the mean proportion of genes shared IBD is the same for concordant and discordant sib pairs. Similarly, the mean for concordantly affected, concordantly unaffected, and discordant pairs are each tested against a value of one-half, which is the expected mean if there is no linkage; in each case a one-sided test is performed. If linkage is present the mean will be larger than one-half for concordant pairs, and smaller than one-half for discordant pairs.

The results of these analyses are often presented in the form of a table of marker loci by trait phenotypes (a "marker–phenotype matrix") with the nominal p-values for each marker-phenotype sib-pair test as entries in the table. Tentative evidence for genetic linkage can be inferred when a p-value for a specific marker–phenotype combination is significant after adjustment for the number of tests performed. If the marker–phenotype matrix is arranged with the marker loci as rows and the trait phenotypes as columns, tentative evidence for oligogenic involvement can be inferred when there are multiple significant p-values in a single column (i.e., more than one marker locus demonstrates significant *p*-values with a single trait phenotype). Similarly, tentative evidence for pleiotropic effects of a single locus can be inferred when multiple significant *p*-values occur in a single row (i.e., a single marker demonstrates significant results with more than one trait phenotype) (Wilson et al., 1991b).

Affected Sib-Pair Methods

In the case of a dichotomous trait, affected versus unaffected, an efficient data collection design is to include only pairs of affected sibs in the sample. This design increases the power of the test at the expense of foregoing the inclusion of discordant pairs in the sample as controls. The Haseman–Elston test then tests whether the mean proportion of alleles IBD for the concordantly affected sib pairs is significantly greater than one-half, the expected mean if there is no linkage. The method of Green and Woodrow (1977) uses a similar approach for sets of affected sibs. Sets of affected relatives other than sibs can also be analyzed using model-free methods (Lange, 1986; Weeks and Lange, 1988), although these tests are based on identity by state (like the original Penrose test).

Heterogeneity, Reduced Penetrance, Variable Expressivity, and Phenocopies

In lod-score linkage studies, the appropriateness of a number of assumptions should be considered, although these issues have been largely ignored in the relatively few lod-score linkage studies of alcoholism to date. It has been shown that inappropriate assumptions lead to loss of power, but not validity, of the linkage tests (Williamson and Amos, 1990).

Typically, each family in a sample is usually ascertained through a proband meeting certain diagnostic criteria and then other relatives in the family are diagnosed according to these same criteria. Although the definition of the clinical phenotype may be quite rigorous, this does not automatically translate into a discrete genetic disorder. One of the strongest assumptions made in a lod-score linkage analysis is that segregation at the same genetic locus underlies the observable clinical variation in *all* the families with a similar clinical phenotype. The lack of *homogeneity* (or presence of *heterogeneity*) seriously affects the results of a lod-score linkage analysis, particularly if an actual linkage between a marker locus and a locus responsible for the phenotype exists only in a small subset of families in the sample. Although methods exist to allow for linkage to a particular marker in only a proportion of the families (Smith, 1961; Ott, 1983), and to test whether the lod scores from a set of families are homogeneous (Morton 1956), these methods have not as yet been applied in lod-score linkage analysis of alcoholism.

A second assumption to be considered is that individuals who carry a gene for alcoholism will necessarily express alcoholism or alcohol abuse. Given that exposure to alcohol is necessary for alcoholism, any unaffected individuals who are not exposed to alcohol for ethical, social, or religious reasons, may in fact be carriers of genes that would contribute to the expression of alcoholism if they were exposed. Reduced *pene-*

trance of alcoholism is often taken to be a function of age in linkage studies, but these studies have not as yet attempted to take into account a measure of exposure such as the quantity of alcohol consumed.

A third assumption is that an individual with a putative gene involved in the expression of alcoholism will necessarily express that gene as alcoholism rather than some other phenotype such as depression, antisocial behavior, other substance abuse, or other psychiatric illness. In linkage analysis, the possibility of such *variable expressivity* has been handled by varying the diagnostic criteria for affection status, for example, from a very narrow definition of alcoholism to a definition that includes alcohol abuse, other substance abuse, and depression (e.g., E. M. Hill et al., 1988).

A fourth assumption is that the same underlying gene is carried by all individuals in a family with a phenotype that meets specific diagnostic criteria. In this situation, individuals with an underlying undiagnosed depression, for example, may be misdiagnosed as having alcoholism because they are self-medicating with alcohol. The possibility of such *phenocopies* should be allowed for in the linkage model used for analysis.

Design of Linkage Studies

For linkage studies in general, the ideal sampling unit is a family containing a large number of sibs, their parents, and grandparents on the side(s) of the family through which the disease is actually inherited. If we assume that a not too common autosomal dominant gene is involved in alcoholism, then only one set of grandparents need be included. Assuming that alcoholism is genetically heterogeneous, i.e., that different loci may be involved in different families, it is preferable to select families to maximize the probability that only one of these loci is segregating in any one family. It is advantageous to study larger, extended families if we can assume that segregation at only one locus accounts for most of the genetic component of alcoholism in each family. This will maximize the power to detect genetic heterogeneity among families by linkage analysis.

Consider a double-backcross mating: in this situation the affected parent is heterozygous at both the trait locus (Aa) and the marker locus (Bb), and the unaffected parent (aa) has at most one marker allele in common with the affected parent (bb). Furthermore, assume that there is marker information available on both parents of the affected parent (one of these grandparents being affected: Aa). Also assume that there is complete penetrance, so that the genotype of each offspring can be unequivocally classified as a recombinant or nonrecombinant. Elston and Bonney (1984) have shown that the equivalent of at least 20 offspring from this type of mating, all segregating at the same locus for alcoholism, are usually required to either accept or reject linkage. If several families are needed to achieve this number, then a larger number of offspring may be required because only a fraction of the families may be segregating at the same locus.

Other factors may also necessitate a larger number of offspring. If the marker is very polymorphic, then nearly every mating of affected by unaffected will be a double-backcross mating. But if the marker is diallelic (with two equally frequent alleles), no more than a one-fourth of the matings are expected to be double-backcross matings and four or more times as many offspring will be required. If there is reduced penetrance, a further increase in the number of offspring is needed: assuming a recombination fraction of 0.1, about 50% more are needed when the penetrance is 0.9, and about three and a half times more when the penetrance is as low as 0.5 (Ott, 1985).

Sib-pair analyses can be performed on the data collected in these same extended families, but the power to detect linkage will be less—this is the price paid to obtain results that do not depend on knowledge of the exact mode of inheritance. If one is willing to study affected sib pairs only, foregoing the advantage of having a control group of discordant sib pairs, then when the recombination fraction is 0.1 and the marker is very polymorphic, 54 sib pairs would be expected to give a result that is as significant as a lod score of 3 ($p < 0.0005$). As before, this number needs to be increased to allow for genetic heterogeneity, a less polymorphic marker, or reduced penetrance. It is not necessary for the sib pairs to be from different sibships. For example 18 sets of affected sib trios, each trio giving rise to three sib pairs, provides approximately the same information. However, the test statistic approaches a normal distribution as the number of *sibships* becomes large, so it is preferable to have at least 30 independent sibships in the sample (Blackwelder and Elston, 1985; Wilson and Elston, 1993).

Review of Linkage Studies of Alcoholism

At the outset it should be acknowledged that direct comparisons between the linkage studies of alcoholism that have been conducted to date are difficult because of the use of different diagnostic criteria, different schemes for classifying individuals as affected, and differences in the methods of analysis used, especially with respect to allowing for age of onset and reduced penetrance. Through 1992, four independent linkage studies have focused specifically on alcoholism.

1. S. Y. Hill et al. (1975) investigated 11 markers in 35 families using the Penrose sib-pair method and suggested a linkage between alcoholism and the Rhesus blood group (RH). The pattern observed, however, was the opposite of that expected under a hypothesis of linkage and so the true *p*-value is taken to be one.

2. S. Y. Hill et al. (1988) studied 6 polymorphic markers in 30 nuclear families, each with two male alcoholics, excluding families with individuals containing other psychiatric disorders. Both DSM-III and Feighner (Feighner et al., 1972) criteria were used to establish diagnoses. An affected sib-pair analysis using the method of Green and Woodrow (1977) suggested evidence of linkage with the MNS blood group, but not with the RH, Duffy (FY), Kidd (JK), or ABO blood group loci. Subsequent maximum likelihood linkage analysis resulted in a lod score of 2.02 at a recombination fraction of 0.01 between alcoholism and the MNS locus. Tight linkage (recombination fraction of 0.0) with the RH and FY loci were excluded in the lod-score analysis. Aston and Hill (1990) expanded the families in the S. Y. Hill et al. (1988) study and reported an increase in lod score between alcoholism and MNS from 2.02 to 2.49.

3. Tanna et al. (1988) investigated 30 polymorphic marker loci in 42 families origi-

nally collected as part of a study on depression spectrum disease. In this study, ascertainment was originally intended to select depression spectrum disease families, i.e., families in which the proband had depression and at least one other first-degree relative had alcoholism or antisocial personality. In the analysis of alcoholism, only those individuals with alcoholism were classified as affected, all other individuals (including those with depression and antisocial personality) were classified as unaffected. The Feighner criteria were used to establish diagnoses. Using the Haseman and Elston method, possible evidence of linkage was found with the esterase-D (ESD) locus on chromosome 13q. The maximum lod score between alcoholism and ESD was 1.644 at a recombination fraction of 0.11. Most of the information for the linkage to ESD came from a single family in which three of eight sibship members were alcoholic and one member was depressed, and this family was fairly typical of the DSD families in general. In the lod-score analysis, linkage could be excluded at a recombination fraction of 0.0 with the following loci: PGM1, RH, ACP1, JK, GC, MNS, GLO1, BF, ORM, AK1, ABO, DB, PR, PA, PI, IGHG (GM), HP, LE, C3, ADA, P1, KEL, and GPT.

Wesner et al. (1991) used an RFLP as a marker at the ESD locus in several of the same families as in the Tanna et al. (1988) study, and excluded linkage between alcoholism and this RFLP at a recombination fraction of 0.0. When using a single liability class with complete penetrance, however, the maximum lod score was 0.986 at a recombination fraction of 0.24, which is similar to the Tanna et al. (1988) finding.

4. E. M. Hill et al. (1988) used the Haseman and Elston method to analyze 25 families for evidence of linkage between various classifications of affective disorders and 24 genetic markers. Probands having either depression or mania and having at least one first-degree relative with either manic disorder, alcoholism, or antisocial personality were ascertained for this study. Diagnoses were made using the research diagnostic criteria of Spitzer et al. (1978). All of these families included individuals with alcoholism, and in this analysis all 25 were classified as alcoholism families. They noted a nominal significance level of 0.04 for linkage between alcoholism and the ABO locus.

Metaanalysis

In this section, we pool the results of the four independent analyses by combining nominal p-values unadjusted for multiple tests. This is done separately for p-values from the sib-pair tests and p-values derived from lod scores. In the latter case p-values were obtained by multiplying the maximum lod score by $2 \cdot \log_e 10$, taking the square root of the product, and comparing the result with the standard normal distribution in a one-tailed test. When the maximum lod score was 0 at a recombination fraction of 1/2, the p-value was taken to be 1. p-Values were then combined using Fisher's (1950) method: $-2 \cdot \Sigma \log_e p$ is compared to a χ^2 distribution, the number of degrees of freedom being twice the number of p-values combined. It is important to note that because large p-values cannot be taken as evidence for the null hypothesis, the p-values provide no information about the consistency of the results from study to study. This is especially true for linkage studies, which typically require large samples to be powerful.

Determining a significance level from a lod-score analysis and then combining p-

values over different studies is a departure from the usual procedure for combining lod scores. The standard procedure is to sum the lod scores at corresponding recombination fractions, and then determine the largest value of the overall summed lod-score curve. This largest lod score can then be converted, if desired, to a p-value for a one-tail test, as just indicated. This is the appropriate procedure to test the null hypothesis of no linkage when the alternative hypothesis of interest is linkage at a *single* recombination fraction, *the same in all studies,* that is less than 1/2. If a p-value is determined for each study and these p-values combined using Fisher's method, the implicit alternative hypothesis is that the recombination fraction is less than 1/2, *but possibly different* in each study. Ideally we should sum lod scores from a model that allows for a proportion of unlinked families that varies from study to study. But because such lod scores were unavailable, we chose to allow for the heterogeneity by using Fisher's method to combine p-values.

Results from these four independent studies are combined in Tables 14-2 and 14-3. Each of the tables includes any published result that was suggestive of linkage (nominal p-value ≤ 0.05 in either sib-pair or lod-score analysis), together with the corresponding results from the other studies even if not significant. For the sib-pair analyses (Table 14-2), only the linkage with ESD (13q14) was significant at the 0.01 level ($p \leq 0.005$) when the three studies were combined. For the lod-score analyses (Table 14-3), both the MNS (4q28) and ESD (13q14) linkages were significant ($p \leq 0.005$). The possible linkage with the ABO locus (9q34) in the E. M. Hill et al (1988) study was not reproduced in any of the other studies.

Conclusions

It is interesting to note that a number of candidate loci are located in the 4q, 9q, and 13q chromosomal regions. On the long arm of chromosome 4, the loci for alcohol dehydrogenase class I (ADH1) and III (ADH3) are located between the GC and MNS loci (4q21–q24). The recombination fractions between the GC and ADH3 loci, and between the ADH3 and MNS loci, are estimated to be about 0.20 and 0.30, respectively (Keats et al., 1989). In addition, Comings et al. (1991) reported that the locus for tryptophan oxygenase (TDO2) has been localized to chromosome 4q31. On the long arm of chromosome 9, the dopamine-β-hydroxylase (DBH) locus has been linked to the ABO locus (9q34) (Wilson et al., 1988; Craig et al., 1988). The recombination fraction between DBH and the ABO locus has been estimated to be between 0.0 and 0.17 (Wilson et al., 1988). Another possible candidate locus, aldehyde dehydrogenase (ALDH1), is also located on the long arm of chromosome 9 (9q21), although it is probably outside the ABO–AK1–ORM linkage group, most likely located between the ORM locus and the centromere. And on the long arm of chromosome 13, Sparkes et al. (1991) have reported that the serotonin 5 HT 2 receptor has been localized to the 13q14-q21 region near ESD.

It should be noted that the controversy over clinical heterogeneity with respect to alcoholism and unipolar depression has not yet been resolved. Wilson et al. (1991a) reanalyzed data from earlier DSD studies. A genometric approach was used to identify

Table 14-2 Nominal Significance Levels from Sib-Pair Linkage
Analyses of Alcoholism

	Marker Locus (Chromosome)		
Reference	MNS (4q28)	ABO (9q34)	ESD (13q14)
S. Y. Hill et al. (1975)	0.5[a]	0.5[a]	—[b]
S. Y. Hill et al. (1988)	0.04	0.88	—
Tanna et al. (1988)	0.98	0.43	0.0003
E. M. Hill et al. (1988)	0.88	0.04	0.37
Overall p-value	>0.1	>0.1	<0.005

[a]Approximated from the results given.

[b]Polymorphism not typed in this study.

genetic components that may underlie unipolar depression and/or alcoholism for a broad spectrum of clinical phenotypes. Four different criteria were used to classify individuals as affected: (1) individuals with any psychiatric disorder as affected, and individuals with no psychiatric disorder as unaffected (any psychiatric disorder); (2) individuals with depression, alcoholism, or antisocial personality as affected, and all other individuals as unaffected (triad DSD) (3) only individuals with depression as affected, and all other individuals as unaffected, including those with alcoholism (depression only); and (4) only individuals with alcoholism as affected, and all other individuals as unaffected (alcoholism only). Analyses based on classifications of any psychiatric disorder and triad DSD suggested linkage to genetic markers on chromosomes 9q34 and 13q14, while analyses based on the depression-only classification suggested linkage to 9q34, and the alcohol-only classification suggested linkage to 13q14. The results of the single- and multiple-marker analyses suggest that genetic loci on two different chromosomes may be independently involved in the expression of affective disorder, either as depression or alcoholism, in these data.

Although the results of the metanalysis are intriguing, particularly with respect to the candidate loci identified in regions implicated in these studies, additional studies

Table 14-3 Nominal Significance Levels from Lod-Score Linkage
Analyses of Alcoholism

	Marker Locus (Chromosome)		
Reference	MNS (4q28)	ABO (9q34)	ESD (13q14)
S. Y. Hill et al. (1988)	0.0014	0.33	—[a]
Tanna et al. (1988)	0.26	1.00	0.003
Overall p-value	<0.005	>0.5	<0.005

[a]Polymorphism not typed in this study.

will be required to either confirm or refute these possible linkages. As with any statistical method, there are situations where these methods will produce spurious results. In addition to chance sampling variations, as reflected in the significance level, these methods can give false indications of linkage when there are undetected errors in the family structure or when the sample exhibits a trait–marker association not due to tight linkage. Linkage studies of alcoholism have been performed in very few families compared to other psychiatric illnesses, and given the rapid growth in the availability of polymorphic DNA markers over the last few years, follow-up studies seem long overdue. The identification of single loci, even if their effects on alcoholism are minor, will have a major impact on the perception of alcoholism as a disease, and on its treatment and prognosis.

References

Agarwal, D. P., Harada, S., and Goedde, H. W. (1981). Radical differences in biological sensitivity to ethanol. *Alcoholism* **5**:12–16.

Amos, C. I., Elston, R. C., Wilson, A. F., and Bailey-Wilson, J. E. (1989). A more powerful test of linkage for quantitative traits. *Genet. Epidemiol.* **6**:435–449.

Amos, C. I., Elston, R. C., Bonney, G. E., Keats, B. J. B., and Berenson, G. S. (1990). A multivariate method for detecting genetic linkage with application to a pedigree with adverse lipoprotein phenotype. *Am. J. Hum. Genet.* **47**:247–254.

Anderson, R. J., Dyer, P. A., Donnai, D., Klouda, P. T., Jennison, R., and Braganza, J. M. (1988). Chronic pancreatitis, HLA and autoimmunity. *Int. J. Pancreatol.* **3**:83–90.

Aston, C. E., and Hill, S. Y. (1990). Segregation analysis of alcoholism in families ascertained through a pair of male alcoholics. *Am. J. Hum. Genet.* **46**:879–887.

Barnard, G. A. (1949). Statistical inference. *J. Roy. Stat. Soc. B.* **11**:115–140.

Billington, B. F. (1956). Note on distribution of blood groups in bronchiectasis and portal cirrhosis. *Aust. Ann. Med.* **5**:20–22.

Blackwelder, W. C., and Elston, R. C. (1982). Power and robustness of sib-pair linkage tests and extension to larger sibships. *Commun. Stat. Theor. Meth.* **11**:449–484.

Blum, K., Noble, E. P., Sheridan, P. J., Montgomery, A., Ritchie, T., Jagadeeswaran, P., Nogami, H., Briggs, A. H., and Cohn, J. B. (1990). Allelic association of human dopamine D2 receptor gene in alcoholism. *JAMA* **263**:2055–2060.

Boerwinkle, E., Chakraborty, R., and Sing, C. F. (1986). The use of measured genotype information in the analysis of quantitative phenotypes in man I. Models and analytical methods. *Ann. Hum. Genet.* **50**:181–194.

Bolos, A. M., Dean, M., Lucas-Derse, S., Ramsburg, M., Vrown, G. L., and Goldman, D. (1990). Population and pedigree studies reveal a lack of association between the dopamine D_2 receptor gene and alcoholism. *JAMA* **264**:3156–3160.

Bosron, W. F., Nagnes, L. J., and Li, T-K. (1983) Human liver alcohol dehydrogenase: $ADH_{Indianapolis}$: result from genetic polymorphism at the ADH_2 gene locus. *Biochem. Genet.* **21**:735–744.

Botstein, D., White, R. L., Skolnick, M., and Davis, R. W. (1980) Construction of a genetic linkage map in man using restriction fragment length polymorphisms. *Am. J. Hum. Genet.* **32**:314–331.

Cadoret, R., and Winokur, G. (1974). Depression in alcoholism. *N.Y. Acad. Sci.* **233**:34–39.

Camps, F. E., and Dodd, B. E. (1967). Increase in the incidence of non-secretors of ABH blood group substances amongst alcoholic patients. *Br. Med. J.* **1**:30–31.

Camps, F. E., Dodd, B. E., and Lincoln, P. J. (1969). Frequencies of secretors and non-secretors of ABH group substances among 1,000 alcoholic patients. *Br. Med. J.* **4**:457–459.

Cannings, C., Thompson, E. A., and Skolnick, M. H. (1978). Probability functions on complex pedigrees. *Adv. Appl. Prob.* **10**:26–61.

Cloninger, C. R., Reich, T., and Wetzel, R. (1979). Alcoholism and affective disorders: Familial associations and genetic models. In *Alcoholism and Affective Disorders: Clinical Genetic and Biochemical Studies.* D. W. Goodwin and C. K. Erikson, eds., New York: SP Medical and Scientific Books, pp. 57–86.

Cloninger, C. R., Bohman, M., and Sigvardsson, S. (1981). Inheritance of alcohol abuse: Cross fostering analysis of adopted men. *Arch. Gen. Psychiatr.* **38**:861–868.

Comings, D. E., Muhleman, D., Dietz, Jr. G. W., and Donlon, T. (1991). Human tryptophan oxygenase localized to 4q31: Possible implication for alcoholism and other behavioral disorders. *Genomics* **9**:301–308.

Corsico, R., Pessino, U. L., Morales, V., and Jmelnisky, A. (1988). Association of HLA antigens with alcoholic disease. *J. Stud. Alcohol* **49**:546–550.

Craig, S. P., Buckle, V. J., Lamouroux, A., Mallet, J., and Craig, I. W. (1988) Localization of the human dopamine beta hydroxylase (DBH) gene to chromosome 9q34. *Cytogenet. Cell Genet.* **48**:48–50.

Demenais, F. M., and Amos, C. I. (1989). Power of the sib-pair and lod-score methods for linkage analysis of quantitative traits. In *Multipoint Mapping and Linkage Based Upon Affected Pedigree Members,* R. C. Elston, J. W. MacCluer, S. E. Hodge, and M. A. Spence, eds. New York: Alan R. Liss, pp. 201–206.

Dumont-Damien, E., and Duyme, M. (1991). Genetic markers and alcoholism: A review. *Psychiatr. Genet.* **2**:73–74.

Elston, R. C., and Bonney, G. E. (1984) Sampling considerations in the design and analysis of family studies. In *Genetic Epidemiology of Coronary Heart Disease: Past, Present and Future,* D. C., Rao, R. C., Elston, L. H., Kuller, M., Feinleib, C. Carter, and R. Havlik, eds. New York: Alan R. Liss, pp. 349–371.

Elston, R. C., and Stewart, J. (1971). A general model for the genetic analysis of pedigree data. *Hum. Hered.* **21**:523–542.

Elston, R. C., and Wilson, A. F. (1990). Genetic linkage and complex diseases: A comment. *Genet. Epidemiol.* **7**:17–19.

Feighner, J. P., Robins, E., Guze, S. B., Woodruff, R. A., Jr., Winokur, G., and Munoz, R. (1972). Diagnostic criteria for use in psychiatric research. *Arch. Gen. Psychiatr.* **26**:57–63.

Fisher, R. A. (1950). *Statistical Methods for Research Workers,* Edinburgh and London: Oliver and Boyd, pp. 99–101.

George, V. T., and Elston, R. C. (1987). Testing the association between polymorphic markers and quantitative traits in pedigrees. *Genet. Epidemiol.* **4**:193–202.

Gilligan, S. B., Reich, T., and Cloninger, C. R. (1987). Etiological heterogeneity in alcoholism. *Genet. Epidemiol.* **4**:395–414.

Goldman, D. (1988). Molecular markers for linkage of genetic loci contributing to alcoholism. *Recent Dev. Alcohol.* **6**:333–349.

Green, J. R., and Woodrow, J. C. (1977). Sibling method for detecting HLA-linked genes in disease. *Tissue Antigens* **9**:31–35.

el-Guebaly, N. (1986). Risk research in affective disorders and alcoholism: Epidemiological surveys and trait markers. *Can. J. Psychiatr.* **31:**352–361.

Haldane, J. B. S., and Smith, C. A. B. (1947). A new estimate of the linkage between the genes for colour blindness and haemophilia in man. *Ann. Eugen.* **14:**10–31.

Haseman, J. K., and Elston, R. C. (1972). The investigation of linkage between a quantitative trait and a marker locus. *Behav. Genet.* **2:**3–19.

Hill, E. M., Wilson, A. F., Elston, R. C., and Winokur, G. (1988). Evidence for possible linkage between genetic markers and affective disorders. *Biol. Psychiatr.* **24:**903–917.

Hill, S. Y., Goodwin, D. W., Cadoret, R., Osterland, C. K., and Doner, S. M. (1975). Association and linkage between alcoholism and eleven serological markers. *J. Stud. Alcohol* **36:**981–992.

Hill, S. Y., Aston, C., and Rabin, B. (1988). Suggestive evidence of genetic linkage between alcoholism and the MNS blood group. *Alcohol.: Clin. Exp. Res.* **12:**811–814.

Hodge, S. E., Morton, L. A., Tideman, S., Kidd, K. K., and Spence, M. A. (1979). Age-of-onset correction available for linkage analysis (LIPED). *Am. J. Hum. Genet.* **31:**761–762.

Keats, B. J. B., Ott, J., and Conneally, P. M. (1989). Report of the committee on linkage and gene order. *Cytogenet. Cell Genet.* **51:**459–502.

Lange, K. (1986). The affected sib-pair method using identity by state relations. *Am. J. Hum. Genet.* **39:**148–50.

Lange, K., and Elston, R. C. (1975). Extensions to pedigree analysis. I. Likelihood calculations for simple and complex pedigrees. *Hum. Hered.* **25:**95–105.

Litt, M., and Luty, J. A. (1989). A hypervariable microsatellite revealed by in vitro amplification of a dinucleotide repeat within the cardiac muscle actin gene. *Am. J. Hum. Genet.* **44:**397–401.

Mendel, G. (1966). *Experiments in Plant Hybridization* (Translation of *Versuche über Pflanzenhybriden,* 1866), Cambridge: Harvard University Press.

Merikangas, K. R., Leckman, J. F., Prusoff, B. A., Pauls, D. L., and Weissman, M. M. (1985). Familial transmission of depression and alcoholism. *Arch. Gen. Psychiatry.* **42:**367–372.

Monteiro, E., Alves, M. D., Santos, M. L., Quintas, I., Baptista, A., Galvao-Telles, A., and Gavaller, J. S. (1988). Histocompatibility antigens: Markers of susceptibility to and protection from alcoholic liver disease in a Portuguese population. *Hepatology* **8:**455–458.

Morton, N. E. (1955). Sequential tests for the detection of linkage. *Am. J. Hum. Genet.* **7:**277–318.

Morton, N. E. (1956). The detection and estimation of linkage between the genes for elliptocytosis and the Rh blood type. *Am. J. Hum. Genet.* **8:**80–96.

Morton, N. E. (1990). Genetic linkage and complex diseases: A comment. *Genet. Epidemiol.* **7:**33–34.

Noble, E. P., Blum, K., Ritchie, T., Montgomery, A., and Sheridan, P. J. (1991). Allelic association of the D2 dopamine receptor gene with receptor-binding characteristics in alcoholism. *Arch. Gen. Psychiatr.* **48:**648–654.

Nordmo, S. H. (1959). Blood groups in schizophrenia, alcoholism and mental deficiency. *Am. J. Psychiatr.* **116:**460–461.

Ott, J. (1974). Estimation of the recombination fraction in human pedigrees. Efficient computation of likelihoods for human linkage studies. *Am. J. Hum. Genet.* **26:**588–597.

Ott, J. (1983). Linkage analysis and family classification under heterogeneity. *Ann. Hum. Genet.* **47:**311–320.

Ott, J. (1985). *Analysis of Human Genetic Linkage.* Baltimore: Johns Hopkins University Press, pp. 1–196.

Ott, J. (1991). *Analysis of Human Genetic Linkage* 2d ed. Baltimore: Johns Hopkins University Press.

Parsian, A., Todd, R. D., Devor, E. J., O'Malley, K. L., Suarez, B. K., Reich, T., and Cloninger, R. (1991). Alcoholism and alleles of the human D2 dopamine receptor locus: Studies of association and linkage. *Arch. Gen. Psychiatr.* **48**:655–663.

Penrose, L. S. (1953). The general purpose sib-pair linkage test. *Ann. Eugen.* **18**:120–124.

Radouco-Thomas, S., Garcin, F., Murthy, M. R. V., Faure, N., Lemay, A., Forest, J. C., and Radouco-Thomas, C. (1984). Biological markers in major psychosis and alcoholism: Phenotypic and genotypic markers. *J. Psychiatr. Res.* **18**:513–539.

Reid, N. C. R. W., Brunt, P. S., Bias, W. B., Maddrey, W. C., Alonso, B. A., and Iber, F. L. (1968). Genetic characteristics and cirrhosis: A controlled study of 200 patients. *Br. Med. J.* **2**:463–465.

Smith, C. A. B. (1953). The detection of linkage in human genetics. *J. Roy. Stat. Soc. B* **15**:153–184.

Smith, C. A. B. (1961). Homogeneity test for linkage data. In *Proceedings, 2nd International Congress on Human Genet* 1, 212–213.

Sparkes, R. S., Lan, N., Klisak, I., Mohandas, T., Diep, A., Kojis, T., Heinzmann, C., and Shih, J. C. (1991). Assignment of a serotonin 5HT-2 receptor gene to human chromosome 13q14-q21 and mouse chromosome 14. *Genomics* **9**:461–465.

Spitzer, R. L., Endicott, J., and Robins, E. (1978). Research diagnostic criteria: Rationale and reliability. *Arch. Gen. Psychiatr.* **35**:773–782.

Swinson, R. P., and Madden, J. S. (1973). ABO blood groups and ABH substance secretion in alcoholics. *Q. J. Stud. Alcohol* **34**:64–70.

Tanna, V. L., Winokur, G., Elston, R. C., and Go, R. C. P. (1976). A linkage study of pure depressive disease: The use of the sib-pair method. *Biol. Psychiatr.* **6**:767–771.

Tanna, V. L., Wilson, A. F., Winokur, G., and Elston, R. C. (1988). Possible linkage between alcoholism and esterase-D. *J. Stud. Alcohol* **49**:472–476.

Wald, A. (1947). *Sequential Analysis.* New York: Wiley.

Weber, J. L., and May, P. E. (1989). Abundant class of human DNA polymorphisms which can be typed using the polymerase chain reaction. *Am. J. Hum. Genet.* **44**:388–396.

Weeks, D. E., and Lange, K. (1988). The affected-pedigree-member method of linkage analysis. *Am. J. Hum. Genet.* **42**:315–326.

Weissman, M. M., and Myers, J. K. (1980). Clinical depression in alcoholism. *Am. J. Psychiatr.* **137**:372–373.

Wesner, R. B., Tanna, V. L., Palmer, P. J., Thompson, R. J., Crowe, R. R., and Winokur, G. (1991). Close linkage of esterase D to unipolar depression and alcoholism is ruled out in eight pedigrees. *J. Stud. Alcohol* **52**:609–612.

Williamson, J. A., and Amos, C. I. (1990). On the asymptotic behavior of the estimate of the recombination fraction under the null hypothesis of no linkage when the model is mis-specified. *Genet. Epidemiol.* **7**:309–318.

Wilson, A. F., and Elston, R. C. (1993). Statistical validity of the Haseman-Elston sib-pair test in small samples. *Genet. Epidemiol.* **10**:593–598.

Wilson, A. F., Elston, R. C., Siervogel, R. M., and Tran, L. D. (1988). Linkage of a gene regulating dopamine-β-hydroxylase activity and the ABO blood group locus. *Am. J. Hum. Genet.* **42**:160–166.

Wilson, A. F., Elston, R. C., Sellers, T. A., Bailey-Wilson, J. E., Gersting, J. M., Deen, D. K., Sorant, A. J. M., Tran, L. D., Amos, C. I., and Siervogel, R. M. (1990). Stepwise oligogenic segregation and linkage analysis illustrated with dopamine-β-hydroxylase activity. *Am. J. Med. Genet.* **35:**425–432.

Wilson, A. F., Elston, R. C., Mallot, D. B., Tran, L. D., and Winokur, G. (1991a). The current status of genetic linkage studies of alcoholism and unipolar depression. *Psychiatr. Genet.* **2:**107–124.

Wilson, A. F., Elston, R. C., Tran, L. D., and Siervogel, R. M. (1991b). Use of the robust sib-pair method to screen for single locus, multiple locus, and pleiotropic effects: Application to traits related to hypertension. *Am. J. Hum. Genet.* **48:**862–872.

Winokur, G., Cadoret, R., Dorzab, J., and Baker, M. (1971). Depressive disease—a genetic study. *Arch. Gen. Psychiatry.* **24:**135–144.

Winokur, G., Cadoret, R., Baker, M., and Dorzab, J. (1975). Depression spectrum disease versus pure depressive disease: Some further data. *Brit. J. Psychiatry..* **127:**75–77.

Yoshida, A., Huang, I -Y., and Ikawa, M. (1984). Molecular abnormality of an inactive aldehyde dehydrogenase variant commonly found in Orientals. *Proc. Natl. Acad. Sci. (USA)* **81:**258–261.

CONTRIBUTORS

Rodney C. Baker
Department of Pharmacology
University of Colorado
Alcohol Research Center
Denver, Colorado

Henri Begleiter
Department of Psychiatry
Neurodynamics Laboratory
SUNY Health Science Center
Brooklyn, New York

Remi J. Cadoret
Department of Psychiatry
University of Iowa
Iowa City, Iowa

David W. Crabb
Departments of Medicine
and of Biochemistry and Molecular
Biology
Indiana University Medical Center
Indianapolis, Indiana

John C. Crabbe
VA Medical Center and
Oregon Health Sciences University
Portland, Oregon

Richard A. Deitrich
Department of Pharmacology
University of Colorado
Health Science Center
Denver, Colorado

Ivan Diamond
Ernest Gallo Clinic & Research Center
University of California, San Francisco
San Francisco, California

Howard J. Edenberg
Departments of Biochemistry and
Molecular Biology
and of Medical and Molecular
Genetics
Indiana University School of Medicine
Indianapolis, Indiana

Robert C. Elston
Louisiana State University Medical
Center
New Orleans, Louisiana

Adrienne Gordon
Ernest Gallo Clinic & Research Center
University of California, San Francisco
San Francisco, California

Andrew C. Heath
Department of Psychiatry
Washington University
St. Louis, Missouri

Michie N. Hesselbrock
Southern Connecticut State University
School of Social Work & Human
Services
New Haven, Connecticut

Victor M. Hesselbrock
Department of Psychiatry
University of Connecticut Health Center
Farmington, Connecticut

Ann E. Kosobud
Department of Physiology and Biophysics
Hahnemann University
Philadelphia, Pennsylvania

Elizabeth Laffan
Institute for Behavioral Genetics
University of Colorado at Boulder
Boulder, Colorado

Ting-Kai Li
Departments of Medicine
and of Biochemistry and Molecular
Biology
Indiana University
Indianapolis, Indiana

Lawrence Lumeng
Departments of Medicine
and of Biochemistry and Molecular
Biology
Indiana University Medical Center
Indianapolis, Indiana

William J. McBride
Department of Psychiatry
Indiana University
Indianapolis, Indiana

Gerald E. McClearn
Center for Developmental and Health
Genetics
Pennsylvania State University
University Park, Pennsylvania

Howard B. Moss
Department of Psychiatry
University of Pittsburgh
Pittsburgh, Pennsylvania

James M. Murphy
Departments of Psychiatry and
Psychology
Indiana University
Indianapolis, Indiana

Robert Plomin
Center for Developmental and Health
Genetics
Pennsylvania State University
University Park, Pennsylvania

Bernice Porjesz
Department of Psychiatry
SUNY Health Science Center
Brooklyn, New York

Ralph E. Tarter
Department of Psychiatry
University of Pittsburgh
Pittsburgh, Pennsylvania

Holly R. Thomasson
Department of Medicine
Indiana University
Indianapolis, Indiana

Michael M. Vanyukov
Department of Psychiatry
University of Pittsburgh
Pittsburgh, Pennsylvania

Alexander F. Wilson
Louisiana State University Medical
Center
New Orleans, Louisiana

James R. Wilson
Institute for Behavioral Genetics
University of Colorado at Boulder
Boulder, Colorado

INDEX

A1 allele, 339
A2 allele, 339
Aalto, J., 175t
Abstainers, risk for alcoholism in, 83
Abstinence: genetic and environmental determinants of, 108–109; versus level of consumption, 109; twin studies on, 24, 85, 87t, 89, 102–103, 110, 111 (Australian NH&MRC twin surveys, 96, 97; U.S. NAS/NRC, 91; Vietnam-Era Twin Surveys, 102; Virginia 30,000 Survey, 99, 100)
Abstinent alcoholics: event-related potentials in, 275, 276–277; stress response in, 283–284
Acetaldehyde, 245: accumulation in blood, 175; in alcohol flush reaction, 206–208, 211; enzymes oxidizing, 205; oxidation of, 155
Acetaldehyde dehydrogenase, atypical, 207
Acetaldehyde dehydrogenase 2 (ALDH2) deficiency: in alcohol flush reaction, 211; molecular basis for, 208–209; population genetics of, association with alcohol-drinking behavior, 209–210; polymorphism, in rats selected for alcohol preference, 212
Acetaldehyde dehydrogenase 2 genes, mutations in, 214
Achievement-related activity in children, 51
Activity, withdrawal measurement by, 230
Adams, M. D., 338
Addictability, high and low (HA, LA), 229
Addictive components in genetic analysis, 330
Addictive genetic model, twin correlations, 84

Adenine, 353
Adenosine, 11: ethanol effects on, 261; receptor system for, 147
Adenylyl cyclase, 262, 337
Adjustment disorder, temperament phenotype and, 304
Adolescent, adolescence: alcohol behavior in, National Merit Twin Study on, 92–93; antisocial personality disorder in, alcoholism related to, 71; attention-span persistence in, 307; early, alcohol and drug use during, 296; emotionality in, 311; excessive use of alcohol by, 42; hyperactive, alcoholism liability related to, 307; maladjustment in, 297
Adoptees, genetic diathesis for alcohol abuse, environmental factors and, 75–76
Adoption studies, 3–4, 340, 342: on childhood hyperactivity and conduct disorder related to alcoholism in adults, 50; on genetic influences on alcohol metabolism, sensitivity and tolerance, 124–130; on heritability of alcoholism, 25–26, 33 (Danish Adoption Study, 26–27; half-sibling studies, 29–30; Iowa Adoption Studies, 28–29; Swedish Adoption Study, 27–28); on heterogeneity of antisocial alcoholics, 77; on neurobiological-based classification of alcoholism, 56–59; on relationship of antisocial personality disorder with alcoholism, 71–73; on schizophrenia associated with alcoholism, 73; on variation in drinking patterns, 83